LAW AND
NURSING

North Cheshire Hospital S

i

For Elsevier:

Commissioning Editor: Steven Black
Development Editor: Catherine Jackson
Project Manager: Joannah Duncan
Designer: Erik Bigland
Illustrations Manager: Bruce Hogarth

LAW AND NURSING

Jean McHale LLB, MPhil
Professor of Law, Faculty of Law, University of Leicester, UK

John Tingle BA Law (Hons), CertEd(Dist), MEd, Barrister
Reader in Health Law, Nottingham Law School,
Nottingham Trent University, UK

THIRD EDITION

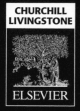

CHURCHILL LIVINGSTONE

ELSEVIER

EDINBURGH LONDON NEW YORK OXFORD PHILADELPHIA ST LOUIS SYDNEY
TORONTO 2007

CHURCHILL
LIVINGSTONE
ELSEVIER

© Reed Educational and Professional Publishing, 1998
© Reed Educational and Professional Publishing, 2001
© 2007, Elsevier Limited. All rights reserved.

First edition 1998
Second edition 2001

ISBN-13: 978 0 7506 8868 0
ISBN-10: 0 7506 8868 8

British Library Cataloguing in Publication Data
A catalogue record for this book is available from the British Library.

Library of Congress Cataloging in Publication Data
A catalog record for this book is available from the Library of Congress.

Note
Knowledge and best practice in this field are constantly changing. As new research and experience broaden our knowledge, changes in practice, treatment and drug therapy may become necessary or appropriate. Readers are advised to check the most current information provided (i) on procedures featured or (ii) by the manufacturer of each product to be administered, to verify the recommended dose or formula, the method and duration of administration, and contraindications. It is the responsibility of the practitioner, relying on their own experience and knowledge of the patient, to make diagnoses, to determine dosages and the best treatment for each individual patient, and to take all appropriate safety precautions. To the fullest extent of the law, neither the Publisher nor the Authors assumes any liability for any injury and/or damage to persons or property arising out or related to any use of the material contained in this book.

The Publisher

PREFACE

It is a truism to say that nurses today practise in challenging times. The law and its relationship with nursing practice is a fast-moving area. From both within and outside the profession nurses have been encouraged to expand their role and also to develop as specialists in nursing practice and as independent prescribers. However such an expanded role brings with it the prospect of enhanced accountability with the risk of consequent litigation should things go wrong. At the same time, nurses are encouraged to act as advocates for their patients, to safeguard standards of care and to speak out where these standards may be at risk. Many nurses have expressed concern regarding the scope of their legal obligations at a time when the structure of health care provision and their own role within it is subject to such changing dynamics.

NHS health care litigation remains, as at the time of the 2nd edition of our book, an acute problem, with the costs of clinical negligence calculated in billions of pounds. Patient safety can be seen to have been given a higher profile through the work of the National Patient Safety Agency. There is a good NHS patient safety infrastructure in place in terms of mechanisms of control, advice and publications. Difficulties remain, however, in ensuring effective engagement with such strategies at a grass roots level. Further challenges face nurses and other health professionals as the NHS is the subject of what seems to be virtually constant restructuring.

This book explores the legal regulation of nursing practice today and sets it in the context of recent developments, from the impact of the Human Rights Act 1998 in cases such as that of Dianne Pretty to the Human Tissue Act 2004 enacted in the aftermath of the Alder Hey inquiry, the Mental Capacity Act 2005 and the expansion of nurse prescribing powers. The volume is not intended to be a substitute for specialist legal advice on specific problems that may arise in individual cases. Furthermore it should be noted that, as this area is so vast, in some areas the account provided must be seen in context as a 'taster' for further more extensive reading of specialist legal sources.

As with previous editions our very special thanks go to the editorial team at Elsevier and in particular Catherine Jackson and Susan Young. John Peysner was involved in the first edition of this text and his inspiration and insight into civil litigation issues provided an invaluable basis for our treatment of these issues in this book. All comments expressed and any errors that remain are, of course, the responsibility of the authors.

The law is as stated at 1 May 2006, although we were able to incorporate certain developments subsequent to this date.

CASE LIST

Page numbers in **bold** refer to pages in this book.

AC	Law Reports, Appeal Cases
All ER	All England Law Reports
BMLR	Butterworths Medico-Legal Reports
CA	Court of Appeal
ChD	Chancery Division Law Reports
CMLR	Common Market Law Reports
Cr App R	Criminal Appeal Reports
DLR	Dominion Law Reports
ECR	European Court Reports
EHRR	European Human Rights Reports
EWCA	England and Wales Court of Appeal
EWCA Admin	England and Wales Court of Appeal Administrative
EWCA Civ	England and Wales Court of Appeal Civil
EWCA Crim	England and Wales Court of Appeal Criminal
EWHC	England and Wales High Court
Fam Law	Family Division Law Reports
FCR	Family Court Reports
FLR	Family Law Reports
KB	Law Reports, Kings Bench
Lloyd's Rep Med	Lloyd's Medical Law Reports
Med LR	Medical Law Reports
NLJR	New Law Journal Reports
PIQR	Personal Injuries and Quantum Reports
QBD	Law Reports, Queen's Bench Division
RTR	Road Traffic Reports
SJ	Solicitors Journal
UKHL	UK House of Lords
WLR	Weekly Law Reports

A, Re [1992] 3 Med LR 303, **237–238**
A, Re [2000] 4 All ER 961, **122–123**
A, Re (children) (conjoined twins: surgical separation) [2001] Fam 147, **222**
A, Re (Medical treatment: male sterilisation) [2000] FCR 193, **196**
A Health Authority v. *X* [2001] 2 FCR 634, **150**
AG Ref (No. 6 of 1980) [1981] QB 715, **105**
Airedale NHS Trust v. *Bland* [1993] AC 879, **227–229**
Att. Gen v. *Guardian Newspaper (No 2)* [1988] 3 All ER 545, **144**

B, Re [1981] 1 WLR 1421, **230**

B, Re [1987] 2 WLR 1212, **194–195**

B, Re (Adult: Refusal of Medical Treatment) [2002] 2 All ER 449, **108**, **179**, **224**

B v. Croydon HA [1995] 1 All ER 683, **133**, **208**

Barnett v. Chelsea and Kensington Hospital Management Committee [1968] 1 All ER 1068, **35–36**

Black v. Forsey [1988] *The Times* 21 May, **132**

Blyth v. Bloomsbury AHA [1987] (1993) 4 Med LR 151 CA, **113–114**

Bolam v. Friern Hospital Management Committee [1957] 1 WLR 582; [1957] 2 All ER 118, **28**, **29**, **31–32**, **36**, **82–83**, **103**, **109**, **207**

Bolitho v. City and Hackney Health Authority (1997) [1998] AC 232; [1998] Lloyd's Rep Med 26, **31–32**, **36**, **83**, **110–111**

Bolitho v. City and Hackney Health Authority (1997) [1998] Lloyd's Rep Med 26, **31–32**, **36**, **83**, **110**

Bravery v. Bravery [1954] 3 All ER 59, **193**

Bull v. Devon Area Health Authority [1989] [1993] 4 Med LR 117, 22 BMLR, 79, **40–41**, **44**

C, Re [1989] 2 All ER 782, **230–231**

C, Re [1994] All ER 819, **100**, **102**, **104**

C, Re [2003] 2 FLR 678, **124**

C, Re (a baby) [1996] FLR 43, **231**

C, Re (a minor) [1997] 40 BMLR, **232**

C, Re (HIV Test) [1999] 2FLR 1004, **121–122**

C v. S [1988] QB 135, **216**

Campbell v. MGN [2004] 2 AC 457 (HL), **145**

Cassidy v. Ministry of Health [1951] 1 All ER 574, **40**, **43**

Cattley v. St John's Ambulance Brigade (1988) QBD (unreported) (but see *Lexis*), **28**

Chatterson v. Gerson [1981] QB 432, **106**, **115**, **178**

Chester v. Afshar [2005] 1 AC 234, **111**, **115**

CR v. Central Birmingham HA ex p Collier [1988] *Lexis* 6 January, **17**

Crawford v. Board of Governors of Charing Cross Hospital (1953) (*The Times*, 8 December 1953), **34**

D, Re [1976] 1 All ER 326, **194**, **195**

D, Re (Medical Treatment) [1998] 1 FLR 411, **233**

Davies v. Johnson [1979] AC 264, **9**

De Freitas v. O'Brien [1995] 6 Med LR 108, **110**

De Freitas v. O'Brien and Another [1993] 4 Med LR, **30**

Djemal v. Bexley Health Authority [1995] 6 Med LR 269, **79**

Duchess of Kingston's case (1776) 20 State Trials 355, **152**

Dwyer v. Roderick [1983] 127 SJ 806, **95**

E, Re (a minor) [1992] 2 FLR 585, **196**

E, Re (minor) (Wardship: Medical Treatment) [1993] 1 FLR 386, **127**, **128**

Early v. Newham Health Authority [1994] 5 Med LR 214, **82–83**

Evans v. Amicus Health Care [2004] 2 FLR 767, **199**

Evans v. UK [2006] Application No 6339/05, Strasbourg, 6 March, **12**, **199–200**

F, Re [1990] 2 AC 1, **102, 103, 146, 181–182, 195–196, 207**
F, Re (in utero) [1988] 2 All ER 193, **204, 206**
Frenchay v. *S* [1994] 2 All ER 403, **229**

G, Re [1995] 2 FCR 46, **228**
Gascoine v. *Ian Shendon and Co. and Lathan* [1994] 5 Med LR 437, **34**
Geraets–Smits v. *Stichting Ziekenfonds VGZ Case 157/99*, **20**
Gillick v. *West Norfolk and Wisbech AHA* [1986] 1 AC 112; [1985] 2 All ER 545;
    [1985] 3 All ER 402; [1986] AC 150, **3, 9, 118–119, 125, 145–146, 180–181,
    194**
Glass v. *Cambridgeshire Area Health Authority* [1995] 6 Med LR 91, **41**
Glass v. *UK* [2004] 1 FLR 1019, **123, 233**
Gold v. *Essex County Council* [1942] 2 All ER 237, **32**
Gregg v. *Scott* [2005] UKHL 2, **38–39**
Grogan [1991] ECR 4685, **11**

H (a health worker) v. *Associated Newspapers Ltd* [2002] EWCA Civ 195, **150**
H, Re (a patient) [1998] 2 FLR 36, **233**
Hefferen v. *The Committee of the UKCC* (1988), **23**
HIV Haemophiliac Litigation, Re [1990] NLJR 1349, **152**
HL v. *UK* [2004] Application No. 45508/99, **129, 133**
Hotson v. *East Berkshire Area Health Authority* [1987] 2 All ER 909, **38, 39**

Inizan Case C-56/-01, **20**

J, Re [1990] 3 All ER 930, **231**
J, Re [2000] FLR 571, **124**
Jannaway v. *Salford AHA* [1988] 3 All ER 1079, **216**
Jepson v. *Chief Constable of West Mercia* [2003] EWCA 3318, **213**
Johnston v. *Bloomsbury AHA* [1991] 2 All ER 293, **78**
Jones v. *Manchester Corporation* [1952] 2 QB 852, **44**

K, W and H (minors) (Medical Treatment), Re [1993] FLR 584, **125–126**
Kay v. *Ayrshire and Arran Health Board* [1987] 2 All ER 417, **36**
Kent v. *Griffiths and Others* [2000] 2 All ER 474, **26**
Kholl/Dekker Case C-158/966, **20**

L, Re (Medical Treatment: Gillick competency) [1998] 2 FLR 810, **127–128**
Luisi and Carbone v. *Ministero del Tesoro* [1984] ECR 377, **19**

M, Re [1999] 2FLR 1097, **126, 240**
M, Re (a minor) (wardship: sterilisation) [1988] 2 FLR 497, **196**
M v. *Calderdale and Kirklees HA* [1998] Lloyd's Rep Med 157, **43**
McKay v. *Essex Area Health Authority* [1982] 2 All ER 771, **211**
Marshall v. *Southampton and SW Hampshire AHA* [1986] ECR 723, **10**
Maynard v. *West Midlands Regional Health Authority* [1984] 1 WLR 634, **30–31,
    110**
MB, Re [1997] FLR 426, **100–101, 108, 206–208, 209**
Muller Faure Case C-385/99, **20**
Murray v. *McMurchy* [1942] 2 DLR 442, **106–107**

Naylor v. *Preston AHA* [1987] 2 All ER 353, **152**
Nettleship v. *Weston* [1971] 2 QB 691, **29**

NHS Trust A v. *M; NHS Trust B* v *H* [2000] 2 FLR 348, **228**
Norfolk & Norwich NHS Trust v. *W* [1996] 2 FLR 613, **206**

O, Re (a minor) (Medical Treatment) [1993] 2 FLR 149, **120**

P, Re (a minor) (wardship: sterilisation) [1989] 1 FLR 182, [1989] Fam Law 102, **196**
Paton v. *British Pregnancy Advisory Authority* [1978] 2 All ER 987, **206**, **213**
Paton v. *UK* [1980] 3 EHRR 408, **11**, **213**
Pearce v. *United Bristol NHS Trust* [1999] PIQR P53 (CA), **110–111**, **114**, **179**
Penney and Others v. *East Kent Health Authority* (*The Times*, 25 November 1999 (CA), **83**
Philips v. *William Whitley Ltd* [1938] All ER 566, **79**
Plon (Societé) v. *France* [2004] Application No 58148/00 18 May, **147**
Portsmouth NHS Trust v. *Wyatt* [2004] EWHC 2243; [2005] 2 FLR 403, **233**
Poutney v. *Griffiths* [1975] 2 All ER 881, **137**
Prendergast v. *Sam and Dee* [1989] 1 Med LR 36, **95**
Pretty v. *UK* [2002] 2 FCR 97, **224**

R, Re [1991] 4 All ER 177 CA, **102**, **124**, **125**
R, Re [1996] 2 FLR 99, **237**
R v. *Adomako* [1994] 3 All ER 79, **45**
R v. *Arthur* (1981) *The Times*, 5 November, **220**
R (Axon) v *Secretary of State for Health* [2006] EWHC 37 (Admin) (QBD), **145–146**, **194**
R v. *BHB Community Healthcare NHS Trust ex parte B* [1999] 1 FLR 106, **138**
R v. *Bingley Magistrates Court ex parte Morrow* 13 April 1994 (unreported), **228**
R v. *Bodkin Adams* [1957] Criminal Law Review 365, **222**
R v. *Bourne* [1939] 1 KB 687, **212**
R v. *Bournewood NHS Trust ex parte L* [1998] 3 All ER 289, **129**, **132–133**
R v. *Brown* [1994] 1 AC 212, **105**
R (Burke) v. *GMC* [2005] EWCA 1003, **234**
R v. *Cambridge District Health Authority ex parte B* [1995] 2 All ER 129, **17–18**, **19**
R v. *Canons Park Mental Health Review Tribunal ex parte A* [1994] 1 All ER 481, **131**
R v. *Cardiff Crown Court ex parte Kellam* [1993] 16 BMLR 76, **152**
R v. *Carr* (1986) *Sunday Times*, 30 November, **219**
R v. *Collins ex parte Brady* [2000] Lloyd's Rep Med 355, **133**
R v. *Department of Health ex parte Source Informatics* [2001] 1 All ER 786, **154**
R v. *Donovan* [1934] QB 638, **105**
R v. *East London and the City Mental Health NHS Trust ex parte Von Brandenberg* [2003] UKHL 58, **137**
R v. *Ethical Committee of St Mary's Hospital, Manchester* [1988] 1 FLR 512, **198**
R v. *Gloucester CC ex parte Barry* [1997] AC 584, **19**
R (H) v. *Mental Health Review Tribunal North and East London Region* [2001] EWCA Civ 415, **12**
R v. *Hallstrom ex parte W* [1986] QB 1090, **138**
R v. *Hamilton* (1983) *The Times*, 16 September, **217**
R v. *Human Fertilisation and Embryology Authority ex parte Blood* [1997] 2 All ER 687, **11**, **200**

R v. *Kelly* [1998] 3 All ER 741, **186**

R v. *Kirklees MBC ex parte C* [1993] 2 FLR 187, **128–129**

R v. *Lowe* [1973] QB 70, **221**

R (Mellor) v. *Secretary of State for the Home Department* [2002] QB 13, **197**

R v. *Misra; R* v. *Srivastava* [2004] EWCA Crim 2375 *The Times*, 13 October 2004, **45**

R (N) v. *M and others* [2003] 1 WLR 562, **134**

R v. *North Derbyshire Health Authority ex parte Fisher* [1997] 8 MedLR 327, **18**

R v. *North West Lancashire Health Authority ex parte A, D and G* [2000] 1 WLR 977, **18–19**

R (on the application of Aston) v. *NMC* [2004] EWCA Admin., para 64, **22**

R (on the application of B v. *Ashworth Hospital Authority* [2005] UKHL 20, **133**

R (on the application of CS) v. *MHRT* [2004] EWCA 2958, **138**

R (on the application of DR) v. *Merseycare NHS Trust* [2002] All ER D 28, **138**

R (on the application of Pretty) v. *DPP* [2002] 1 All ER 1, **12, 223–224**

R (on the application of S) v. *Plymouth City Council* [2002] EWCA Civ 388, **146**

R (on the application of Smeaton) v. *Secretary of State for Health* [2002] 2 FLR 146, **216**

R v. *P&O European Ferries (Dover) Ltd* [1991] 93 CR App R 72, **45**

R v. *Portsmouth Hospital NHS Trust ex parte Glass* [1999] Lloyd's Rep Med 367, **232**

R (ex parte Quintavelle) v. *Secretary of State for Health HL* [2003] 2 All ER 113, **202, 203**

R v. *Rothery* [1976] RTR 478, **186**

R v. *Secretary of State for Health ex parte Pfizer Ltd* [1999] Lloyd's Rep Med 289, **18**

R v. *Secretary of State for Social Service ex parte Hincks* [1980] [1979] 123 SJ 436, **17**

R v. *Senior* [1989] 1 QB 283, **221**

R v *Sheffield Health Authority ex parte Seale* [1994], **198–199**

R v. *Welsh* [1974] RTR 478, **186**

R (Wilkinson) v. *Broadmoor Special Hospital Authority* [2002] 1 WLR 419, **134**

R v. *Wilson and Williamson* [1995] *The Independent* 19 April, **130**

R v. *Woolin* [1999] AC 82, **222**

RCN v. *DHSS* [1981] AC 800, **215**

Reid v. *Secretary of State for Scotland* [1999] 1 All ER 481, **131**

Rice v. *Connolly* [1966] 2 QB 416, **151**

Rickard v. *Rickard* [1989] 2 All ER 193, **9**

Riverside Mental Health Trust v. *Fox* [1994] 2 Med LR 95, **133**

Rochdale NHS Trust v. *C* [1997] 1 FCR 274, **206**

Roe v. *Ministry of Health and Others, Woolley* v. *Same* [1954] 2 All ER 131, **33**

S, Re [1992] 4 All ER 671, **206**

S, Re [2000] 3 WLR 1288, **101, 103**

S, Re (a minor) [1993] 1 FLR 376, **120**

S v. *McC, W* v. *W* [1972] AC 24, **118**

St George's NHS Trust v. *S* [1998] 3 All ER 673; 3 WLR 936, **134, 208–210**

Secretary of State for Health v. *R on the application of Yvonne Watts* [2004] EWCA Civ 166, **20**

SG, Re [1991] 6 BMLR 95 (Fam Div), **214**

Sidaway v. *Bethlem Royal Hospital Governors* [1985] 1 All ER 643, **109–110**, **111**, **112**, **113**, **178–179**

Sims v. *Sims and an NHS Trust* [2002] EWHC 2743, **182**

Slater v. *UKCC* 18 May 1988 (QBD) (unreported), **23**

Smith v. *Littlewood* [1987] 1 All ER 710, **157**

Smith v. *Tunbridge Wells Health Authority* [1994] 5 Med LR 334, **110**

South Glamorgan CC v. *and B* [1993] 1 FLR 574, **125**

T, Re [1992] 4 All ER 649, **102**, **107–108**, **234**

T, Re [1997] 1 WLR 242, **120–121**, **231–232**, **240**

Tameside and Glossop Acute Hospital Trust v. *CH* [1996] 1 FLR 762, **208**

Tameside v. *Glossop* [1996] 1 FCR 753, **206**

Thake v. *Maurice* [1986] 1 All ER 497, **193**

The Queen on the application of Yvonne Watts Case C-372/04, **20**

Vo v. *France* [2005] 40 EHRR 12; 2 FCR 577, **11**, **213**

W, Re (a minor) [1992] 3 WLR 758, **125**, **240**

W v. *Egdell* [1990] ChD 359, **148–149**, **156–157**

W v. *L* [1974] QB 711, **130**

Wainwright v. *Home Office* [2003] UKHL 53, **145**

Walker v. *Northumbria County Council* [1985] 1 All ER 737, **78**

Watson v. *McEwan* [1905] AC 480, **152**

Watts v. *Bedford PCT* [2006] QB 667, **11**, **19–20**

Wilsher v. *Essex Area Health Authority* [1986] 3 All ER 801,833, **29**, **30**, **36**, **44**, **78–79**

Woolgar v. *Chief Constable of the Sussex Police* [1999] 3 All ER 604, **150–151**

Wyatt, Re [2005] EWHC 2293, **233**

X v. *Y* [1988] 2 All ER 648, **144**, **150**

Y, Re [1996] 2 FLR 791, **240**

Z, Re (An adult's capacity) [2004] EWMC 2817, **226**

Z v. *Finland* [1997] 25 EHRR 371, **145**

Australian cases
  Chappel v. *Hart* [1998] HCA 55, **115**
  Rogers v. *Whittaker* [1993] 4 Med LR 79, **110**

Canadian cases
  Halushka v. *University of Saskatchewan* [1965] 53 DLR (2d) 436 at 438, **178**
  Malette v. *Schumann* [1990] 67 DLR (4th) 321, **107**
  Marshall v. *Curry* [1933] 3 DLR 260, **106**
  Re Eve [1986] DLR (4t) 1, **195**
  Vancouver General Hospital v. *McDaniel* [1934] 152 LT 56,57, **43–44**

European cases
  Van Gend en Loos v. *Netherlands Belastingensadministratie* [1963] CMLR 105, **11**

USA cases

Canterbury v. *Spence* [1972] 464 F 2d 772, **109**

Moore v. *University of California* [1990] 793 P 2d 479, **187**

Norwood Hospital v. *Munoz* [1991] 564 NE 2d 1017, **210**

Re AC [1990] 573 A.2d 1235 at 1240, **206**

Tarasoff v. *Regents of the University of California* [1976] 551 P 2d 344, **156**

Health Service Ombudsman decisions

E.189/97–98, **64**

E.2775/02–03, **64**

S.104/93–94, **64**

W.232/90/91, **63**

STATUTES AND STATUTORY INSTRUMENTS

Page numbers in **bold** refer to pages in this book.

ACTS OF PARLIAMENT

Abortion Act 1967	**8, 212–216**
s1(1)	**213**
s1(1)a	**212**
s1(1)b	**212–213**
s1(1)c	**213**
s1(1)d	**213**
s1(3)	**214–215**
s1(4)	**213**
s4	**215–216**
s5(2)	**213**
Access to Health Records Act 1990	**163–164, 166**
Access to Justice Act 1999	**13, 14**
Access to Medical Reports Act 1988	**163**
s(2)	**163**
s(5)	**163**
s(17)	**163**
Administration of Justice Act 1970	**152**
s32	**152**
Animals Scientific Procedures Act 1986	**172, 173**
Births and Deaths Registration Act 1953	**217–218, 238**
Children Act 1989	**119–120, 125, 210**
s1(1)	**122**
s2	**117**
s3(5)	**117**
s4	**117**
s8	**125–126**
s12	**117**
s33	**117**
Children and Young Persons Act 1933	**221**
Chronically Sick and Disabled Persons Act 1970, s2	**19**
Civil Liability (Contribution) Act 1978	**43**
Civil Procedure Act 1997	**5**
Compensation Act 2006	**35**

Computer Misuse Act 1990	**166**
Congenital Disabilities (Civil Liability) Act 1976	**211**
s1(3)	**211**
s2	**211**
s4(2)	**211**
Consumer Protection Act 1987	**44**
s3(2)	**44**
s4(1)	**44**
Courts and Legal Services Act 1990	**13–14**
Criminal Justice Act 1994	**151**
Data Protection Act 1998	**163–166**
s1(1)	**164**
s7	**164**
s7(2)(a)	**165**
s7(4)	**165**
s7(5)	**165**
s7(8)	**164**
s7(10)	**164**
s10	**164**
s14	**164**
s31(2)(a)(iii)	**165**
s31(4)(a)(iii)	**165**
s31(4)(b)	**165**
s33	**165**
s68(2)	**164**
s69	**164**
Disability Discrimination Act 1995	**155**
Employment Rights Act 1996	
s42(H2)	**162**
s43(B)	**161**
s43(B)(1)	**161**
s43(F)	**161, 162**
s43(H)	**162**
s43(J)	**163**
s43(K)	**161**
s46	**161**
s47(B)	**162**
s48(2)	**162**
s98	**159**
s100	**161**
s103	**162**
European Communities Act 1972	**10**
Article 152	**10**
s2(1)	**10, 11**
Family Law Reform Act 1969	**240**
s8	**117, 125, 180**

Health Act 1999

    s18   **15**

    s26   **15**

Health and Safety at Work Act 1974 — **8, 78**

Health and Social Care Act 2001 — **90**

    s57 — **134**

    s60 — **153**

    s63 — **93**

Health and Social Care (Community Health and Standards) Act 2003

    s1(1) — **15**

    s14(2) — **15**

    s41 — **15**

Human Fertilisation and Embryology Act 1990 — **8, 157–158, 165, 172, 185, 197, 199–200, 201, 202–203, 204, 212**

    s3(3) — **172, 197**

    s13(5) — **197, 198, 203**

    s33 — **157**

    s33(6B) — **157**

    s33(6c) — **157**

    s36(1) — **204**

    s38 — **200**

    s40(1)(5) — **157**

Human Organ Transplants Act 1989 — **238, 239, 241**

Human Reproductive Cloning Act 2001 — **202**

Human Rights Act 1998 — **11–12, 18–19, 122, 126, 186, 197, 213, 228, 233**

Human Tissue Act 1961 — **238**

Human Tissue Act 2004 — **9, 185–186, 238–239, 240, 241**

    s1 — **185, 186**

    s2 — **185, 239**

    s4 — **185, 239**

    s5 — **185**

    s6 — **185, 239**

    s8 — **185**

    s26 — **186**

    s27 — **239**

    s32 — **239**

    s33 — **241**

    s45 — **185**

Infant Life Preservation Act 1929 — **211, 216**

Legal Aid Act 1988 — **13**

Medicinal Products (Prescription by Nurses) Act 1992 — **85, 90**

Medicines Act 1968 s58(2)(b) — **85**

Mental Capacity Act 2005	104, 183, 196, 214, 229
s1	104
s2(1)	104
s3(1)	104
s3(4)	104
s3(5)	104
s4	104–105
s4(6)	105
s9	236
s10	236
s11	236
ss24–26	234, 235
s30	183
s31	184
s32	184
s62	234–235
Mental Health Act 1983	12, 125–126, 128–139
s1(2)	130
s1(3)	131
s2	130, 131, 208, 209
s3	131, 137–138
s3(2)	131
s4	131
s5(2)	133
s5(4)	132–133
s7(2)	137
s8	137
s11(1)	137
s11(3)	130
s19	209
s23	136
s23(2)(a)	136
s24(4)(5)	136
s25A–H	138
s57	134, 135
s58	134–135
s62	135
s63	133–134, 208, 209
s66	136
s68	136
s120(1)	138–139
s131	129
s132	133
s135	129–130
s136	130
s139	137

Mental Health (Patients in the Community) Act 1995   138
Misuse of Drugs Act 1971   89

National Assistance Act 1948 s48   108
National Assistance (Amendment) Act 1951 s1(1)   108
National Health Service Act 1977   14
   s1   16
   s3   16–17
   s5(1)b   193
   s16A   15
   s16b   15
   s124   217
National Health Service and Community Care Act 1990   15

Offences Against the Person Act 1861
   s18   105
   ss58-59   211, 216

Police and Criminal Evidence Act 1984
   s9–s11   151
   schedule 1   151
Prevention of Cruelty to Children Act 1896   221
Prohibition of Female Circumcision Act 1985   118
Public Health (Control of Diseases) Act 1984   108
   s11   153
   s37   108
Public Interest Disclosure Act 1998   161–162, 163

Still Birth Definition Act 1992   217, 218
Suicide Act 1961   222, 223
   s2(1)   223
Supreme Court Act 1981, ss33–34   152
Surrogacy Arrangements Act 1985   204

Terrorism Act 2000   151

AUSTRALIAN ACTS

Rights of the Terminally Ill Act 1995   225

EC DIRECTIVES

Clinical Trials Directive (2001/20/EC)   10, 172, 184
Nursing qualifications (77/452/EEC) and 77/453/   10
EEC OJ 1977 L 176

NETHERLANDS ACTS

Termination of Life on Request and Assisted Review   225–226
   Procedure Act 2001

USA ACTS

Death with Dignity Act 1997 — 225
Pain Relief Promotion Act 1999 — 225

INTERNATIONAL TREATIES AND DECLARATIONS

Convention on Human Rights and Biomedicine — 183, 239
Declaration of Helsinki 1964 — 171
European Convention on Human Rights — 11, 12
   Article 2 — 199, 213, 223, 224, 228, 234
   Article 3 — 126, 134, 223, 228, 234
   Article 5(1) — 129
   Article 5(4) — 129
   Article 6 — 234
   Article 8 — 122, 123, 126, 143, 144–145, 146, 150, 199, 223, 224, 234
   Article 9 — 126, 223
   Article 10 — 147, 150
   Article 12 — 199
   Article 14 — 199, 223–224, 234
Nuremberg Code 1949 — 171
Treaty of European Union — 10
Treaty of Amsterdam — 10
Treaty of Rome — 10

SECONDARY LEGISLATION: SIS AND REGULATIONS

Data Protection Act 1998 (Commencement) Order 2000 SI 2000/183 — 164
Data Protection (Subject Access) (Fees and Miscellaneous Provisions) Regulations 2000 SI 2000 No 191 — 165
Data Protection (Subject Access Modification) (Health) Order 2000 SI 2000 No 413 — 165
Data Protection Tribunal (Enforcement Appeals) Rules 2000 SI 2000 No 189 — 164
Health Service (Control of Patient Information Regulations SI 2002/1438, reg 4 — 153
Human Fertilisation and Embryology Research Purposes Regulations 2001 SI No 188 — 202
Medicines for Human Use (Clinical Trials) Regulations SI 2004/1031 — 172, 173, 174, 175, 184–185
Medicines and Human Use (Prescribing) (Miscellaneous Amendments) Order May 2006 — 91

Medicines for Human Use (Prescribing Order) 2005,   93
  SI 2005, No 765
Medicines (Pharmacy and Sale) Exemptions Order 2000   87
Medicines (Products Other Than Veterinary Drugs)   85
  (Prescription Only) Order 1983 SI 1983 No 1212
  as amended
Mental Health Act 1983, Remedial Order 2001   137
  SI 2001/3712
Mental Health Nurses Order 1998, SI 1998/265   132
Midwives Supply Order   85
Miscellaneous Provisions (Amendment) Regulations 2000   87
National Health Service (Complaints) Regulations 2004,   57
  SI No 1768
National Health Service Venereal Disease Regulations   158
  (SI 1974 No 29)
NHS Pharmaceutical Services (Amendment)   85
  Regulations SI 1996 No 698 r8
Notification of Births and Deaths Regulations 1982;   217
  SI 1982 No 286
Nursing and Midwifery Order 2001 (SI 2002/253)   21, 22–24
Nursing and Midwifery Rules 2004   21, 22
Prescription Only Medicines (Human Use)   87, 93
  Amendment Order 2000
Transplant Regulations 2006 SI 2006 No 1659   241

MISCELLANEOUS

Civil Procedure Modification of Supreme Court   3
  Act 1981 Order 2004; SI 2004, 1133
Civil Procedure Rules   5–6
Mental Capacity Act Draft Code of Practice 2006   105
Mental Health Act Code of Practice   128, 132, 133, 136

CONTENTS

Preface v
Case list vi
Statutes and statutory instruments xiii

Chapter **1** Introduction: the nurse and the legal environment 1
Jean McHale

Chapter **2** Nursing negligence: general issues 25
John Tingle

Chapter **3** Patient safety, litigation and complaints in the National Health Service 49
John Tingle

Chapter **4** Legal aspects of expanded role, clinical guidelines and protocols, and nurse prescribing 69
John Tingle and Jean McHale

Chapter **5** Consent to treatment I: General principles 99
Jean McHale

Chapter **6** Consent to treatment II: Children and the mentally ill 117
Jean McHale

Chapter **7** Privacy, confidentiality and access to health-care records 143
Jean McHale

Chapter **8** Clinical research and the nurse 171
Jean McHale

Chapter **9** Reproductive choice 193
Jean McHale

Chapter **10** The end of life 219
Jean McHale

Appendix The NMC code of professional conduct: standards for conduct, performance and ethics 247

Index 255

Introduction: the nurse and the legal environment

Jean McHale

The role of the nurse is the subject of constant evolution. Today, nurses perform tasks that would in the past have been undertaken by doctors, an initiative encouraged by the government (NHS Executive 2000). Many nurses are developing their practice to become clinical nurse specialists, emergency care practitioners and nurse prescribers. At the same time the nurse–doctor dynamic has been changing. There are new models of collaboration and of cooperation (Davies 2000, Salvage & Swift 2000). Further challenges face nurses from the fast-changing nature of health-care provision (Norris 2006). Modern electronic technologies are already transforming health-care delivery. The development of genetic technology has incredible potential but also gives rise to new dilemmas such as enhanced genetic screening and the development of personalised medicines. Demographic changes such as the rising number of older people in the population will give rise to new challenges for health-care provision in a community setting.

At the same time, nurses are also being encouraged to act as advocates for their patients, to safeguard standards of care and to speak out where those standards may be at risk. Such an expanded role is accompanied by enhanced responsibilities, and some considerable debate and indeed controversy (see Ch. 4). In recent years, legal issues in relation to the nurse's role have never been far from the headlines: 'Nurse performs operation'; 'Nurse blows the whistle on poor standards of care'; 'Nurses to prescribe drugs'. Many nurses have expressed concern regarding their legal obligations at a time when the structure of health-care provision and their own role within it is subject to such shifting dynamics.

The legal environment affects nurses in many ways, from the law of negligence concerning breaches of the legal duty of care to patients and others to the nursing professions' governing body, the Nursing and Midwifery Council. Aside from the specific issues concerning nursing practice, the last few years in health care have been characterised by controversy and resultant considerable legal change. Major inquiries were instigated into events at Bristol Royal Infirmary and the deaths in the cardiac paediatric unit at that hospital (Department of Health 2001). Controversy was further generated by the revelation of the unauthorised retention of human material at hospitals up and down the country, leading notably to the 'Alder Hey' inquiry (Redfern 2000). These inquiries led both to legislation in relation to clinical governance and also to new legislation regulating the use of human material. The courts have been faced with many issues relating to health-care practice, from the decision to withdraw treatment from patients in persistent vegetative state, to consent to treatment from negligence actions brought when patients have suffered harm during operations, to whether to sanction assisted suicide in the case of the terminally ill patient.

The structure of health-care provision has been affected by legislation, and the pace of change of law in this area has been rapid. Recent developments considered in this book include the expansion of nurse prescribing, the changes to the law concerning the use of tissue and organs in the Human Tissue Act 2004 and the new statutory decision-making framework for adults lacking mental capacity under the Mental Capacity Act 2005. There has been an increase in the number of negligence actions brought against health-care practitioners. The scope of liability in negligence is considered below. Accompanying this has been the development of risk management practices aimed at reducing the prospect of litigation.

This book attempts to provide nurses with an account of their legal obligations, whether studying law as part of a diploma or degree course or as a busy practitioner seeking clarification of her or his legal position. This is a book on nursing law written by lawyers for nurses. Although many ethical issues do arise in relation to the health-care law matters in this book, the ethical debate is not addressed specifically; for that the reader is referred to the many health-care ethics texts available (e.g. Tingle & Cribb 2000). While it illustrates some of the legal dilemmas that arise, this book should not be seen as a substitute for the need to obtain specialist legal advice if particular problems occur.

This introductory chapter considers the framework of law and regulation within which the nurse practices. First, the structure of the English legal system and the nature of law, legal proceedings and the court system are considered, then the structure of the National Health Service (NHS) and finally the role of the nurse in relation to her or his professional body. The professional obligations of the nurse have been affected by recent guidance upon the scope of the nurse's professional practice. This guidance is considered in detail in this book and reproduced in the appendices.

LAW AND THE LEGAL SYSTEM

Types of law

The legal system is divided into two main branches: criminal and civil law. Criminal law is a system for the state punishment of offences. In a criminal law case the action is usually brought by the Crown against the defendant. An individual may bring a private prosecution, but in practice these are very rare. A criminal law case is referred to as Regina versus Smith, which means the Crown against Smith or, as it is usually written, *R* v. *Smith*.

Civil law is the term given to an action brought by a person who has suffered some harm or loss – known as the claimant (after 1 April 1999; before this date they were referred to as the 'plaintiff') – against another person or organisation – the defendant. A civil law case is normally referred to as *Bloggs* v. *Smith*. The types of civil law action with which the nurse is most likely to be concerned are claims for breach of contract and actions in 'tort'. A tort is a civil wrong. Examples of torts include undertaking surgery without obtaining any form of consent from the patient (a battery) and failing to monitor oxygen levels during an operation with the patient as a consequence suffering brain damage (negligence). Other civil law actions include the action for breach of confidence in which the patient claims that there has been unauthorised disclosure of confidential information entrusted to another in confidence. In civil law actions the claimant seeks a remedy, usually in the form of financial compensation – damages. In addition, s/he may claim an 'injunction' to stop a particular type of conduct. An injunction is an order stopping the party performing the unjustified act. A contract is a legally enforceable promise, enforceable because both parties have given something of value. Examples include contracts of employment and contracts for sale of goods.

Public law

In some situations a person may want to challenge a decision of a government body, NHS trust or other public body. S/he may claim that the body went beyond powers given to it by statute or that it has wrongly exercised a discretion granted under statute. Claims against public bodies in such situations should usually be brought through a special procedure known as 'judicial review'. Judicial review is not an appeal: the court cannot substitute its own view as to how the public body should have behaved. Instead, the court determines whether the public body has acted legally.

A number of special remedies are available against public authorities through judicial review. An action can be brought seeking a 'declaration' from the court – asking the court to declare the law on a specific point. So for example, in *Gillick* v. *West Norfolk and Wisbech AHA* ([1986] 1 AC 112), Mrs Victoria Gillick went to court to ask for a declaration as to whether guidance given to health authorities that doctors could give contraceptive advice and treatment to girls under 16 years of age without parental consent was lawful. The court also has the power to grant a number of statutory orders, the mandatory order, the quashing order and the prohibiting order (Civil Procedure Modification of Supreme Court Act 1981 Order 2004; S1 2004, 1133). These are discretionary orders.

The nurse in the courtroom

When is the nurse likely to appear in court? S/he may be a party to an action; so, for example, the nurse may be a claimant in a civil claim bringing an action for damages against her or his employer on the grounds of the employer's negligence. In a claim brought by a patient, the nurse may be called to give evidence; this may be as to what the nurse saw happen to a patient claiming that s/he was given negligent treatment. In addition, the nurse may be called to give expert evidence, for example in a negligence action as to the standard of practice that would be expected of a responsible nursing professional in that situation (see below).

Types of court

Criminal courts

The magistrates court is a local court. Magistrates try minor criminal offences. In addition, they hear evidence in relation to more serious criminal offences before committing these cases for trial at the Crown Court. In the Crown Court cases are heard by a judge, usually sitting with a jury of 12 lay persons selected at random from persons drawn from the electoral register in the local community.

Civil courts

The court in which a civil law case is heard usually depends upon the amount of damages claimed, which relates to the degree of harm caused and to the complexity of the case, as we shall see below. Use of juries in civil cases is very rare today, the most notable exception is that of libel cases. The whole civil justice system was subject to radical reform in 1999 following the report of Lord Woolf (Woolf 1996).

Court structure – the upper courts

High Court

There are three divisions of the High Court: the Chancery and Family Divisions hear exclusively civil law matters; and the Queen's Bench Division hears criminal law and public law matters. Each division is headed by a senior judge: in the case of the Chancery Division, the Vice-Chancellor, in the case of the Family Division, the President, and the Lord Chief Justice for the Queen's Bench Division. These judges also sit in the Court of Appeal. The High Court may hear cases taken on appeal from the lower courts. Alternatively, cases may be heard for the first time in the High Courts. As noted above, such cases would include serious negligence cases.

Court of Appeal

Above the High Court is the Court of Appeal. This is composed of senior judges known as Lord Justices of Appeal. It hears appeals in both civil and criminal cases. The civil division is headed by the Master of the Rolls, the criminal division by the Lord Chief Justice.

House of Lords

The highest court within the United Kingdom is the House of Lords. It is composed of senior judges known as Law Lords. The Lord Chancellor presides over the House of Lords. He is a political appointment and also is a member of the Cabinet. This court bears the same name as the second chamber of Parliament, the House of Lords. Peers who have a right to sit in the House of Lords do not have the right to sit as judges in the court, but the Law Lords may participate in parliamentary debates.

Civil procedure and the Woolf reforms

The legal system has long been criticised for its antiquated procedure, delays and use of complex language. In 1995 Lord Woolf was given the task of looking at the operation of the civil procedure rules. This led, however, to a wide-ranging enquiry into the operation of the civil justice system itself. Lord Woolf recommended that the civil justice system should:

- Be just in results delivered
- Be fair in the way in which litigants are treated
- Offer appropriate procedures at reasonable cost
- Deal with cases at reasonable speed
- Be understandable to those who need it
- Be responsive to the needs of those who use it
- Provide as much certainty as the particular case allows
- Be effective/adequately resourced/organised.

The government accepted the majority of Lord Woolf's recommendations and these were implemented with the bulk of the reforms becoming operational on 1 April 2000.

A new body, the Civil Justice Council, was created with the task of keeping civil justice under review. It considers how to make the civil justice system more accessible, fair and efficient. It advises the Lord Chancellor and the judiciary on the development of the civil justice system, and refers proposals for changes in the civil justice system to the Lord Chancellor and the Civil Procedure Rules Committee. It also makes proposals for research. New civil procedure rules were brought into operation alongside practice directions, forms and protocols (Civil Procedure Act 1997) such as the pre-action protocol for the resolution of clinical disputes. As a result of the reforms the use of legal language has been considerably amended. For example the word 'plaintiff' was replaced by the term 'claimant'.

Using alternative dispute resolution

Parties are encouraged to resolve their differences through the use of alternative dispute resolution mechanisms. There is a new power to stay (or halt) proceedings pending the parties being referred to alternative dispute resolution (Civil Procedure Rules, rule 1.4. (2) (e)). This has the aim of removing many issues from the scope of the courtroom and to encourage parties to resolve their differences. The aim of the hearing is that matters are dealt with 'justly'. According to rule 1 (1) (2) of the Civil Procedure Rules:

" Dealing with a case justly includes, so far as is practicable –

    a. Ensuring that the parties are on an equal footing
    b. Saving expense
    c. Dealing with the case in ways which are proportionate –
    d to the amount of money involved
    e. to the importance of the case

f. to the complexity of the issues; and

g. to the financial position of each party.

h. ensuring that it is dealt with expeditiously and fairly; and

i. allotting to it an appropriate share of the Court's resources while taking into account the need to allot resources to other cases.

The division of civil litigation

Civil proceedings today fall into three broad categories. The first is the 'small claims' track. There is a limit of £5000 on such cases and of £1000 in personal injury cases. These cases are allocated to what were known as the 'small claims' courts. This referred to the procedure used in county courts for claims of low value. Cases regarded as suitable for such hearings are consumer disputes, accident claims, disputes regarding the ownership of goods and most landlord and tenant disputes other than those for possession. Secondly, there is what is known as the 'fast-track', where there is a limit of cases of value of up to £15 000. Such cases will usually be heard in the county court. Here claims will be subject to a fixed timetable, judicial monitoring and only limited use of oral evidence. Failure to comply with case management directions will be the subject of sanctions. Cases involving claims of larger value- and of greater complexity are dealt with under the 'multi-track', where these are cases not on another track (CPR rule 26. 6 (6)). Here there is greater flexibility given to the court in the way in which a case will be managed appropriate to the particular needs of that case. A major feature of the reforms is the role of the procedural judge in 'managing' the case – guiding the proceedings through the court (CPR part 3). Timetables are used and costs controlled. Failure to comply with the rules/protocols may result in the parties being subject to sanctions so, for example, the defence may be struck out or this may have an impact upon the costs to be awarded.

Medical negligence litigation and Woolf – some specific issues

In chapter 15 of his report Lord Woolf directed considerable attention to medical negligence litigation (Woolf 1996). The report identified a number of problems in such litigation. There was disproportion between the costs awarded and the damages given. In many instances there were unacceptable delays in resolving cases. The success rate was lower in medical negligence actions than in other personal injury cases. The report also commented that there was a perceived lack of trust and openness between health-care professionals and patients and that doctors/hospitals were traditionally unwilling to admit negligence.

Lord Woolf believed that patients had a number of aims. They wanted impartial information and advice, including independent medical assessment. They also wanted fair compensation for losses suffered. Patients also wanted the dispute to be resolved quickly by fair and independent adjudication and (sometimes) a day in court. Health-care professionals also wanted speedy resolution and discreet (private) adjudication. They wanted an expert of their own/solicitor's choice. They also wanted an economical system that did not encourage trusts to settle disputes over their heads regardless of liability. Lord Woolf considered the possibility of a new non-pecuniary remedy from the courts – a formal statement from the hospital explaining the incident of alleged negligence. The need for more open communication between the parties was emphasised in the report.

The Woolf Report and the subsequent civil justice reforms suggest that professionals and patients should adopt a constructive approach to complaints and claims. Guidance is now provided to the parties in the conduct of such cases through the operation of pre-action protocols and in particular the pre-action protocol for the resolution of clinical disputes. The aim of protocols is to maintain/restore the patient–health-care provider relationship and to resolve as many disputes as possible without litigation. Sufficient information should be disclosed by the parties to enable each of them to understand the other's viewpoint. While the guidance in the protocols does not make specific reference to adverse outcome reporting it provides that health-care providers should have procedures in place for this. The role of clinical risk management is acknowledged in the pre-action protocol but is left as a matter for specific health authorities. It is suggested that clinical risk management systems should be established and also that health-care providers should ensure that key staff are trained in an appropriate manner with some knowledge of health-care law and of complaints procedures. Information regarding adverse incidents and complaints should be used in a positive manner. Patients should be advised as to an adverse outcome and should be given on request information on what actually happened and also information on other steps that could be taken.

Role of expert evidence

One of the major generators of costs in civil litigation which Woolf identified was in the use of expert evidence. (See Ch. 13 of the Woolf Report and also Ch. 15, paras 63 onwards.) The Woolf reforms are concerned to reduce the use of expert evidence to where it is necessary. Today, calling experts requires the permission of the court. There is great emphasis placed upon the use of written evidence. Where experts are to be called then experts from the opposing sides will be encouraged to meet prior to trial to identify the pertinent issues where consensus may be achieved and those issues where there is disagreement between the parties. In some areas there is provision for the use of a single expert, although in practice it appears to be the case that use of the single expert is unlikely in the majority of clinical negligence cases. This is because of the operation of the *Bolam* principle and the fact that the test for negligence is that of the responsible body of professional practice, which necessitates the calling of evidence regarding professional practice regarding that particular issue (see the discussion in Ch. 2). Nonetheless, the Woolf Report did identify various areas in clinical negligence actions where the use of a single expert might indeed be appropriate – for example:

- the assessment of quantum of damages such as future care costs
- in relation to those medical issues that are uncontroversial, such as the precise nature of a tumour
- in relation to such matters as condition and prognosis in straightforward claims
- on matters of liability in claims under £10 000.

It will be interesting to see how restrained parties become through judicial intervention in reducing the number of experts called before the courts.

Specialist courts/tribunals

In addition to the two main categories of court outlined above there are also a number of specialist courts dealing with issues such as family law or, in the case of coroners' courts, examinations into unexplained deaths. Hundreds of different bodies known as tribunals hear matters ranging from unfair dismissal claims in the context of employment tribunals to immigration appeals. A tribunal chairperson is normally legally qualified. For instance, in employment tribunals the chairperson usually sits to decide the case along with two other persons; one person is drawn from an employers' organisation and the other from a trade union. Tribunals are less formal than the courts, with more flexible procedures in relation to calling witnesses and hearing evidence. There is also no automatic right to legal representation or to legal aid.

Sources of law

There are a number of sources of law: first, Acts of Parliament (also known as statutes); second, case law (derived from cases decided in the courts of law). In addition, English law is in some situations governed by laws laid down in Europe through our participation in the European Union (see below, p. 10).

Statutes

English law is to be found in Acts of Parliament. There are many Acts of Parliament relevant to nursing practice, such as the Human Fertilisation and Embryology Act 1990 regulating infertility treatment, or the Abortion Act 1967. In addition, the nurse is affected by those statutes that apply more generally to the population as a whole, such as the Health and Safety at Work Act 1974. Statutes are being continually passed to govern new problems as they arise. A new statute may repeal an earlier statute, or it may amend it either in whole or in part. Statutes may also codify a particular area of law that was previously to be found in a large number of cases, or consolidate both earlier statute law and later case law in one statute.

To become an Act of Parliament, legislation must receive the approval of both Houses of Parliament (Lords and Commons) and it must also receive Royal Assent. A statute is presented to the House of Commons as a Bill. These take two forms. The first category involves Bills sponsored by the government, which will almost certainly result in legislation if the government has a majority. MPs are generally constrained to vote along party political lines. In addition, government-sponsored legislation is allocated a greater amount of parliamentary time. Alternatively, there may be Bills on which the government allows its supporters a free vote so that they can make their decision on a point of conscience. An example is the Abortion Act 1967. The second main category are Private Members' Bills. These, as the name suggests, are Bills introduced into Parliament that do not have the sponsorship of the government. These Bills usually only become law if they have government support.

A statute may provide an outline of the legal position but then leave provisions to be defined by later secondary legislation known as 'statutory instruments'. This enables the legislation to have a more rapid passage through Parliament. So, for example, the Human Tissue Act 2004 set down a regime for undertaking transplants from living organ donors, but the detailed procedure for undertaking those transplants is to be subject to subsequent statutory instruments (see further Ch. 10).

Government departments, such as the Department of Health, issue circulars. While such documents do not have the force of law, they may provide guidance as to what conduct constitutes accepted practice.

Statutory interpretation

A statute may state general legal obligations but where disputes later arise the statute will require interpretation. A court will examine the statute to see how it applies in a particular situation. A word or phrase within the statute may be ambiguous and require construction by the court. There are a number of rules of statutory interpretation that the court may apply. The court may look at the words of the statute and apply them literally. However, it is more likely that the court will construe a word or phrase in the light of the 'purpose' of the statute.

Common law

In some situations there is no legislation governing a particular area, or if there is room for interpretation of the statute then it may be necessary to look elsewhere for guidance as to what is the current law. The relevant law may be found in common law, the term given to describe law that has arisen from previous decisions of the courts on that issue.

Precedent

Some cases are more important than others. Case law operates through a system of 'precedent'. A later court may be obliged to follow the decision of an earlier court. The decisions of the highest court of the land, the House of Lords, are binding on all lower courts (*Davies* v. *Johnson* [1979] AC 264). The House of Lords may depart from its own previous decisions where it 'is appropriate to do so' ([1966] 3 All ER 77). Decisions of the Court of Appeal are also very important and generally bind lower courts. The Court of Appeal itself is normally bound by its previous decisions but it may depart from them in circumstances of 'manifest error' (*Rickard* v. *Rickard* [1989] 2 All ER 193).

Where a case arises involving a very important point of law it may be referred up to the House of Lords in order to obtain a definitive ruling as to the legal position in this area. For example, the famous case of *Gillick* v. *West Norfolk and Wisbech AHA*, which concerned the legality of providing children under 16 years of age with contraceptive advice and treatment without parental consent, was heard in the High Court, the Court of Appeal and then in the House of Lords ([1985] 2 All ER 545).

The decisions of some lower courts do not act as binding precedents, for example, decisions at magistrates' court level. As far as tribunals are concerned, in theory each case is decided on its own facts. However, tribunal decisions are frequently reported and as a consequence general principles have become established.

Interpreting cases

While there may not be a previous case with precisely the same facts, that does not mean that there are no previous cases that can be followed. Lawyers, when trying to discover the current law from previously decided cases, are primarily concerned not with the facts of a particular case but with the point of law that was decided in that case – the ratio decendendi. They then use that point of law in order to argue by analogy to the particular case before them. In a particular case a judge may make a suggestion as to his or her view of the law, a statement that is not directly related to the decision in that case. That statement, known as the obiter dictum, does not bind lower courts. However, an obiter statement may be referred to in a later case as providing a helpful judicial view on the point of law in question.

European law

In 1973 the UK signed the Treaty of Rome and entered the European Economic Community (EEC). Since then UK law has been increasingly affected by European law. In 1993 the Treaty of European Union was passed, which created a new body – the European Union. This is comprised of the states of the European Community but is broader in scope than the EEC.

The European Community Act 1972 provides that rights created by or arising out of the Community Treaties shall have effect in UK law (s2 (1) European Communities Act 1972). There is no general competence to regulate health matters as such across the European Union but there is an explicit legal basis for health in the public health area (Hervey & McHale 2004). So, for example, Article 152 EC, which was introduced by the Treaty of Amsterdam, provides that

> " A high level of human health protection shall be ensured in the definition and implementation of all Community policies and activities. Community action which shall complement national policies shall be directed towards improving public health preventing human illness and diseases and obviating sources of danger to human health.

A number of particular health matters are included, for example, major health scourges and research into the cause and transmission of those diseases. Also included is the provision of information and education relating to health. In addition, UK citizens are affected by European secondary legislation; this is made up of regulations, directives and decisions. Regulations are binding and they are directly applicable in English law, which means that the English courts are required to apply such regulations in English cases. Directives are binding but generally each state is left to determine the manner in which they apply. However, directives do apply to state authorities without further incorporation and this includes NHS bodies (*Marshall v. Southampton and SW Hampshire AHA* [1986] ECR 723). There are many directives that have had a considerable impact upon nursing practice, such as the mutual recognition of nursing qualifications (Directives 77/452/EEC and 77/453/EEC OJ 1977 L 176.) and the Clinical Trials Directive (see further Ch. 8).

The European Court of Justice sits in Luxembourg. If in an English case point of law arises and a UK statute appears to be in conflict with European law, European law is supreme (*Van Gend en Loos* v. *Netherlands Belastingens-administratie* [1963] CMLR 105 ECJ). If there is uncertainty as to the extent to which, for example, a European directive applies in English law then a reference can be made to the European Court of Justice under a procedure known as Article 177, asking for their opinion on this case. Decisions made by the European Court of Justice may be directly binding on English courts and at the very least English courts will take notice of them (s2 (1) European Communities Act 1972). Provisions of EU law have been used in litigation concerning access to health-care services – so, for example, free movement principles under Article 49 EC have been successfully argued in relation to abortion services by EU citizens (*Grogan* [1991] ECR 4685) and in relation to access to infertility services by Diane Blood, who sought to travel to Belgium in order that she could be artificially inseminated by her deceased husband's sperm (*R* v. *Human Fertilisation and Embryology Authority ex parte Blood* [1997] 2 All ER 687) (see further discussion in Ch. 9, and on EU and health see Hervey & McHale 2004). Most recently, as this book goes to press, in *Watts* v. *Bedford PCT* [2006] QB 667 the European Court of Justice has held that patients may use free movement principles to bypass NHS waiting lists and instead travel to another EU country and then claim reimbursement of the cost of treatment from the NHS.

European Convention on Human Rights

We are also party to the European Convention of Human Rights (ECHR). This is totally separate from our membership of the European Union. The ECHR came into force on 3 September 1953. Individual citizens of the UK have had a right to petition under the Convention since 1966. The Convention contains a list of what are regarded as fundamental human rights. If a person believes that one of his or her fundamental rights has been violated and the claim is not upheld in the English courts, s/he can seek to bring the case before the European Commission of Human Rights in Strasbourg. Actions have been brought, for example, challenging a woman's decision to have an abortion (*Paton* v. *UK* [1980] 3 EHRR 408; *Vo* v. *France* [2005] 40 EHRR 12). Where a claim is upheld before the European Court of Human Rights the English courts were in the past not able to follow it, nor has Parliament been bound to change the law on that matter. However the role of human rights changed radically following the enactment of the Human Rights Act 1998, which came into force in October 2000.

Human Rights Act 1998

The Human Rights Act 1998 is the first comprehensive bill of rights to be enacted in the UK. It incorporates rights contained in the European Convention of Human Rights into English law. As noted above, individuals were able to bring claims direct to the European Court of Human Rights in Strasbourg but this was a protracted process. Bringing such a claim would take several years and ultimately, while the British government might decide to act upon the findings of the Court, this was not invariably the case. The Human Rights Act 1998 therefore enacts a radical change (McHale & Gallagher 2003).

From October 2000, where an English court is determining a matter 'in connection with' a right under the Convention, then it must, as far as is applicable, take account of Strasbourg case law (s.2). All primary and secondary legislation must be construed consistently with the 1998 Act (s.3). Where subordinate legislation (e.g. statutory instruments) are inconsistent the court may disapply it. This applies as long as the legislation doesn't debar this (s.3 (2)). What the court cannot do is strike down primary legislation – in effect act as a 'Supreme Court'. The word of Parliament, as expressed through statute, ultimately prevails. Certain courts, such as the House of Lords, High Court and County Court, have the power to make what is called a 'declaration of incompatibility' (s.4). This does not effect the continuing validity of the legislation itself (s4 (6)), however, as a consequence of such a declaration of incompatibility a government minister may make a 'remedial order' in relation to a particular piece of legislation, which may also lead to remedial action in a particular case, although this is not automatic. The first such declaration of incompatibility in health-care law was in the case of *R (H)* v. *Mental Health Review Tribunal North and East London Region* [2001] EWCA Civ. 415. This case concerned a patient detained under the Mental Health Act 1983 after having been convicted of manslaughter. He applied for discharge to a Mental Health Review Tribunal. At that time section 72 of the Mental Health Act placed the burden of proof on the patient to show that he no longer suffered from a disorder that warranted his continued detention. The Court of Appeal held that this provision contravened Article 5 (4) of the ECHR and an infringement of an individual's liberty and made a declaration of incompatibility. The government subsequently amended this specific provision in the light of the declaration. There is also new right of action provided against a public body acting in a public capacity, such as an NHS body, that acts in a manner that is incompatible with a right under the ECHR. (ss6 (1),7 (1) Human Rights Act 1998).

While the Human Rights Act has been used in a number of notable cases its impact in the context of health care has been to a certain extent muted to date. Some of this is due to the fact that applying broad principles such as those stated in the ECHR may prove practically problematic, and because many Convention rights are subject to exceptions and in addition a margin of appreciation is employed. As we shall see in later chapters in relation to issues such as end-of-life decision-making (*R (on the application of Pretty)* v. *DPP* [2002] 1 All ER 1), abortion and in vitro fertilisation (IVF) treatment (*Evans* v. *UK* [2006] Application No. 6339/05, Strasbourg, 6 March 2006), application of ECHR principles, despite an impact in areas such as mental health and donor identity in relation to IVF (see Ch. 9), has not in practice led to any radical alteration of the current legal position generally.

Access to justice

One of the main restrictions upon use of the court process is that of the cost involved in bringing a case. For many years there has been a system of state-funded legal advice, assistance and representation known as legal aid ((s1) Legal Aid Act 1988). Generally, applicants seeking legal aid are subject to a means test of their income and disposable capital to determine their eligibility. There was considerable criticism of the scheme and it was argued that the threshold for disposable income and capital above which there was no entitlement to free legal aid was very low. In a situation in which a person's income and disposable capital are higher than the levels of eligibility, then s/he could be required to make contributions in accordance with income levels. The levels of those eligible to receive legal aid gradually decreased. Many cases were funded by legal expense insurance, for example individuals involved in road accident cases, and trade union members have access to legal support.

The operation of the funding system was altered by the Access to Justice Act 1999. (Legal Aid Board 1999) This established a new Legal Services Commission, which is a non-departmental public body. It has the task of creating and developing the Community Legal Service and the Criminal Defence Service (ss1–3). There are regional legal services committees, which work to ensure that needs for legal services and regional priorities are correctly identified. The previous civil and family legal aid budget was replaced by a Community Legal Services Fund. The changes in funding in legal services were partly driven by a concern that unmeritorious claims were being funded, that the previous system had been too heavily biased towards court-based solutions and that, because lawyers were paid according to the amount of work that was undertaken, they had no incentive to undertake cases expeditiously.

The Fund is obliged to obtain the best value for money. It contracts for legal services with solicitors' firms. This is an extension of the scheme of legal aid franchising under which firms who wanted to obtain legal aid work had to satisfy various quality control thresholds before they obtained a legal aid franchise, which gave them the ability to obtain more work. There is a 'quality mark', and applications for this can be received not only from solicitors' firms but also from other advice agencies, etc. The government has also encouraged the development of 'community legal service partnerships' between bodies such as local authorities, charities and advice providers. The aim is to widen access to legal advice.

Persons making applications to the Fund must satisfy the Funding Code (s8 and 9). This replaces the civil merits test. The Code is more restrictive than the previous system. Applicants for funding from the scheme are subject to a 'funding assessment'. Factors that are relevant are whether there is an alternative way of resolving the dispute and whether there are alternative sources of funding for litigation, and in addition whether a reasonable person would be prepared to spend their own funds to pursue the litigation. The majority of personal injury claims are now be funded through what is known as a 'conditional fee' system rather than through state aid.

Conditional fees

'Conditional fees for civil law cases' were introduced by the Courts and Legal Services Act 1990 (s58). These allow lawyers to take on cases without the client incurring any costs for representation, but the lawyer can recover a higher fee offset against the damages awarded in a successful action. These are different from the scheme of contingency fee common in the USA. That system operates by a lawyer taking on a client's case without requiring the client to make any initial financial contribution to the legal fees, but, if the client's case succeeds, the lawyer can recover an agreed percentage of the damages. The scope of conditional fees was extended in 1998 to apply to a range of civil litigation, although not in relation to family proceedings. Following the 1999 reforms the conditional fee has an enhanced importance because state-funded legal assistance will not be available to those persons who are bringing personal injury actions (although clinical negligence actions are excluded from this restriction). The conditional fee system has been amended so that successful litigants can recover success fees and insurance fees from their opponents (Access to Justice Act 1999). Although in principle such an approach may widen access to litigation and provide enhanced financial incentives for lawyers to undertake litigation, for litigants the danger is that those cases where there is considerable uncertainty may never be pursued, as lawyers do not want to take the risk; one reason why clinical negligence actions still receive state-funded assistance.

Criminal Defence Service

In criminal cases there is no set budget for funding litigation and the crucial issue is rather the merits of the case. There is a 'Criminal Defence Service' that has the aim of ensuring that persons 'have access to such advice, assistance and representation as the interests of justice require'. As with civil procedure, if solicitors wish to provide this service they must 'contract' to do so with the Legal Services Commission. Some lawyers are directly employed by the Commission to undertake representation in criminal cases. One of the criticisms made is that this scheme is leading to a reduction in the availability of legal services because far fewer law firms will be offering this type of representation.

Settlements

While a dispute may lead to parties seeking legal advice and beginning legal proceedings, that does not mean that a case will ultimately go to court. The majority of cases are settled before proceedings in court have begun. Indeed, the threat of legal proceedings may operate as a negotiating tool, encouraging parties to settle their differences.

THE STRUCTURE OF THE NATIONAL HEALTH SERVICE

Most health care provided in England is provided by the NHS, although nurses may of course work outside the NHS, for example in nursing homes and residential care homes. The Secretary of State for Health is accountable to Parliament for the operation of the health service. S/he has statutory obligations to promote a 'comprehensive health service' (s1 (1) NHS Act 1977). S/he controls NHS expenditure through the use of cash limits. Day to day management of the Health Service is undertaken by the Department of Health. Below the Secretary of State are Strategic Health Authorities (SHAs) (s8 NHS Act 1977, as amended). Currently there are around 30 such bodies but the number is presently being reduced to eight as part of the most recent NHS reorganisation.

Below SHAs are Primary Care Trusts (PCTs) (s16 A and s16 B NHS Act 1977, as amended). These commission primary care services, which include ' personal medical services' (s29 NHS Act 1977, as amended). This includes GP services.

In addition, PCTs purchase hospital care. These may be from private hospitals or from NHS trusts. NHS trusts were created under s5 (1) of the National Health Service and Community Care Act 1990, which provides that they can be created by the Secretary of State by order.

Services may also be purchased from new bodies known as Foundation Hospital Trusts. (s1 (1) Health and Social Care (Community Health and Standards) Act 2003). These are bodies that are given much greater autonomy than standard NHS trusts. They are accountable to a new independent regulator, the Monitor (s14 (2) Health and Social Care (Community Health and Standards Act 2003), the Commissions, the Healthcare Commission and the public. Only NHS Trusts that reach three-star rating can apply to be Foundation Trusts (see s26 Health Act 1999, as amended by Health and Social Care, Community Health and Standards Act 2003, and Newdick 2005).

Clinical governance

Emphasis is being placed upon the need to maintain standards in health care. An early example of such emphasis on standards was the Patient's Charter. While this document is essentially a list of guidelines and breach of Patient Charter requirements are not directly enforceable in the courts, the movement towards stating acceptable standards of health care has continued in recent years. In the White Paper *The New NHS* the concept of clinical governance was discussed. This was further explored in the consultation paper on quality that was issued by the Department of Health in 1998 (Department of Health 1998). This defined 'clinical governance' as being 'a framework through which NHS organisations are accountable for continuously improving the quality of their services and safeguarding high standards of care by creating an environment in which excellence in clinical care will flourish'. The Health Act 1999 made provision, in section 18, for the NHS trusts and primary care groups to be placed under a new statutory duty of quality. Clinical governance will be promoted through the operation of the Healthcare Commission and the National Institute for Health and Clinical Excellence (NICE). The former has a role in providing oversight and inspection of health quality issues. The latter plays an important role in providing guidance on promotion of good health and the prevention and treatment of ill health. Guidance is provided in relation to public health, health technologies and clinical practice.

The Healthcare Commission

The Healthcare Commission was established in 2004 (under s41 of the Health and Social Care (Community Health and Standards) Act 2003). It replaces the Commission for Health Improvement. The Healthcare Commission is headed by Professor Sir Ian Kennedy. From 2005 it has undertaken annual 'health checks'. The Commission inspects NHS organisations – PCTs and hospitals – also independent health-care services, private doctors and hospitals, and hospices. It examines seven categories – safety, clinical and cost-effectiveness, governance, is it patient focused, is the care accessible and responsive, the environment and amenities, and public health. Organisations are measured to ascertain whether they meet basic standards and then whether they are improving.

The Healthcare Commission also plays a role at the second stage of the NHS complaints process, undertaking independent reviews of complaints (see further Ch. 4).

It also has powers to undertake serious investigations where concerns are expressed regarding the levels of NHS care, and to undertake audit and make unannounced inspections.

The Healthcare Commission works alongside the Commission for Social Care Inspection, particularly in respect of care of children and of the elderly. The government's aim is that these two bodies will merge in 2008 as part of a broader governmental review of health and social care. In addition, the intention is that the functions of the Mental Health Act Commission will be transferred to this body (see further Ch. 6).

National Institute for Health and Clinical Excellence

The National Institute for Clinical Excellence has also been established. This is a special health authority and provides guidance to patients, health professionals and the public as to 'best practice'. Such guidance covers the clinical management of specific conditions and also individual health technologies such as medicines, diagnostic devices and procedures. NICE is involved in the development of clinical audits with the aim of enabling health professionals to monitor their practice and will be involved in assessing how a particular technology has been used nationally through the merger of clinical audit findings. NICE's important role in the development of clinical guidelines, is discussed further in Chapter 4. Nurses need to be aware of the role and operation of such organisations and of the increasing emphasis on both clinical accountability and upon quality in health-care practice (discussed further in Ch. 4.)

Challenges to failure to provide health services

The Secretary of State for Health has various statutory duties. Section 1 of the National Health Service Act 1977 states:

“ It is the Secretary of State's duty to continue the promotion in England and Wales of a comprehensive health service designed to ensure improvement:

(a) in the physical and mental health of the people of those countries and
(b) in the prevention, diagnosis and treatment of illness and for that purpose to provide or secure effective provision of services in accordance with the Act.

Section 3 of that Act states:

“ It is the Secretary of State's duty to provide throughout England and Wales to such extent as he considers necessary to meet all reasonable requirements – (a) hospital accommodation… (c) medical, dental, nursing and ambulance services… (f) such other services as are required for the diagnosis and treatment of illness.

Can the Secretary of State be held liable if services are not provided? In a number of cases persons have challenged a failure to provide health-care services in the courts. For example, patients in Birmingham challenged the health authority's refusal to provide a unit for orthopaedic services (*R* v. *Secretary of State for Social Service ex parte Hincks* [1980] [1979] 123 Sol J 436). The application failed. In the Court of Appeal, Lord Denning, agreeing with the judge at first instance, stated that the Secretary of State's duty needed to be read in the light of the financial resources that he had available. Subsequently, in two cases, both concerning surgery required on an infant, the courts again rejected the claim that in refusing to provide these facilities, the Secretary of State had acted in breach of duty. *CR* v. *Central Birmingham HA ex p Collier [1988] Lexis* 6 January.

In the second case Stephen Brown L.J. stated that

❝ this is a hearing before a court. This is not the forum in which a court can properly express opinions upon the way in which national resources are allocated or distributed. [There] may be very good reasons why the resources in this case do not allow all the beds in the hospital to be used at this particular time. We have no evidence of that and indeed… it is not for this court or for any other court to substitute its own judgment for the judgment of those who are responsible for the allocation of resources.

It might have been thought that the advent of the NHS internal market would have led to more parties 'chancing their arm' and challenging resource allocation decisions. However, litigants have not been flocking to the courts.

The question of allocation of resources arose in the context of a well publicised case involving a young child. B, a 10-year-old child, suffered from leukaemia. Treatment was undertaken involving chemotherapy and a bone marrow transplant, which was initially successful; however, the cancer re-urred. Cambridgeshire Health Authority refused to authorise a further course of treatment. Doctors stated that a third course of chemotherapy and a further transplant would not be in the child's best interests and that, overall, the success rate of the procedure was 1–4%. The child's father sought to challenge the decision to refuse treatment. The case was heard first in the High Court and then on appeal in the Court of Appeal (*R* v. *Cambridge District Health Authority ex parte B* [1995] 2 All ER 129). Both hearings took place on the same afternoon.

At first instance in the High Court, Laws J. said that, in determining whether to give treatment, the health authority must act reasonably. This meant that, in making the decision, the health authority should have regard to all relevant considerations. In this case he said the health authority had not taken into consideration the views of B's family. He was also of the view that in a situation where, as here, a patient was at risk of death, the health authority had to explain why it had decided not to fund the treatment.

However, his judgment was overturned in the Court of Appeal. Sir Thomas Bingham, the Master of the Rolls, held that, while the finance director of the health authority had not spoken directly to the family, he had noted the interests of the family. In addition, difficult issues concerning resource allocation had to be weighed in the balance. He stated that

> ❝ Difficult and agonising judgments had to be made as to how a limited
> budget could best be allocated for the maximum advantage of the
> maximum number of patients. That was not a judgment for the court.

Sir Thomas Bingham held that the health authority had weighed up the various factors in reaching the decision and had not acted unreasonably. Relevant factors were that the treatment was untested and that it could almost be regarded as being experimental in its nature. There was only around a 1–4% success rate. In addition, the court noted the fact that there were potentially debilitating side-effects. The court held that in these circumstances the decision of the health authority was not unreasonable.

However, subsequently the courts have indicated greater willingness to scrutinise decisions concerning the allocation of resources. In *R* v. *North Derbyshire Health Authority ex parte Fisher*, ([1997] 8 MedLR 327) High Court judge held that North Derbyshire Health Authority had acted unlawfully in that a patient with multiple sclerosis had been denied treatment with an expensive new drug, interferon. The Authority adopted a policy to the effect that the drug would not be made available outside a clinical trial and this was even though they were informed of the fact that clinical trials of this drug had been the subject of indefinite postponement. Dyson J. held that the health authority had imposed what amounted to a blanket ban on the drug although there was NHS guidance in existence regarding its use. He said that 'a blanket ban was the very antithesis of national policy, whose aim was to target the drug at patients who could most benefit from the treatment'.

In *R* v. *North West Lancashire HA ex parte A, D and G* ([2000] 1 WLR 977) Lancashire Health Authority's refusal to fund gender reassignment surgery for transsexuals was challenged successfully. The Authority had a policy that stated that they would not fund such treatment unless there was overriding clinical need or other exceptional circumstances. The Court of Appeal held that, while the Authority was entitled to establish a policy, they had applied the policy such as to allow only individually determined exceptions; rather it was closer to the blanket allocation of a policy in a particular situation.

The issue of guidelines in relation to GP prescribing of Viagra was challenged successfully in *R* v. *Secretary of State for Health ex parte Pfizer Ltd* ([1999] *Lloyds Rep. Med.* 289). Here the Secretary of State issued a health service circular with the aim of limiting the prescription of Viagra by general practitioners. The NHS terms of service for general practitioners had provided that 'a doctor shall order any drugs or appliances which are needed for the treatment of any patient to whom he is providing treatment under these terms of service by issuing to that patient a prescription form'.

The action for judicial review succeeded. It was held that the doctor was entitled to give such treatment as was considered necessary and appropriate.

The advent of the Human Rights Act has to date had little impact in this area. In *R* v. *North West Lancashire HA ex parte A, D and G* ([2000] 1 WLR 977) the human rights claims were unsuccessful. Here, Auld L.J. held that Article 8, which protects the right to privacy of home and family life, was not applicable here. In addition the Court of Appeal also held that Article 3 – the prohibition on torture and inhuman and degrading treatment – was inapplicable in a situation, such as here, that concerned resource allocation.

On what basis should such matters be left to the courts? The approach taken by Laws J. in the Child B case has considerable relevance for those who are arguing for health rights and exploring this in the context of litigation deriving from the Human Rights Act 1998. It is undeniable that resources are, and indeed always will be, limited. In analogous area, the provision of care under the Chronically Sick and Disabled Persons Act 1970, section 2, the House of Lords confirmed that, when assessing needs under that Act, this could not be divorced from the costs that were involved in the supply of those needs (*R v. Gloucester CC ex parte Barry* [1997] AC 584).

European Union law and resource allocation

Recently litigants have been attempting to use EU law as a means of bypassing NHS waiting lists. In *Watts v. Bedford PCT*, Mrs Watts, who was on a waiting list in the UK, went to France for a hip operation and then claimed the cost of reimbursement of the operation from the NHS. She relied on her rights under EU law. EU provides 'free movement' rights under the Treaty and these include the right to travel to receive medical services. Article 49 of the EC Treaty provides that:

" Restrictions on the freedom to provide services within the Community shall be prohibited in respect of nationals of Member States who are established in a State of the Community other than that of the person for whom the services are intended.

Article 50 further provides that:

" Services shall be considered to be 'services' within the meaning of this Treaty where they are normally provided for remuneration….

" 'Services' shall in particular include… (d) activities of the professions.

Treatment has long been regarded by the ECJ as a 'service' (*Luisi and Carbone v. Ministero del Tesoro* (joined cases 286/82 and 26/83) [1984] ECR 377). Litigants have sought to combine their claims under Article 49 with Article 22 of Regulation No. 1408/71, which concerns social security provisions. Article 22 provides states with discretion to determine whether treatment is reimbursed. However it also provides that this authorisation

" may not be refused where the treatment in question is among the benefits provided for by the legislation of the Member State on whose territory the person concerned resides and where he cannot be given such treatment within the time normally necessary for obtaining the treatment in question in the Member State of residence, taking account of his current state of health and the probable course of the disease.

The issue that arose in this case is the extent to which these rights also enable a person to bypass an NHS waiting list by receiving treatment in another member state. It had been clear from earlier decisions that if a person was subject to 'undue delay' they could seek treatment abroad and claim reimbursement but this applied in the context of EU countries with a social insurance system (*Kholl/Dekker Case C-158/96*; *Geraets–Smits* v. *Stichting Ziekenfonds VGZ Case 157/99*; *Muller Faure Case C-385/99*; *Inizan Case C-56/01*). Here the difference was that this related to a state national health service and it was unclear as to, first, whether the case law applied to the UK NHS and, second, if it did whether Mrs Watts could reclaim the cost of the operation because there had been undue delay. At first instance Mumby J. said Yes to the first question but rejected the second issue on the facts. The Court of Appeal then referred this issue for a preliminary ruling to the European Court of Justice to obtain a clarification of this issue (*Secretary of State for Health* v. *R on the application of Yvonne Watts* [2004] EWCA Civ 166). The matter was referred to the European Court of Justice (*The Queen on the application of Yvonne Watts* Case C-372/04). In an initial opinion the Advocate General expressed his view that the free movement cases did apply in the context of the NHS. In May 2006, the European Court of Justice held that these cases did indeed apply in the context of the NHS. Moreover, in considering what amounted to 'undue delay', the fact that a particular health authority had complied with waiting list times was not sufficient. It was the task of PCTs to ensure that the waiting time 'does not exceed the period which is acceptable in the light of an objective medical assessment' of clinical need. Factors that will be taken into account include the degree of pain suffered and level of disability. Furthermore it was the case that waiting list times were to be set 'flexibly and dynamically' and they should also be reassessed if there was a deterioration in condition. The issue has been remitted to the English courts for a final determination of the facts of the case.

The involvement of EU law raises the prospect of individuals who believe that waiting list times are too long bypassing them and being treated abroad and reclaiming the cost from the NHS. How far will this change resource allocation? Despite concerns as to the impact on NHS resources it is possible that it may prove a 'middle-class solution', since patients will need to have sufficient resources to pay 'up front' for the treatment abroad and then to reclaim the cost. In addition, it will almost certainly only arise in situations of elective surgery as opposed to emergency treatment.

Even if they are prepared to intervene, it is arguable that the courts do not provide an appropriate forum for such scrutiny. The whole question of rationing in health care needs to be addressed at national level rather than on a case-by-case basis as matters are referred to the courts. We may profit from consideration of the model adopted in one USA state, Oregon, where rationing has been put on a statutory footing (Newdick 2005). Here, public consultation was undertaken before a list of treatment priorities was enacted in statute. The role of NICE in the public prioritisation of health-care resources is thus likely to prove of some considerable importance here in the future.

PROFESSIONAL ACCOUNTABILITY

The Nursing and Midwifery Council

The work of nurses in the UK is overseen by their professional governing body, the Nursing and Midwifery Council (NMC), which was established by the Nursing and Midwifery Order 2001 (SI 2002/253). (This replaces the previous regulatory system under the Nurses, Midwives and Health Visitors Act 1997.) The principle function of the Council is to establish standards of education, training, conduct and performance for nurses and midwives and to ensure that these standards are maintained. The Council has four Committees established under regulations: the Investigating Committee, the Conduct and Competence Committee, the Health Committee and the Midwifery Committee.

The professional register

The Nursing and Midwifery Council is required to establish a register of qualified nurses and midwives (Nursing and Midwifery Order 2001 (SI 2002/253, reg. 5)). It establishes rules regarding entry, removal and reinstatement from the register. Qualifications obtained in other European Union countries will be recognised and the NMC also recognises other qualifications obtained outside the UK (article 9). Nurses may be entered on the register if they hold an approved qualification awarded either within 5 years, or before that if they have also obtained additional education, training and experience and in addition have satisfied the Registrar in accordance with the Council's requirements that they are capable of safe and effective practice as a nurse or midwife (article 9). The NMC is also concerned with standards of nurse education and training, both at entry into the profession and post-qualification (articles 15–19).

Code of conduct

The NMC is required to establish standards of conduct, performance and ethics (article 21). Failure to comply with the code of practice is something that may be taken into account in deciding whether fitness to practice is impaired (article 22 (4) 2001 Order; rules 31 (7) of 2004 Rules). As we will see later, the nurse may face a difficult dilemma if her/his obligations under the professional ethical code and under the contract of employment are at variance.

Impairment of fitness to practice

The Council deals with situations in which fitness to practice is impaired.

- Misconduct
- Lack of competence
- Conviction for a criminal offence or a caution in the UK for a criminal offence
- Physical or mental health
- Or a decision by a health regulatory body that fitness to practise is impaired, or a determination by a licensing body elsewhere to the same effect (article 22)

Investigation of allegations that fitness to practice is impaired

The Order sets out the procedure to be followed in investigating whether the fitness to practise of a registrant is impaired. The Council has power to appoint 'screeners', although to date this has not been done (article 22).

The Investigating Committee

Allegations may be referred to the Investigating Committee (article 26). It shall inform the person of the allegation and invite them to submit written representations within the period. The hearing is in private (r4 (1) NMC Rules 2004). If having investigated the allegation it finds that there is a case to answer; or an entry in the register has been fraudulently procured or incorrectly made, then it shall notify in writing both the person concerned and the person making the allegation, if any, of its decision, giving its reasons. If the Committee finds there is a case to answer it has several options. It may undertake mediation. Alternatively, a reference may be made to the Health Committee or to the Conduct and Competence Committee (art 26.6 of 2001 Order).

The Conduct and Competence Committee and the Health Committee

The Conduct and Competence Committee has the task of advising the Council on standards of conduct, performance and ethics expected of registrants and prospective registrants (article 27). In addition, it advises on requirements as to good character and good health to be met by registrants and prospective registrants, and the protection of the public from people whose fitness to practise is impaired.

In addition, it considers any allegation referred to it by the Council, the Investigating Committee or the Health Committee, and also any application for restoration referred to it by the Registrar. Matters may also be referred for consideration by the Health Committee.

Procedure

The procedure for the Committees is set out in Part 5 of the 2004 Rules (NMC 2004). The practitioner will be informed of the allegation and written representations will be invited. Notice of the referral to the Committee must be given to the employer and to the relevant government department. The person against whom the allegation has been made may be invited to undergo an assessment of competence or a medical examination. A hearing may be undertaken where requested by the person subject to the allegation or where the Committee is of the opinion that a hearing would be desirable (r10 (2) NMC Rules 2004).

In deciding whether an allegation is 'well founded', in the past a criminal standards of proof – beyond all reasonable doubt – has been used (*R (on the application of Aston)* v. *NMC* [2004] EWCA Admin., para 64).

The Conduct and Competence Committee and Health Committee have a wide range of options (article 29). They may undertake mediation, or decide that it is not appropriate to take any further action. They also have considerable sanctions, in that they may make a 'striking off' order requiring the Registrar to strike the person concerned off the register. Alternatively, they may suspend registration for a period that must not exceed 1 year – the 'suspension order'. A further option is the imposition of a 'conditions of practice order', which can impose conditions with which the person must comply for a period that does not exceed 3 years. They may also make a 'caution order'. This means that they caution the person concerned and make an order directing the Registrar to annotate the register accordingly for a specified period, which shall be not less than 1 year and not more than 5 years. There is also provision for further review of the orders while they are in force (article 30) and they can confirm, extend or reduce the orders. Where the allegations concern physical or mental health or lack of competence, then a striking-off order may not be made in respect of an allegation of the kind mentioned in article 22 (1) (a) (ii) or (iv) unless the person concerned has been continuously suspended, or subject to a conditions of practice order, for a period of no less than 2 years immediately preceding the date of the decision of the Committee to make such an order.

Appeal

There is provision for an appeal to the High Court in the case of England and Wales against the order made (article 30 (9)) and this must be made within 28 days beginning on the date at which such an order is served. The court has wide-ranging powers to terminate a suspension or in the case of conditions of practice orders to revoke or vary any condition imposed by the order.

However, in practice the court is unlikely to overturn the decision, as they are more prepared to accept the professional judgment (*Slater* v. *UKCC* unreported 18 May 1988 (QBD)). In addition, the conduct of proceedings of the committee may be subject to judicial review. The committees are under a duty to act fairly and must give nurses an opportunity to present their case and to answer the charges made against them. If they fail to do so, this may lead to a challenge that the conduct of the hearing was contrary to the rules of natural justice (*Hefferen* v. *The Committee of the UKCC* (1988); *The Independent*, 11 March).

Restoration to the register

There are provisions enabling a nurse to be reinstated to the register under article 33 of the 2001 Order. Applications can only be made after 5 years have passed since the striking-off order took effect. If they fail at that point then they must wait another year before reapplying. If that further application is unsuccessful, the Committee has the power to make an order of indefinite suspension subject to providing that this should be reviewed at regular intervals (articles 33 and 10, 2001 Order). If a restoration to the register order is made, a 'condition of practice' order may also be imposed, which, as the name suggests, stipulates conditions regarding the conduct of the nurse's practice (article 33 (7) b, 2001 Order).

Special provisions also relate to midwives. There is a Midwifery Committee (article 41). The role of the Committee is to advise the Council on midwifery matters. Specific rules also relate to midwifery determining suspension from practice, to give notice of their intention to practice and also require them to attend training courses (article 42). There is also provision for local supervising authorities (LSA) of midwives (article 43). The LSA must report to the Council the fact that the fitness to practise of a midwife in its area is impaired. In addition it has powers to suspend midwives from practice.

CONCLUSIONS

This chapter has set out the framework of legal regulation within which the nurse undertakes her/his practice. In subsequent chapters the operation of the law is considered in a number of areas that are particularly pertinent to nursing practice.

REFERENCES

Davies C 2000 Getting health care professionals to work together. British Medical Journal 321: 698

Department of Health 1998 A first class service – quality in the new NHS. Department of Health, London

Department of Health 2001 Learning from Bristol: the report of the Public Inquiry into children's heart surgery at the Bristol Royal Infirmary 1984–1995. Stationery Office, London

Hervey TK, McHale JV 2004 Health law and the European Union. Cambridge University Press, Cambridge

Legal Aid Board 1999 Modernising justice. HMSO, London

McHale JV, Gallagher A 2003 Nursing and human rights. Butterworth Heinemann, Edinburgh

Newdick C 2005 Who should we treat?: rights, rationing, and resources in the NHS, 2nd edn. Oxford University Press, Oxford

NHS Executive 2000 Modernising regulation: the new Nursing and Midwifery Council. NHS Executive, London

Norris R 2006 The next nursing century. Nursing Times 102(18): 14–16

Nursing and Midwifery Council 2004 NMC Code of professional conduct: standards for conduct, performance and ethics. NMC, London

Redfern M 2001 The Royal Liverpool Children's Inquiry. HMSO, London

Salvage J, Smith R 2000 Doctors and nurses: doing it differently. British Medical Journal 320: 1019–1020

Tingle J, Cribb A (eds) 2000 Nursing law and ethics. Blackwell Scientific Publications, Oxford

Woolf H 1996 Access to justice: final report, by the Right Honourable the Lord Woolf, Master of the Rolls. HMSO, London

Nursing negligence: general issues

John Tingle

2

INTRODUCTION

Nurses are not only professionally accountable to patients through the Nursing and Midwifery Council (NMC) *Code of Professional Conduct: Standards for Conduct, Performance and Ethics* (the Code) (Nursing and Midwifery Council 2004) but, like all other professionals, they are accountable in law, and malpractice may lead to a civil action or a criminal prosecution. A nurse is under a legal duty to act carefully towards the patient. If a nurse fails to exercise sufficient care and by so doing causes injury or harm to the patient, s/he will be held liable in the tort of negligence.

The next section considers liability in tort for negligent conduct; later sections consider liability in criminal law where actions are gravely negligent, and some issues regarding reform of the law of negligence. The present chapter focuses upon general principles of liability. Various related negligence issues are examined in later chapters, including liability under certain statutes for negligence. Questions of liability in relation to childbirth and conception are considered in Chapter 9.

LIABILITY IN TORT FOR NEGLIGENT CONDUCT

Accidents sometimes happen

A nurse is not negligent if s/he acts in accordance with a practice accepted as proper by a responsible body of nursing opinion. The nurse is not expected to take precautions against unforeseeable risks and even if risks are foreseeable they may still be justified in the particular circumstances of the case. Accidents, untoward incidents or adverse treatment outcomes may occur without any findings of fault being made against the nurse. The following two examples illustrate this point.

> A competent nurse, following the correct procedure for venepuncture, may still cause the patient to develop a haematoma, or bleed after the removal of the needle if the patient is on anticoagulant therapy. This may happen occasionally even though the nurse has ascertained that the patient is taking anticoagulants and has applied pressure to the site of venepuncture him/herself. Bruising can be reduced if pressure is applied by the nurse or phlebotomist but bruising can still occur in the older patient and, occasionally, slight pain and discomfort.

> Ribs have been known to fracture when a patient receives external cardiac massage even though the nurse has carried out the procedure correctly.

Elements of the tort of negligence

Generally speaking, the claimant (the person bringing the court action) must prove negligence against the nurse or the nurse's employers. The claimant will normally have to prove his/her case on the 'balance of probabilities'. The elements of the tort of negligence must be established.

The basic elements are as follows:

- Duty
- Breach
- Damage
- Remoteness.

Duty

The claimant must first establish that the defendant (nurse or health authority, Trust) owed him/her a legal duty of care. In the health-care context this is usually not a problem as Jones (1992) has commented when defining the tort:

" In cases of medical negligence the existence of a duty owed to the patient is usually regarded as axiomatic, and attention normally focuses on whether there has been a breach of duty or whether the breach caused damage.

However, the issue of duty could be problematic where a nurse acts as a 'good Samaritan' and causes further injury by negligently administering first aid to the accident victim. The duty issue in relation to accident victims was raised in the Court of Appeal in *Kent* v. *Griffiths and Others* ([2000] 2 All ER 474). It was held that, in appropriate circumstances, an ambulance service could owe a duty of care to a member of the public on whose behalf a 999 call was made if, through carelessness, it failed to arrive within a reasonable time. The acceptance of the call by the ambulance service established the duty of care. The ambulance in this case was delayed through no good reason, taking 40 minutes to arrive. The claimant, an asthmatic, suffered an asthma attack and eventually went into respiratory arrest. Had the ambulance arrived in a reasonable time there was a high probability that the arrest would have been averted. The delay caused the claimant further injuries. The defendant's appeal was dismissed.

The courts are unlikely to find an express legal duty to rescue a stranger: the nurse could walk past the victim with legal impunity (Tingle 1991). However, if the nurse stops and acts then a legal duty of care will flow from his/her actions. The nurse now could be sued if s/he practices first aid negligently and causes further injury. In contrast, it appears that the NMC would expect the nurse to act as a good Samaritan and assist if s/he could easily do so. Clause 8.5 of the NMC Code provides:

" In an emergency, in or outside the work setting, you have a professional duty to provide care. The care provided would be judged against what could reasonably be expected from someone with your knowledge, skills and abilities when placed in those circumstances.

Examples 2 and 3 given by the predecessor regulatory body to the NMC, the United Kingdom Central Council for Nursing, Midwifery and Health Visiting (UKCC), in their advisory document (United Kingdom Central Council for Nursing, Midwifery and Health Visiting 1996), provide useful illustrations of the UKCC approach to the nurse as good Samaritan, and the NMC approach would probably be the same. In example 3 a distinction is made between legal and professional duties. A nurse would be expected to make some response in the emergency situation postulated, at the very least comforting and supporting the injured patient. There is a risk, however, that if s/he does act and makes a mistake, then legal consequences may follow. However, it should be remembered that the likelihood of a good Samaritan being sued is fairly remote and that the public interest is better served by doing and encouraging good Samaritan acts.

Duty questions

The first issue is whether a person has in fact become a patient of a health-care professional or a hospital. This question is discussed in sections 11–14 of UKCC (United Kingdom Central Council for Nursing, Midwifery and Health Visiting 1996) and some useful illustrations are given. The NMC Code now provides in Clause 1.2:

> As a registered nurse, midwife or specialist community public health nurse, you must:
>
> - protect and support the health of individual patients and clients
> - protect and support the health of the wider community
> - act in such a way that justifies the trust and confidence the public have in you
> - uphold and enhance the good reputation of the profession.

Clause 1.4 provides:

> You have a duty of care to your patients and clients, who are entitled to receive safe and competent care.

Patient and client are defined in the glossary in the Code as 'Any individual or group using a health service'.

The following situation may also help to explain the issue:

An injured confused man wanders into a hospital after a road traffic accident and is unable to locate the Accident and Emergency Department. He requires urgent medical treatment. A hospital security guard passes him in a corridor in the hospital and does not challenge or question him. A nurse hurrying home after finishing her shift also passes him without stopping. Should the guard and the nurse have stopped and questioned him?

Can the guard and the nurse be said to have owed a duty of care to the accident victim that would have required such action? Furthermore, what about the position of the hospital? Were there any organisational failures, such as failure to erect a signpost properly or to man a reception desk, that would make the hospital directly liable for any negligence?

Much will depend on the circumstances of the case and on answers to factual questions such as: How ill did the victim look? What was the time of the incident? and so on. It will be seen that Example 2 of section 14 in United Kingdom Central Council for Nursing, Midwifery and Health Visiting 1996 is similar in facts to the problem discussed. The UKCC states that in its example the nurse would be expected to take some action, comforting and supporting the patient and calling for expert help. Clause 8.5 of the NMC Code would now govern this situation.

An issue does arise of how generally competent nurses are in first aid: not every nurse will necessarily be good at first aid; it will be an acquired skill. A case that is instructive in this area is *Cattley* v. *St John's Ambulance Brigade* (1988) QBD (unreported) (but see *Lexis*). This case involved an allegation of negligence against two members of the St John's Ambulance Brigade. It was alleged that the plaintiff's spinal injuries were made worse by the negligent way he was treated by the St John's members immediately after his fall from a motor cycle at a schoolboy motor scrambling event. The judge in the case, Judge Prosser, applied the '*Bolam*' test and stated that the St John's ambulance men were not negligent because the volunteers had observed the procedures laid down in the Brigade's *First Aid Manual*. The judge stated:

> " In my judgment the test to be applied to determine whether negligence has been proved against the first-aider, like Mr Nicholson, or the St John's Ambulance Brigade, is the test set out in *Bolam* and approved in subsequent cases. Mr Nicholson or any other person holding himself out as a first-aider trained in accordance with the manual I referred to would be negligent if he failed to act in accordance with the standards of the ordinary skilled first-aider exercising and professing to have that special skill of a first-aider.

> " To adapt the words of Lord President Clyde to a first-aider, the true test for establishing negligence in a first-aider is whether he has been proved to be guilty of such failure as no first-aider of ordinary skill would be guilty of, if acting with ordinary care.

> " If in any situation the first-aider acts in accordance with the First-Aid Manual and does so with ordinary skill, then he has met the test and he is not negligent.

Good Samaritans such as the St John's Ambulance Brigade can be sued. The court would probably expect more from the good Samaritan nurse assisting in an emergency than from a member of the public. A nurse administering first aid would be holding him/herself out ostensibly as somebody who knows what they are doing and the court would probably adopt the conventional wisdom of members of the public generally or, to use a modern phrase, the 'urban myth' that all nurses are trained in first aid, which of course they are not. By stopping and assisting at a first aid event the nurse creates a legal duty of care situation and can be sued personally if negligence and damage results.

Breach

We have mentioned about breach of the standard of care above but will now go into some more detail about the topic (Jones 2004). The second step is for the claimant to prove that the nurse was negligent in breach of his/her legal duty of care. The nurse's conduct would be viewed from the perspective of what 'the ordinary skilled nurse in her/his speciality would have done in the circumstances of the case'. The nurse would also have been expected to take precautions against reasonably known risks only.

Legal standard of nursing competence

In determining the legal standard of care if litigation was being brought, lawyers would have to take advice from other nurses in the same speciality. If the case went to trial, the judge would hear expert evidence and would draw conclusions from this as to the standard of professional practice. The legal principles stated come from the well known *Bolam* case (*Bolam* v. *Friern Hospital Management Committee* [1957] 1 WLR 582). In the case, the Judge, Mr Justice McNair, stated what has become known as the *Bolam* test:

> " The test is the standard of the ordinary skilled man exercising and professing to have that special skill. A man need not possess the highest expert skill; it is well established law that it is sufficient if he exercises the ordinary skill of an ordinary competent man exercising that particular art... .

The judge went on to say that a professional would not be liable in negligence:

> " if he has acted in accordance with a practice accepted as proper by a responsible body of medical men skilled in that particular art... . Putting it the other way round, a man is not negligent, if he is acting in accordance with such a practice, merely because there is a body of opinion who would take a contrary view.

Clause 1.4 of the NMC Code applies here: 'You have a duty of care to your patients and clients, who are entitled to receive safe and competent care'. 'Competent' and 'reasonable' are defined in the Glossary in the NMC Code. The *Bolam* and *Bolitho* cases, to be discussed below, are mentioned.

Sections 15 and 16 of United Kingdom Central Council for Nursing, Midwifery and Health Visiting 1996 provide a useful discussion of the concept of reasonableness with reference to the *Bolam* principle (see above):

> " The case of *Wilsher* v. *Essex AHA* (1988) set the standard of reasonable care to be expected of students and junior staff. The standard is that of a reasonably competent practitioner and not that of a student or junior. You have a duty to ensure that the care which you delegate is carried out at a reasonably competent standard. This means that you remain accountable for the delegation of the work and for ensuring that the person who does the work is able to do it.

If a nurse is a trainee s/he is still expected to accord with the standard of a qualified practitioner (*Nettleship* v. *Weston* [1971] 2 QB 691). Nurses who are unsure of what to do should get advice from a more experienced practitioner. By doing so, not only are they acting in accordance with good practice but this is likely to absolve them of liability in negligence (*Wilsher* v. *Essex AHA* [1986]3 All ER 801).

Reasonable differences of opinion

There may be legitimate differences as to what constitutes a body of responsible professional practice. Take, for instance, the issue of nurses using cot-sides. One nurse may decide to use cot-sides while another nurse may refuse to have them on his/her ward because it is known that patients can roll over the sides and fall from a higher level. Another nurse may decide not to take any of these courses of action and to nurse the patient on a mattress on the floor. Nursing experts advising lawyers and the court would say that, generally speaking, all the above nursing actions are reasonable and that there are competent bodies of nursing opinion that would support such practices. Applying the *Bolam* test the courts would usually accept the nursing experts' views and would not choose between competing views and practices. A small number of medical practitioners could constitute a responsible body of medical opinion (*De Freitas* v. *O'Brien and Another* [1993] 4 Med LR 281).

The courts have not handed over totally the task of determining the standard of care to the nursing and medical professions. While expert evidence as to nursing or medical practice will usually be accepted, the courts could still overrule a body of professional practice. Nevertheless, the courts would not easily condemn accepted nursing or medical practice as negligent (Jones 2003). The question of what happens when professional opinion differs was considered by the House of Lords in a case involving a nurse plaintiff (*Maynard* v. *West Midlands Regional Health Authority* [1984] 1 WLR 634). Staff Nurse Maynard consulted a physician and a surgeon experienced in the treatment of chest diseases. Tuberculosis was considered to be her most likely diagnosis but there were symptoms that also suggested Hodgkin's disease, carcinoma and sarcoidosis. Unless Hodgkin's disease was treated early it would prove fatal (as treatment was understood in 1970). The doctors decided upon a mediastinoscopy, which would provide them with a biopsy that they could have examined immediately. The operation involved a risk of damage to the left laryngeal nerve even if carried out correctly. Unfortunately, the nerve was damaged despite the fact that the operation was carried out carefully. The biopsy proved negative and it was later confirmed that the plaintiff was suffering from tuberculosis and not Hodgkin's disease. She sued in negligence, alleging, among other things, that it was a negligent decision to carry out the mediastinoscopy rather than to await the results of the sputum test. Her action failed. Lord Scarman stated:

> " A case which is based on an allegation that a fully considered decision of
> two consultants in the field of their special skill was negligent clearly
> presents certain difficulties of proof. It is not enough to show that there is
> a body of competent professional opinion which considers that theirs was
> a wrong decision, if there also exists a body of professional opinion,
> equally competent, which supports the decision as reasonable in the

circumstances. It is not enough to show that subsequent events show that the operation need never have been performed, if at the time the decision to operate was taken it was reasonable in the sense that a responsible body of medical opinion would have accepted it as proper… . Differences of opinion and practice exist, and will always exist, in the medical as in other professions. There is seldom any one answer exclusive of all others to problems of professional judgment.

These legal principles can be applied to another controversial nursing issue; the Edinburgh University solution of lime (Eusol) wound care dressing debate (Tingle 1990). Many nurses are reluctant to use Eusol, some arguing that they have a professional duty not to do so as they say it is ineffective as a promoter of wound healing. Some consultants like to use Eusol and ask nurses to use it. There have been a number of publicised disputes, as nurses face a conflict between the consultant's request and their own professional view on Eusol. Applying the principles set out in *Bolam* and *Maynard* it can be seen that, generally speaking, it is not negligent to use Eusol because there is a competent body of medical opinion that would support its use (Burton 1993).

Developments in health-care practice generally may influence the manner in which the *Bolam* test may operate and assist in defining what amounts to a responsible body of professional practice. It is interesting to speculate the extent to which concepts such as evidence-based medicine/nursing and clinical guidelines and protocols will push the standard of care from reasonable practice, in the *Bolam* sense, to best practice. Evidence-based medicine is practice based on a clear body of research and agreed principles. The *Bolitho* case can be seen to revamp the notion of 'evidence-based health-care practice', giving judicial credence to the concept. The courts now seem to expect more from practitioners: just coasting along on outdated nursing practices that have no evidence base is no longer a tenable practice.

The Bolitho case, Bolitho v. City and Hackney Health Authority (1997) ([1998] Lloyd's Rep Med 26)

In this case a 2-year-old boy was being treated for breathing difficulties in hospital. He suffered, on one day, two episodes of acute shortness of breath and a doctor was urgently summoned by the ward sister. The doctor failed to attend or arrange for another doctor to attend. Later that day, the boy suffered a respiratory and cardiac arrest. He was resuscitated and was found to have brain damage. The health authority was sued for negligence. It was alleged that the plaintiff's brain damage was caused by the negligent failure of medical staff to attend. Negligence was admitted by the defendant's medical staff, who should have attended when summoned, but that was not the end of the matter. Intubation of an infant is not an easy or completely safe procedure. The doctor who had been summoned and failed to attend said that she would not have intubated him even if she had attended. Expert opinion was divided on the necessity of intubation. This case was referred to the House of Lords and the issues of breach of duty and causation were key issues of discussion. The *Bolam* case was discussed and Lord Browne-Wilkinson's speech contains the contemporary view on how Bolam will be applied. To an extent, we can see a movement away from reasonable to best or evidence-based practice as the legal benchmark for standard of care to be looked for:

> " The use of these adjectives responsible, reasonable and respectable all show that the court has to be satisfied that the exponents of the body of opinion relied upon can demonstrate that such opinion has a logical basis. In particular in cases involving, as they so often do, the weighing of risks against benefits, the judge before accepting a body of opinion as being responsible, reasonable or respectable, will need to be satisfied that, in forming their views, the experts have directed their minds to the question of comparative risks and benefits and have reached a defensible conclusion on the matter.

Expert reports in cases must be evidence-based. We will see in Chapter 4, in *Penney and Others* v. *East Kent Health Authority* (*The Times*, 25 November 1999 (CA)) how the courts can approach national clinical guidelines and the *Bolitho* and *Bolam* cases. It is also unclear whether nurses will be subject to the same degree of scrutiny as doctors, or indeed whether the courts would be willing to undertake a more rigorous review than is the case regarding medical decision-making. (See also the discussion of *Bolitho* in Chapter 5.)

Departing from accepted practice

A nurse would not necessarily be viewed as being negligent if s/he departed from accepted nursing practice in a particular situation. For example, a wound care specialist might decide, on the basis of a recent research study, to mix two types of topical wound care solution together and apply them to a patient's wound, arguing that recent research had shown that when the solutions are mixed together they became more effective. This is not, however, the conventional way to apply the solutions. If problems did occur and the patient then took legal action, the nurse would have to justify the departure from conventional practice. There is a clear danger in accepting claims made by one research paper only. There is a need for confirmation and exploration of the implications of changing practice. There must be critical appraisal of new research.

If a nurse is given instructions by a doctor but is of the view that these are wrong, what should s/he do? It is suggested that it would be good practice to raise the concerns with the doctor. But if the doctor disagrees and the nurse goes along with the doctor's instructions, then if harm results the nurse may be held not to be negligent because s/he was acting on doctor's orders (*Gold* v. *Essex County Council* [1942] 2 All ER 237; Montgomery 1995, 1997), although this may be an approach that the courts are less willing to take as the nurse's role in clinical practice increases still further.

Assessing risk

The nurse in the above example might have felt that there were no real significant adverse risks to the patient in his/her proposed course of action, the benefits outweighing any treatment risks. Whether the nurse was correct in his/her assessment would be an important issue for the experts to determine in their reports to the lawyers.

The defendant's conduct in a negligence case is viewed from the date the incident occurred and not from the time of the court hearing. The defendant would be expected only to guard against events that could be reasonably foreseen at the time of the alleged negligence. *Roe* v. *Ministry of Health and Others, Woolley* v. *Same* ([1954] 2 All ER 131) illustrates this point. Two patients underwent an operation. Prior to the operation a spinal anaesthetic consisting of Nupercaine was administered to the patients by lumbar puncture. The plaintiffs developed spastic paraplegia after the operation and were paralysed from the waist down. Their injuries were caused by the injection of contaminated Nupercaine. The Nupercaine was in glass ampoules, which, prior to administration, were immersed in a phenol solution. Unknown to the anaesthetist, the phenol had percolated into the glass ampoules by means of invisible cracks or molecular flaws in the glass. At the time of the incident, the risk of percolation in the manner that occurred was not generally appreciated by competent anaesthetists. It was an unforeseeable occurrence. The defendants were not legally expected to anticipate the danger. Denning L.J. expressed the following sentiment in the case, which can equally be said to be applicable to all health-care professionals today:

" Every surgical operation is attended by risks. We cannot take the benefits without taking the risks. Every advance in technique is also attended by risks. Doctors, like the rest of us, have to learn by experience; and experience often teaches in a hard way. Something goes wrong and shows up a weakness, and then it is put right. That is just what happened here… we must not look at the 1947 accident with 1954 spectacles.

Legal duty to keep up to date

A nurse could breach his/her legal duty of care by not keeping up to date with major developments in his/her speciality. Consider the following example:

A new wound care dressing has been created that is very effective and is becoming widely used. A district nurse is unaware of the new dressing because she feels she has no time to read the professional journals or attend study days that are put on by her employer at regular intervals. One of her patients has a wound that will not heal. Another district nurse attends the patient and uses the new dressing and the wound heals very quickly. The patient asks why the new dressing was not used before by the regular district nurse.

This issue is addressed by the NMC Code; clause 6, 6.1–6.5 is instructive here:

" 6   As a registered nurse, midwife or specialist community public health nurse, you must maintain your professional knowledge and competence

6.1 You must keep your knowledge and skills up-to-date throughout your working life. In particular, you should take part regularly in learning activities that develop your competence and performance.

6.2 To practise competently, you must possess the knowledge, skills and abilities required for lawful, safe and effective practice without direct supervision. You must acknowledge the limits of your professional competence and only undertake practice and accept responsibilities for those activities in which you are competent.

6.3 If an aspect of practice is beyond your level of competence or outside your area of registration, you must obtain help and supervision from a competent practitioner until you and your employer consider that you have acquired the requisite knowledge and skill.

6.4 You have a duty to facilitate students of nursing, midwifery and specialist community public health nursing and others to develop their competence

6.5 You have a responsibility to deliver care based on current evidence, best practice and, where applicable, validated research when it is available.

The nurse in the wound care example, as well as possibly being in breach of her duty of care to her patient, could also be viewed as being in breach of clause 6 of the NMC Code: blind indifference to her professional duty of personal updating and development. She should try to keep reasonably up to date.

The issue of professional updating has been considered by the Court of Appeal in *Crawford v. Board of Governors of Charing Cross Hospital* (1953) (*The Times*, 8 December 1953). The plaintiff, Mr Robert Joseph Crawford, was admitted to the Charing Cross Hospital for an operation for the removal of his bladder. The plaintiff's left arm was extended at an angle from his body so that a blood transfusion could be given. After the operation the plaintiff complained of paralysis in his left arm; brachial palsy had developed. He sued, alleging negligence. The main issue was whether the anaesthetist was negligent in missing an article that appeared in *The Lancet* in January 1950; the operation was performed in July 1950. The article warned about the risk of brachial palsy when the arm was kept in an extended position. The plaintiff did not succeed, as no negligence was found. Denning L.J. states that all reasonable care was taken by the hospital and that it would amount to imposing too high a burden on the doctor to require that he read all articles in the medical press.

The judgment on the facts makes sense: nobody can read all the professional articles that appear in the numerous journals. Nonetheless, while ignorance of one warning in the professional press may be acceptable, missing a number of warnings could well lead to a finding of negligence. Mason & Laurie (2006, p. 311), referring to the *Crawford* case, feel that a less charitable view would be taken if the same facts occurred today:

" The practice of medicine has, however, become increasingly based on principles of scientific elucidation and report – the so-called 'evidence-based medicine' – and the pressure on doctors to keep abreast of current developments is now considerable. It is no longer possible for a doctor to coast along on the basis of long experience; such an attitude has been discredited not only in medicine but in many professions and callings.

The courts have affirmed the health-care professional's obligation to keep him/herself up to date by familiarity with mainstream literature (*Gascoine v. Ian Shendan and Co. and Lathan* [1994] 5 Med LR 437).

The nurse must thus remember the professional and legal duty to keep up to date with developments in nursing practice.

The Compensation Act 2006

'The Compensation Act 2006' is an important piece of legislation which will help deal with the perception held by many, of a 'compensation culture', where schools ban conker matches, etc. and where normal everyday activities are banned because of fear of litigation and where there is too much of a risk management culture in place. The Act's provisions on negligence and breach of statutory duty make clear that courts considering what standard of care is reasonable in a claim for negligence or breach of statutory duty can take into account whether requiring particular steps to be taken to meet the standard of care would prevent or impede a desirable activity from taking place. There is also a provision to the effect that in the above type of claims, an apology, offer of treatment or other redress shall not in itself amount to an admission of liability; saying 'sorry' does not mean that you are admitting liability and apologies can diffuse a potential legal claim.

Damage

The plaintiff must prove that the defendant's breach of duty caused or materially contributed to his/her damage. A direct link has to be made between the two elements of breach and damage. The plaintiff must be 'able to prove that the negligence has made a difference, that it has adversely affected the condition in some way'. A first step is to prove factual causation: the cause in fact of the plaintiff's condition.

Causation in fact

Lawyers use a test known as the 'but for test'. Jones (2002) summarises this test as follows:

" The first step is to eliminate irrelevant causes, and this is the purpose of the 'but for test'. If harm to the plaintiff would not have occurred 'but for' the defendant's negligence then that negligence is a cause of the harm. It is not necessarily the cause because there may well be other events which are causally relevant. Putting this another way, if the loss would have been incurred in any event, the defendant's conduct is not a cause.

The application of this principle can be illustrated by the case of *Barnett* v. *Chelsea and Kensington Hospital Management Committee* ([1968] 1 All ER 1068). The plaintiff, William Barnett, was a night-watchman at a college hall of residence. He was drinking some tea with two other night-watchmen. Soon afterwards they all started vomiting and went to the defendant's casualty department. They were seen by a nurse who telephoned the casualty officer, Dr Banerjee, who unfortunately was not feeling well himself. He did not see the men, saying that they should go home and see their own doctors. Mr Whittall, one of the men, was asked by Dr Banerjee to stay for an X-ray. He had seen Dr Banerjee on another matter some time before. All the men went away and, some hours later, the plaintiff died. It was discovered later that the cause of death was arsenical poisoning. His widow claimed that the hospital had been negligent in not treating her husband. The casualty officer was found by the court to be in breach of his legal duty of care in not examining and treating Mr Barnett but the legal action failed. Element 3, causation in fact, had not been proved: death had been inevitable for Mr Barnett. Had he been seen and admitted to hospital he would have died before the antidote could have been given. The defendant's breach of duty had, therefore, not caused his death; the hospital could not have done anything to save him in time.

The claimant has the burden of proving that the defendant's actions or omissions have caused or materially contributed to the damage s/he has suffered. This can be a difficult task in medical and nursing negligence cases where there can often be a number of biological causes, natural causes of a plaintiff's condition. The burden of proof is on the claimant to establish that the breach of duty was a material contribution to the damage caused (*Wilsher* v. *Essex Area Health Authority* ([1986] 3 All ER 801). A nurse who is expert in the relevant speciality would be called to give evidence. A number of reported cases involve allegations of both medical and nursing negligence and in such circumstances both types of experts will be used.

Nursing negligence: general issues

The case of *Kay* v. *Ayrshire and Arran Health Board* [1987] 2 All ER 417 illustrates key causation principles. Andrew Stuart Kay was aged 2 years and 5 months when he was admitted to the Seafield Children's Hospital, Ayr. His GP admitted him because she thought that he might be suffering from meningitis and this diagnosis was later confirmed by the hospital. The consultant paediatrician in charge of the case instructed that 10 000 units of penicillin be administered intrathecally. By mistake, a senior house officer injected 300 000 units of penicillin instead of the required 10 000 units. Andrew went into convulsions and later developed a degree of paralysis on one side of his body. Immediate action was taken to remedy this negligent mistake. Andrew recovered and appeared to suffer no immediate ill-effects of the overdose. He made a rapid recovery from meningitis.

However, some time after his discharge from hospital his parents noticed that he appeared to be suffering from deafness; this was later confirmed. An action for negligence was commenced alleging that the overdose of penicillin had caused his deafness. The action failed because factual causation was not established: it could not be proved that the overdose caused or materially contributed to Andrew's deafness. The weight of evidence in the case pointed to the deafness being caused by the meningitis.

As well as being instructive on the issue of experts and evidence-based health care, *Bolitho* is also a leading authority on causation. The facts of *Bolitho* were stated earlier. A key issue in the litigation was the possible relationship of the *Bolam* principle to causation. Lord Browne-Wilkinson in the case said that there were two questions for the judge at first instance to decide on causation:

" (1) What would Dr Horn have done, or authorized to be done, if she had attended Patrick? and (2) If she would not have intubated, would that have been negligent? The *Bolam* test has no relevance to the first of those questions but is central to the second.

Bolam therefore does seem to have some relationship to causation.

Jones (2002) argues:

> In reality *Bolitho* is about whether the failure to intubate, for whatever reason (non-attendance or conscious professional judgment), was negligent. The defendant's evidence that she would not have intubated simply moved the focus of the argument about negligence, i.e. breach of duty, from the non-attendance to the non-intubation.

Remoteness

Having established what factually caused the claimant's damage, there may still be a need to consider the cause for attributing legal responsibility, often termed remoteness, causation in law or proximate cause. A defendant generally cannot be held liable for everything that happens to a claimant: the damage may be too remote, outside the bounds of what can be legally recovered. Instances would be where the damage would be much more extensive, or of a different type, or occur in a different way, than would normally have been expected.

Example

A district nurse makes regular visits to an elderly patient to change dressings. The elderly patient lives alone and looks forward to the nurse's regular visits. The nurse gives her company and spends some of her time talking generally to the patient. As a result of promotion the nurse needs to move districts, with another nurse taking over her visits. The patient appears to take this news well but the next day is found dead, leaving a suicide note. The patient, unable to face the change in nursing routine, has committed suicide. The patient's relatives blame the nurse, saying that she should have anticipated the patient's reaction and taken preventative steps.

A key issue would be the foreseeability of the patient's action. Was there any existing evidence of psychiatric illness and was this passed on to the nurse? If there was no such evidence then it could be argued that the patient's actions could not have been reasonably foreseen by the nurse. She would not have been expected to act to prevent the suicide. The event would have been legally too remote.

In some situations there is more than one cause of harm that a patient suffers. Consider a patient who has been negligently knocked off his motorbike by a motorist. He is seriously injured, with damage to the spine. The doctor in casualty causes further injury and paralysis through negligent medical treatment. In ascertaining legal liability, the court would have to consider evidence as to what caused the ultimate injury. It may be the case that both the motorist and doctor could be negligent and liable to some extent.

Where there are two or more defendants liable for the same damage to the plaintiff, the Civil Liability (Contribution) Act 1978 allows them to claim contributions from each other for any damages awarded.

What if there is a delay in providing treatment and the patient later seeks to bring an action, claiming that it was this delay that resulted in her/him not having a full recovery? In effect, the claim is that the negligence led to the 'loss of a chance' of recovery in that situation. This issue arose in the case of *Hotson* v. *East Berkshire Area Health Authority* ([1987] 2 A11 ER 909). The plaintiff was 13 years of age when he injured his hip in a fall. He had sustained an acute traumatic fracture of the left femoral epiphysis but this condition was not diagnosed at the hospital when he attended and he was sent home. He was in severe pain for 5 days. He returned to the hospital and his condition was correctly diagnosed. He suffered avascular necrosis of the epiphysis. At the age of 20 years he had a major permanent disability.

The plaintiff claimed damages for negligence against the health authority, which admitted a breach of duty but denied that the resulting delay had adversely affected the plaintiff's long-term condition. When the action was tried the trial judge found that, even if the hospital medical staff had correctly diagnosed and treated the plaintiff on his first visit to the hospital, there would still have been a 75% risk of the disability developing. The medical staff's breach of duty had turned that risk into an inevitability. The plaintiff was in effect denied a 25% chance of a good recovery. Damages were awarded, which included an amount that represented 25% of the full value of the damages awardable for the disability. The Court of Appeal affirmed the judge's decision. The health authority successfully appealed to the House of Lords and the Court of Appeal's decision was reversed. The appeal was allowed on the narrow ground that the plaintiff failed to establish a cause of action in respect of the avascular necrosis and its consequences. The trial judge's finding of fact was that, on the balance of probabilities, the injury caused by the plaintiff's fall left insufficient blood vessels intact to keep the epiphysis alive. The fall was the sole cause of the avascular necrosis.

This case again graphically illustrates the practical difficulties in establishing causation.

The broad issue raised by the case of the possibility of claiming for loss of chance in tort was left open by the House of Lords and revisited in *Gregg v Scott* [2005] UKHL 2. The claimant, Mr Gregg, consulted Dr Scott in November 1994 about a lump under his arm. Dr Scott assumed that it was benign and failed to refer the claimant to hospital for tests. Dr Scott told the claimant that the most likely explanation was a collection of fatty tissue. Mr Scott visited another GP, who immediately referred him to hospital, and in January 1996 he was found to be suffering from non-Hodgkin's lymphoma. The effect of the delay in diagnosis was that the cancer had spread to his chest. The trial judge held that, on the expert evidence, the delay in diagnosis had reduced Mr Gregg's chances of surviving for more than 10 years from 42% to 25%. He dismissed the claim because the delay had not deprived Mr Gregg of the prospect of a cure, meaning surviving more than 10 years, because, at the time of his misdiagnosis, Mr Gregg had less than a 50% chance of surviving more than 10 years anyway. The Court of Appeal dismissed Mr Gregg's appeal and he appealed to the House of Lords. The House of Lords also dismissed his claim, Lords Nicholls and Lord Hope dissenting. Mason & Laurie (2006) state on the case:

> " Lord Nicholls, in particular, argued forcefully that the 'all-or nothing' approach to what would have happened but for the negligence – that is, the application of the 49/51% rule from Hotson – was premised on a falsehood and led to arbitrary and unjust outcomes.... And Lord Hope opined that the principle on which a patient's loss as a result of negligence is to be calculated and, presumably, recompensed is the same whether the prospects were better or worse than 50%. The majority, however, rejected the appeal and did so largely to protect the integrity of legal principle.

Legal policy considerations can be seen to be very much at work in this case and they did firmly influence the majority of Law Lords' speeches in the case. The majority decisions are largely pragmatic and policy-driven in nature and look to the practicalities of deciding these types of case. Causation issues in clinical negligence cases can be notoriously difficult cases to resolve. The traditional balance of probability test used by the courts was recognised as being robust and as producing a form of rough justice that was preferable to a test that allowed recovery for loss of chance, which would have been difficult if not impossible to apply with confidence in practice. In any event, the claimant was still alive and this factor was an important consideration in the case.

On the balance of probability the majority concluded that the delay in commencing the claimant's treatment had not affected his prospects of being a survivor but had caused him all the adverse events.

Gregg v. *Scott* according to Stauch et al (2006)

> " is undoubtedly a complex and difficult case, and one may well agree with Lord Phillips's assessment that it did not provide a suitable vehicle for recognising 'loss of chance' claims in medical negligence. A fundamental problem, as their Lordships noted, was that the claimant was still alive nearly 10 years after the original misdiagnosis. Thus (ignoring, for present purposes, the more painful treatment he had to undergo and his increased mental suffering) he had quite possibly lost nothing, not even a chance.

The issue of loss of chance in medical negligence cases still awaits appropriate resolution and on balance, subject to appropriate statistical analysis, it would do no harm to accept it in the *Hotson* type of case. Stauch et al (2006) state:

> " Reverting to the classical 'loss of chance' scenario illustrated by *Hotson* – where the claimant's injury has already occurred – it is submitted that such claims, based upon statistical evidence as to the typical progress of the condition that led up to it, should be permitted'

Res ipsa loquitur

There are circumstances when the courts are prepared to infer from the facts that a defendant was negligent. Under this evidential rule the burden of proof is not formally reversed and the inference of negligence can be rebutted.

Generally speaking, the principle will apply where it is obvious that there has been negligence, for example, where the doctor has amputated the wrong leg or a swab or forceps has been left in a patient, etc. An extreme example of res ipsa loquitur was noted in the *Yorkshire Evening Post* on 14 October 1982: 'An enquiry has begun at a hospital in Vienna into how a man, suffering from a broken leg, was mistakenly given a heart pacemaker' (Dixon, 1984). Further examples of situations in which res ipsa loquitur may be pleaded are to be found in the following cases cited by Action for Victims of Medical Accidents (AVMA) 1984–85:

> " Foreign bodies were as varied as ever – ranging from swabs (14), insoluble sutures (5), clips (4), metal thread/wool (3), packs (3), bits of catheter apparatus (3), needles (2), clamps (2), gauze (2), scissors (1), forceps (1), and even part of a glass test tube. Most of these arose from abdominal surgery – 13 from gastroenterology cases.

The Medical Defence Union (1993) noted a case where a patient received approximately £27 000 in compensation for an overlooked swab. This, in common with the other examples of the situation in which res ipsa loquitur might be used, can be seen to be of particular relevance to theatre nursing.

A number of conditions must be satisfied before the res ipsa loquitur principle can apply. The event, when it occurred, must have been under the control, supervision or management of the defendant. The event would not normally have happened unless there was negligence. The whole circumstances of the case would be considered. The lawyers and the judge would consider, as a matter of common sense and common experience, whether such events could have occurred without negligence. The defendant must have offered no reasonable explanation of what had happened.

The principle has worked in a number of health-care cases. *Cassidy* v. *Ministry of Health* ([1951] 1 All ER 574) and *Bull* v. *Devon Area Health Authority* ([1989] [1993] 4 Med LR 117, 22 BMLR, 79) are just two cases where the principle has been used. In *Cassidy* the plaintiff was operated on for Dupuytren's contracture. He was suffering from a contraction of the third and fourth fingers of the left hand. After the operation, a nurse bandaged the plaintiff's hand and arm to a splint. The bandage was tested by a doctor to see if it was too tight; circulation was judged to be satisfactory. The patient subsequently complained of exceptional pain and was seen on occasions by medical staff. The splint and bandage were left intact and morphia was administered. The plaintiff continued to complain about excessive pain until the removal of the splint, when he discovered that he had lost the use of all four fingers. He sued for negligence in regard to the postoperative treatment he received. Even though he could not identify who in particular was negligent, the principle of res ipsa loquitur was applied. The evidence showed a prima facie case of negligence and this evidence was not rebutted by the defendants who were responsible for the medical and nursing staff.

Bull v. *Devon Area Health Authority* ([1989] [1993] 4 Med LR 117) demonstrates a controversial application of the principle, not all the judges in the case agreed to it being used. The case concerned the negligent organisation of maternity services. Mrs Bull was in premature labour carrying uniovular twins. The twins were sharing the same placenta. The first twin, later named

Darryl, was spontaneously delivered at 7.27 pm; he was born healthy. The second twin, later named Stuart, was born 68 minutes later with severe brain damage; he suffers from cerebral palsy, and is a quadriplegic spastic. Experts at the trial agreed that he should have been born as soon as reasonably practical after his brother and in any event within 20 minutes. Stuart did receive £750 000 compensation (Miles 1990). The delay in securing the attendance of senior medical staff capable of dealing with the emergency situation was too long and therefore there was a breach of duty. The call system had broken down.

Lord Justice Slade agreed with the submission made by counsel for the appellants and the judge at first instance: that the health authority had to justify the delays if it could under the res ipsa loquitur principle. He said:

> " In my judgment, however, all the most likely explanations for this failure point strongly either (i) to inefficiency in the system for summoning the assistance of the registrar or consultant… or (ii) to negligence by some individual or individuals in the working of that system. This is, in my judgment, accordingly a case where the res ipsa loquitur principle had to be applied…. ([103] 22 BMLR)

Dillon L.J. did not expressly deal with the desirability of using the principle. Mustill L.J. did not see the case as warranting the application of the principle.

On the issue of res ipsa loquitur the case is notable for a number of reasons. The fact that the judges in the case were not united in their view over the application of the principle illustrates the degree of uncertainty that can surround it. Furthermore, the principle was being used in a novel situation: in the organisation of health-care services. In practice res ipsa is thus only likely to be applicable in exceptional situations. For example, in *Glass* v. *Cambridgeshire AHA* ([1995] 6 Med LR 91) where the plaintiff suffered brain damage consequent upon a heart attack under general anaesthetic. It was held that this was not something which would normally be expected to occur in all the circumstances. As a consequence of this the burden moved to the defendant to explain that this was consistent with an absence of negligence.

WHO PAYS THE COMPENSATION?

The law of tort can be seen as the legal mechanism for the recovery of compensation by the patient. The issue of who is actually responsible for the payment of the compensation is important for nurses. Many worry that if they are negligent that they may be personally liable to pay the patient compensation. Others worry that if their employers pay the compensation to the injured patient their employers may seek to recover the money from them personally. In the NHS damages are paid by the employer of the negligent nurse. Clause 9 of the NMC Code deals with indemnity insurance and provides some useful advice in the area:

> " 9:1 The NMC recommends that a registered nurse, midwife or specialist community public health nurse, in advising, treating and caring for patients/clients, has professional indemnity insurance. This is in the interests of clients, patients and registrants in the event of claims of professional negligence.

9.2 Some employers accept vicarious liability for the negligent acts and/or omissions of their employees. Such cover does not normally extend to activities undertaken outside the registrant's employment. Independent practice would not normally be covered by vicarious liability, while agency work may not. It is the individual registrant's responsibility to establish their insurance status and take appropriate action.

9.3 In situations where employers do not accept vicarious liability, the NMC recommends that registrants obtain adequate professional indemnity insurance. If unable to secure professional indemnity insurance, a registrant will need to demonstrate that all their clients/patients are fully informed of this fact and the implications this might have in the event of a claim for professional negligence.

A number of schemes and organisations help trusts and health authorities deal with clinical negligence damages claims. The National Health Service Litigation Authority (NHSLA) (2005) describe these schemes as follows:

" The Clinical Negligence Scheme for Trusts (CNST) is a voluntary membership scheme, to which all NHS trusts and Primary Care Trusts (PCTs) in England currently belong. It covers all clinical claims where the allegedly negligent incident took place on or after 1 April 1995. The costs of meeting these claims are met through members' contributions. Only NHS bodies are eligible to become members of CNST. However, Independent Sector Treatment Centres treating NHS patients may benefit from CNST cover via their referring Primary Care Trust.

" The Existing Liabilities Scheme (ELS) is centrally funded by the Department of Health and covers clinical claims against NHS bodies where the incident took place before April 1995.

" The Ex-RHAs Scheme is a relatively small scheme covering clinical claims made against the former Regional Health Authorities, which were abolished in 1996. Like the ELS it is centrally funded by the Department of Health. It differs from the NHSLA's other schemes in that the NHSLA is the legal defendant in any action.

" The Liabilities to Third Parties Scheme (LTPS) and the Property Expenses Scheme (PES), known collectively as the Risk Pooling Schemes for Trusts (RPST), are two voluntary membership schemes covering non-clinical claims where the incident occurred on or after 1 April 1999. Costs are met through members' contributions.

In 2004/2005, the NHSLA made payments totalling £528.01 million in respect of all five schemes.

The NHSLA co-ordinates these schemes. It also looks at proposals to settle cases and has an advisory role in cases in which the claim is of a high value or will have policy implications across other NHS bodies.

Vicarious liability

Employers are liable, along with their employees, for non-authorised acts done in the course of their employment. This principle is known as 'vicarious liability' and it makes the employer jointly and severally liable even when not at fault; it is a form of strict liability. It is a necessary condition that the employees were acting in the course of their employment when they committed the tort and that the action complained of was one that the employee was authorised to undertake. The injured patient can sue the nurse, or both the hospital and the nurse, or just the hospital.

Whatever course is taken, the nurse who committed the negligent act always remains personally responsible and accountable for his/her negligence and it is possible that the employer could seek to recover from the nurse the compensation that has been paid out. However, NHS guidance states that attempts should not be made to recover costs from employees in this manner (NHS Executive 1996). The nurse has broken an implied term in the contract of employment that s/he will exercise reasonable care and skill. There is also a statutory provision that would allow the employer to recover any compensation paid out on the negligent nurse's behalf (Civil Liability (Contribution) Act 1978).

Generally speaking, lawyers proceed against the employer and not the employee. If, however, the employer can establish that the nurse was not acting in the course of employment when s/he was negligent, then the lawyers acting for the injured patient could bring an action against the nurse directly. However, in practice such an action is unlikely to go ahead, because it is questionable whether the individual nurse would have the financial resources to pay the compensation. It is not an easy legal task to determine what constitutes action taken in the course of employment. There are many cases on the point and some are quite difficult to reconcile; there is no definitive test.

Direct liability

If a patient was injured not by the acts or omissions of a nurse but because of a defect in machinery or because the system of care in the hospital failed, then the hospital could be held directly liable to the injured patient (*Cassidy* v. *Minister of Health* [1951] 1 All ER 574). This is because of what is termed a 'non-delegable duty'. The issue of a health authority or trust's direct liability for medical or nursing negligence is a controversial one but one that has been affirmed by the court in recent years in *M* v. *Calderdale and Kirklees HA* ([1998] Lloyds Rep. Med. 157). Here the plaintiff underwent an abortion performed by a private clinic that was acting under contract to the defendant health authority. It was held that the health authority had a non-delegable duty in this situation for the actions of the private clinic. The health authority had not taken steps such as ensuring that there was indemnity insurance, ensuring the competence of the staff of the clinic, etc. This is a decision of Judge Garner at first instance at Huddersfield County Court. Nonetheless the concept of direct liability may yet have a greater effect as more services are contracted out to the private sector. Where negligence is alleged the injured patient could proceed against the NHS body, claiming that it was directly liable for the injury that was caused. As (Jones 2002) states:

" a hospital authority may be directly liable in negligence for some failure in the organisation of its services to patients, such as an inadequate system for preventing cross-infection (*Vancouver General Hospital*

v. *McDaniel* (1934) 152 LT 56,57), an unreliable system for summoning expert assistance in an emergency (*Bull* v. *Devon Area Health Authority* (1989), [1993] 4 Med LR117) or employing inexperienced staff without proper supervision (*Jones* v. *Manchester Corporation* [1952] 2 QB 852; *Wilsher* v. *Essex Area Health Authority* [1986] 3 All ER 801,833).

PRODUCT LIABILITY

If a nurse is injured when a piece of equipment s/he is using fractures or a patient claims that s/he has been harmed through the administration of a defective drug, s/he may bring an action claiming damages for the harm suffered under the Consumer Protection Act 1987. This statute allows an action to be brought against producers and suppliers of defective products where the defect in the product led to damage. The legislation was introduced following a European Directive on product liability. Trusts may be liable as producers of medicines, appliances or pharmaceutical products. Second, they may be liable unless the producer or supplier can be identified. Finally, they may be liable as a 'keeper' if the supplier or producer shows that the product has not been used according to instructions or not sufficiently maintained.

The important difference between the 1987 Act and a negligence action at common law, as outlined above, is that fault does not have to be shown. It is sufficient to establish that the defect caused the damage. In considering what amounts to a defect, section 3(2) outlines a number of factors to be taken into account:

> " the manner in which, and the purposes for which, the product has been marketed, its get-up, the use of any mark in relation to the product and any instructions for, or warnings with respect to, doing or refraining from doing anything with or in relation to the product.

If the injured nurse had, for example, not followed the instructions then s/he could not bring an action under the statute.

An action may only be brought against a producer of the product within 10 years of the product having been supplied. There is a defence to actions under the legislation if, at the time the product was produced, scientific and technical knowledge was not such that 'a producer of products of the same description as the product in question might have been expected to have discovered the defect' (s4(1)).

While use of this statute remains theoretically possible, establishing liability may be practically difficult. The fact that the product is defective needs to be shown, which can be as difficult as establishing negligence in a standard common law claim (see Jones 2003).

CRIMINAL LIABILITY AND NEGLIGENT CONDUCT

While in most situations grave carelessness by the nurse will lead to civil proceedings, in some instances a criminal prosecution may result. If a nurse's actions are gravely careless and if death ultimately results then s/he may be prosecuted for manslaughter. While there have been no notable prosecutions of nurses for gross negligence or manslaughter, there have been criminal prosecutions of doctors. In *R v. Adomako* ([1994] 3 All ER 79), a patient died after an anaesthetist, during an eye operation, failed to notice that the endo-tracheal tube assisting the patient's breathing had become disconnected. Evidence at the hearing was to the effect that the conduct of the plaintiff was 'abysmal' with 'gross dereliction of duty'. He was found guilty of manslaughter. Lord MacKay set out in his judgment the basic test for manslaughter in criminal law:

> " the principles of the law of negligence apply to ascertain whether or not
> the defendant has been in breach of a duty of care towards the victim
> who has died. If such a breach of duty has been established the next
> question is whether that breach of duty caused the death of the victim.
> If so, the jury must go on to consider whether that breach of duty should
> be characterised as gross negligence and therefore as a crime. This will
> depend on the seriousness of the breach of duty committed by the
> defendant in all the circumstances in which the defendant was placed
> when it occurred. The jury will have to consider whether the extent to
> which the defendant's conduct departed from the proper standard of care
> incumbent upon him, involving as it must have done a risk of death to the
> patient, was such that it could be judged criminal.

Application of this test is unlikely to be easy; in effect assessment of what amounts to culpability has been left in the hands of the jury. It is not clear whether the same principles apply to situations in which the defendant has failed to act as those that apply when the defendant has acted. There is a further issue where a nurse makes a mistake and a death of a patient results but the nurse claims that the negligence results from working in a situation in which there are severe financial constraints and underfunding. Where does liability lie? One possibility is that the Trust could be held to be liable on the basis of what is known as 'corporate manslaughter'. This means that the managers are held responsible for the actions of the organisation (see *R v. P&O European Ferries (Dover) Ltd* [1991] 93 Cr App R 72). Mason & Laurie (2006) argue that the ruling in *Adomako* has remained controversial in the decade since it was delivered, that there have been various attempts to have the House of Lords revisit its decision and that each attempt has failed, the most recent attempt being *R v. Misra; R v. Srivastava* [2004] EWCA Crim 2375, *The Times*, 13 October 2004. Two doctors who had been convicted of manslaughter by gross negligence appealed. One of their arguments was that the offence lacked certainty and was therefore incompatible with Articles 7 and 6 of the European Convention on Human Rights. The Court of Appeal rejected this argument. Stating that the requirement for legal certainty was 'sufficient' certainty rather than absolute certainty. This requirement had not been changed by the European Convention.

REFORM

Concern over the increase in litigation involving health-care professionals has led to discussions of alternatives that could be proposed. The Chief Medical Officer, Professor Sir Liam Donaldson, published a key report into clinical negligence in the NHS. The report, *Making Amends* (Department of Health

2003) set out proposals for consultation intended to fundamentally reform the way clinical negligence cases are handled in the health service – including the establishment of an NHS redress scheme to speed up the process and offer care and compensation under certain circumstances without the necessity to go to court. The report made a total of 19 recommendations.

A comprehensive no-fault scheme was rejected, although these schemes exist in other countries.

One approach adopted in Sweden and New Zealand is to enable individuals to claim compensation through a no-fault scheme (Brazier 1993, McLean 1993). Under such a scheme claimants would not have to establish fault by a health professional, merely that the actions of the health professional caused the harm suffered. The high likely costs of the no-fault scheme made it an unlikely candidate for adoption in the UK. Many are concerned as to the costs of such a compensation scheme both in its initial establishment and subsequent operation, pointing to the experience of New Zealand, which prompted various limitations to be imposed on the scheme (Oliphant 1996).

However there is increasing emphasis in the UK upon settling matters without recourse to litigation (see Ch. 1). The reforms introduced consequent upon the Woolf report (Woolf 1996) into civil procedure have had a considerable impact upon the conduct of clinical medical negligence litigation. As noted in Chapter 1 (p. 6), cases are more tightly managed by the judge and parties are encouraged to settle their differences prior to trial and to make use of alternative dispute resolution mechanisms. Expert evidence and experts are encouraged to narrow down their differences prior to trial through the use of pre-trial meetings. An NHS Redress Bill has been published (HL Bill 22) and stands a good chance of becoming enacted and providing patients with an alternative mechanism for resolving their disputes. See Chapter 3 for a more detailed discussion of these and other related issues.

CONCLUSIONS

Nurses do not have to practice to an impeccable standard, only as ordinary skilled nurses would have acted in the circumstances of the case. The legal accountability of the nurse is set by the *Bolam* test as modified by *Bolitho*. In Chapter 3, some specific questions of liability in relation to negligence are considered.

REFERENCES

Action for Victims of Medical Accidents (1984–85) Annual Report. AVMA, London, (i) p. 7

Brazier M 1993 The case for a no-fault compensation scheme. In: McClean S (ed.) Compensation for damage: an international perspective. Dartmouth, Aldershot

Burton J 1993 Skin complaint. Nursing Times 89(7): 76

Department of Health 2003 Making amends: a consultation paper setting out proposals for reforming the approach to clinical negligence in the NHS. Department of Health, London

Dixon E 1984 The theatre nurse and the law. Croom Helm, London

Jones MA 1992 Medical negligence. In: Dyer C (ed.) Doctors, patients and the law. Blackwell Scientific Publications, Oxford

Jones MA 2002 Textbook on torts, 8th edn. Oxford University Press, Oxford.

Jones MA 2003 Medical negligence, 3rd edn. Sweet & Maxwell, London

LAW AND NURSING

Jones MA 2004 Breach of duty. In: Grubb, A (ed.) Principles of medical law. Oxford University Press, Oxford

Kennedy I, Grubb A 1993 Commentary, *Bolitho* v. *City and Hackney Health Authority* (1993). Medical Law Review 1: 241

McLean S (ed.) 1993 Can no-fault analysis ease the problem of medical injury litigation? In: Compensation for damage: an international perspective. Dartmouth, Aldershot

Mason JK, Laurie GT 2006 Mason and McCall Smith's law and medical ethics, 7th edn. Oxford University Press, Oxford

Medical Defence Union 1993 Case histories: Delay in diagnosis of retained surgical swab. Journal of the Medical Defence Union 9: 6

Miles K 1990 Health authority liable for negligent organisation of maternity services – *Bull* v. *Devon Health Authority*. AVMA Medical and Legal Journal 1: 11

Montgomery J 1995 Negligence. In: Tingle J H, Cribb A (eds) Nursing law and ethics. Blackwell Science, Oxford

Montgomery J 1997 Health law. Oxford University Press, Oxford

National Health Service Litigation Authority 2006 Our schemes. Available online at: http://.nhsla.com/Claims/Schemes/NHSLA, London

NHS Executive 1996 NHS indemnity arrangements for clinical negligence claims in the NHS. 96 HR 0024. Department of Health, Leeds

Nursing and Midwifery Council 2004 The NMC code of professional conduct: standards for conduct, performance and ethics. Standards 07.04. NMC, London

Oliphant K 1996 Defining medical misadventure: lessons from New Zealand. Medical Law Review 4: 1–31

Stauch M, Wheat K, Tingle J 2006 Text, cases and materials on medical law. Routledge Cavendish, Abingdon

Tingle JH 1990 Eusol and the law. Nursing Times 86(38): 70–72

Tingle JH 1991 First aid law. Nursing Times 87(35): 48–49

United Kingdom Central Council for Nursing, Midwifery and Health Visiting 1996 Guidelines for professional practice. UKCC, London

Woolf H 1996 Access to justice: final report, by the Right Honourable the Lord Woolf, Master of the Rolls. HMSO, London

Nursing negligence: general issues

Patient safety, litigation and complaints in the National Health Service

John Tingle

In this chapter the topics of patient safety, litigation and National Health Service (NHS) complaints will be discussed. The nurse may become directly involved in each of these areas, so a knowledge of them is important. Patient problems do occur and it is important for the health-care professional to know and understand what can be done to avoid the problems happening again. Reflective practice is safe practice and learning the lessons of the past is an essential prerequisite for safe care.

Every day over 1 million people are treated successfully in NHS acute, ambulance and mental health trusts (National Audit Office 2005). For the vast majority of patients, treatment and care goes smoothly and without incident. This care does take place in an increasingly complex health-care environment, an environment where good-quality and safe care is highly dependent on the successful interaction of professional skills, drugs and medical technologies. This is a complex interaction to try and manage as there are many variables and, given the necessary dependence on the human factor, it is always going to be inevitable that some mistakes will be made. Human beings do not always practise their skills to perfection. The challenge for nurses and other health carers today is to try to minimise the possibility of errors occurring by effectively managing risk and more broadly by helping to develop an ingrained NHS patient safety culture and also learning how to handle patient complaints properly.

In this chapter the topics of health-care litigation, patient safety initiatives and handling NHS complaints will be discussed. The role of nurses and others within the patient safety and complaints agenda will be identified.

PATIENT SAFETY: THE SCOPE OF THE PROBLEM

Nobody knows exactly how many patients are injured or killed in the NHS by nursing or medical accidents. It is only in relatively recent times that the NHS has started to count errors and has had the necessary infrastructure to do this with the advent of the National Reporting and Learning System (NRLS) run by the National Patient Safety Agency (NPSA). To date there have still been no major studies in the UK of the incidence and effects of patient safety adverse incidents in the NHS, although there are some smaller-scale studies and other indicators, which will be discussed later in this chapter. What we do know for certain is that patient safety is an acute problem in the NHS and enhancing patient safety has for some years been a central plank of government health policy, along with the development of NHS strategies to reduce patient complaints and clinical negligence claims. The first NHS organisations were connected to the NRLS in November 2003 and all NHS organisations have had the capacity to report incidents to the NRLS since December 2004. The NRLS is the first comprehensive compulsory national reporting system for patient safety incidents in the world.

The NPSA estimate the incidence of errors as follows: 'On the best available data in England, extrapolating from a small study in two acute care trusts, it is estimated that around 10% of patients (900 000 using admission rates for 2002/3) admitted to NHS hospitals have experienced a patient safety incident and that up to half of these incidents could have been prevented' (National Patient Safety Agency 2004).

In 2005 the NPSA provided the first public analysis of national patient safety data in England and Wales. Up until the end of March 2005, 85 342 patient safety incidents were reported. Most of these incidents (68% of the total) resulted in no harm to the patients. Of the reported incidents, about one in 100 led to severe harm or death. In acute hospital settings, about three in every 1000 reported incidents resulted in death:

" Based on incidents and deaths reported over a three month period by 18 trusts, the NPSA has estimated that each year there would be approximately 840 deaths and 572 000 incidents reported in acute trusts in England.... Further work is needed to arrive at a more precise figure. The most common types of incidents reported are patient accidents (in particular falls) and incidents associated with treatment, procedure and medication.... Insufficient communication, education or teamwork are associated with many of the reported patient safety incidents across all settings and types of incidents.

National Patient Safety Agency 2005

Steps are being taken to deal with the issues identified in the reports and from other sources. The NPSA have developed an impressive armoury of publications and tools, which can be viewed from their website. A key NPSA publication is *Seven steps to patient safety* (National Patient Safety Agency 2004). The steps provide a simple checklist to help health-care staff plan their activity and measure performance. Following the steps will help ensure that the care provided is as safe as possible. The steps are:

" 1 **Build a safety culture**
   Create a culture that is open and fair
2 **Lead and support your staff**
   Establish a clear and strong focus on patient safety throughout your organisation
3 **Integrate your risk management activity**
   Develop systems and processes to manage your risks and identify and assess things that could go wrong
4 **Promote reporting**
   Ensure your staff can easily report incidents locally and nationally
5 **Involve and communicate with patients and the public**
   Develop ways to communicate openly with and listen to patients

6 **Learn and share safety lessons**
   Encourage staff to use root cause analysis to learn how and why
   incidents happen
7 **Implement solutions to prevent harm**
   Embed lessons through changes to practice, processes or systems

" For any system as complex as the NHS to achieve all of the above requires
a significant shift in culture and a high level of commitment across the
service over many years. We recognise that some NHS organisations are
further down this path than others, and that you may need to prioritise
the steps you take next.

The NPSA works from the premise that the best way of reducing error rates is
to target the underlying systems failures.

Adjusting patient expectations

Patient expectations about what can be achieved in an NHS struggling to
balance its books (Hawkes & Charter 2006) are today perhaps a tad unrealistic
and a programme of re-education needs to take place. As we have seen,
government policy has been directed towards making the NHS revolve around
the interests of the patient; perhaps it is now time for a new strategy – a
strategy directed towards viewing patients as equal or equity partners in a
common enterprise. Partners have responsibilities and cannot simply function,
as some patients do, just as vitriolic recipients of care. The NHS is becoming
a safer place as a developed patient safety infrastructure is being slotted into
place, although it must be acknowledged that we are still a long way off from
developing an ingrained patient safety culture. Only incremental progress is
being made. The National Audit Office state (NAO 2005):

" The safety culture within trusts is improving, driven largely by the
Department's clinical governance initiative and the development of more
effective risk management systems in response to incentives under
initiatives such as the NHS Litigation Authority's Clinical Negligence
Scheme for Trusts.... However, trusts are still predominantly reactive in
their response to patient safety issues and parts of some organisations still
operate a blame culture.

Powers (2004) brings an interesting perspective to risk management and the
audit regulatory focus of organisations and his comments can equally apply
to the NHS:

" The risk management of everything, and the specific growth of secondary
risk management, has a dark side which is threatening the state,
regulatory bodies, corporations and the individual experts on which so
many individuals in society rely. If we must act as if we know the risks we
face, then we must also create forms of risk management, and a related
politics of uncertainty, which allows us to do this in more, rather than less,
intelligent ways.

To avoid developing an NHS culture that could be termed 'ossified' and 'risk-
obsessed', and to allow organisations and professions to exercise at least

some degree of professional autonomy, we may need to try and educate the public to accept that failure is possible and that nurses and doctors cannot always guarantee a perfect treatment outcome. Patient expectations may have to be adjusted downwards.

As Powers (2004) states:

" the new politics of uncertainty must generate legitimacy for the possibility of failure. Indeed, in contrast to a 'spin-' or 'reputation-culture', such a political discourse would generate public trust precisely because an explicit discourse of possible failure is embedded in innovatory processes. The purpose would not be to defend individuals from blame, but to enrol the wider public in the benefits and excitement of innovation.

The NHS may need to think less about regulation and audit and try to guard against its seemingly natural reactive tendency to create new organisations whenever a new major crisis happens. As Powers (2004) argues: 'the test of good governance would not necessarily be the speed of their reaction to failure; on the contrary, it might be their ability, in Peter Senge's phrase, "to take two aspirin and wait".'

The political policy drivers who control and manage the NHS may not yet be ready for 'Politics of Uncertainty' (Powers 2004), but thought should be given to the concept, particularly in the consent to treatment process and in communication with patients generally. NHS policy makers also need to think more proactively and guard against their natural centralist regulatory tendencies.

LITIGATION CLAIMS

Costs and claims in clinical negligence in the NHS have increased significantly. The National Audit Office states (2001) that 'The rate of new claims per thousand finished consultant episodes rose by 72% between 1990 and 1998'. Figure 8 of their report (Fig. 3.1) places the issue in some perspective.

More recent figures are provided by the National Health Service Litigation Authority (NHSLA) (National Health Service Litigation Authority 2006):

" In 2004–05, 5609 claims of clinical negligence and 3766 claims of non-clinical negligence against NHS bodies were received by the NHSLA. This compares with 6251 claims of clinical negligence and 3819 claims of non-clinical negligence in 2003–04.

" … The NHSLA estimates that its total liabilities (the theoretical cost of paying all outstanding claims immediately, including those relating to incidents which have occurred but have not yet been reported to us) are £6.89 billion for clinical claims and £0.11 billion for non-clinical claims.

The costs and claims of clinical negligence are reported in billions of pounds sterling. Patient complaints to the Health Service Ombudsman (HSO) reach record levels each year: 'This year we have handled a higher workload than ever. We received a record 4703 new complaints – an increase of 18% on the previous year, which had itself seen a huge rise in new complaints, many relating to continuing care' (Health Service Ombudsman 2004).

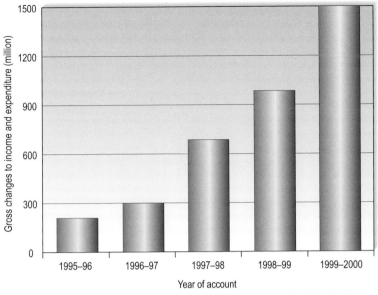

Fig. 3.1 Total charges to income and expenditure accounts for provisions for clinical negligence. Reproduced with permission from National Audit Office 2001 (author Karen Taylor).

To complain or not to complain

A patient may wish to complain and asks a nurse about appropriate channels. To function effectively as a patient advocate, the nurse must have a reasonable working knowledge and understanding of the complaints system and protocols (Tingle 1990), in particular his/her own local hospital complaints procedure. Minor complaints can often be handled by the nurse as they arise, and this is encouraged by Department of Health guidance. More significant complaints should be referred to the nurse's line manager.

A rise in complaints or clinical negligence claims may not necessarily be directly attributable to a general deterioration in the quality of the health service, but rather to a much more informed, consumer orientated and less deferential public which maintains high expectations, (albeit perhaps unrealistic expectations) of the health service and what can be achieved. It is clear that a more vocal public is increasingly holding all types of professionals to account. Initiatives such as the Patient's Charter (Department of Health 1995) and the Government's health quality reforms (Department of Health 1997, 2000), which are intended to forge a quality-driven NHS, have raised patient expectations and helped draw attention to the patient's right to complain. Government health policy has been in recent years to put the patient firmly at the centre of the NHS (*The NHS Plan,* Department of Health 2000) *The NHS Plan* worked from a pure patient focussed premise:

" 10.1 Patients are the most important people in the health service. It doesn't always appear that way. Too many patients feel talked at, rather than listened to. This has to change. NHS care has to be shaped around the convenience and concerns of patients.

The Shipman case (Beecham 2000) and the Wisehart Bristol heart surgery scandal (Dyer 1999), widely reported by the media, have also kept medical and nursing matters well in the public eye, have inevitably driven up care expectations and, along with other medical scandals, have caused the government to reflect on complaint systems and other matters. Berrington & Barnwell (1995) discuss the Central Statistical Office publication *Social Trends* (vol. 25) and note: 'Britons have become healthier, sometimes wealthier and more likely to own their own homes; higher expectations mean we are also increasingly dissatisfied'.

Health complaints and litigation can be seen in a much broader and more generalised context: we live now in a much more complaining and litigation-conscious society. The mantle of infallibility exuded by many health carers seems to have been largely eroded in the minds of many patients today. We hold our health carers to account, like any other professionals involved in providing professional services. Health professionals may in some respects be at a disadvantage in that complaints made against them are more likely to attract media attention because of the 'human interest' factor. Finally, it must be remembered that, where a complaint is made in the context of health care, it is not simply a matter of ensuring that a fault is remedied. There is an important issue of public accountability in the context of the NHS (Simanowitz 1985).

Health-care provision is a matter of public funding and of public concern. There is an expectation that health-care providers should be accountable. Nurses need to be aware of the complaints process and the fact that they may be the subject of complaints made, whether at informal or formal level. It is also important that the nurse is aware of what rights patients have in this area regarding his/her role as patient advocate. Nurses also need to be aware of the mechanisms that have been developed to enhance patient safety as this is also an aspect of professional accountability.

Hill (1991) of the Medical Defence Union also offers some useful guidance on complaint handling: 'When dealing with patients' complaints remember the four S's: complaints should be handled SPEEDILY, with SYMPATHY, to the patient's SATISFACTION, and (if indicated) with an expression of SORROW. Conciliation, not confrontation should be the goal'.

It is important to remember that a complaint could result in litigation.

Complaints should be analysed for trends.

Complaints and patient confusion

Frequently a patient's complaint, or the commencement of a legal claim, may arise from his/her confusion, anxiety and frustration at not receiving a satisfactory explanation of why something has gone wrong; frustration that may result in anger and trigger off a complaint (Medical Defence Union 1993). Litigation or a formal complaint might never have taken place had the patient been given an understandable explanation of what had gone wrong and the steps being taken to remedy matters. Vincent and colleagues (1994) surveyed 227 patients and relatives who were taking legal action through five firms of plaintiff solicitors. They found that the decision to take legal action was determined not only by the original injury but also by insensitive handling and poor communication after the original incident. The following four main factors were identified in the analysis of reasons for litigation:

- Accountability
- Explanation
- Standards of care
- Compensation and admission of negligence

Patients and relatives wished to see staff disciplined and called to account. They wanted an explanation and felt ignored or neglected after the incident. They also wanted to make sure that the same problem did not happen to anybody else.

Complaints can arise from what may seem to the health carer to be trivial matters. The diabetic clinic may have been very busy and short-staffed at a particular time. As a result the patient may have had a long wait for treatment. An overworked nurse may have been a little abrupt when the patient asked how much longer he was going to have to wait. The patient takes offence at what he sees as a personal insult and complains. But some matters are more complex and may raise issues of such gravity that monetary compensation is required as well as an explanation.

Complaints may or may not have a reasonable basis. Truelove (1985) states:

" Some people complain only reluctantly and as a last resort, when prompted by a deep emotion. Some complain reasonably on reasonable grounds. Some complain 'unreasonably' on reasonable grounds. Some complain 'reasonably' on unreasonable grounds. A few (usually with a history of psychological disturbance) complain unreasonably on unreasonable grounds. A few seem to be 'born complainants' who relish a battle and will complain on any grounds whatsoever.

THE COMPLAINTS SYSTEM

Unfortunately there are a number of weaknesses with the present NHS complaints system, the HSO states (Health Service Ombudsman 2005):

" complaints systems are fragmented within the NHS, between the NHS and private health care systems, and between health and social care; the complaints system is not centred on the patient's needs; there is a lack of capacity and competence among staff to deliver a quality service; the right leadership, culture and governance are not in place; just remedies are not being secured for justified complaints.

This is quite a condemning catalogue of complaints on the NHS complaints system, and although reform is taking place, it is rather slow and piecemeal. The complaints system as presently constituted is confusing and there is a lot of scope for improvement. We are still some way off from having a full and comprehensive system.

The HSO is not alone in noting problems. The Healthcare Commission (2005) has seen a doubling in the numbers of people demanding that an NHS complaint should be independently reviewed because it was not resolved locally. They are sending one in three cases back to the NHS because the NHS has not dealt with the issues adequately.

The Department of Health response, in January 2002, to the report of the public inquiry into children's heart surgery at the Bristol Royal Infirmary (Department of Health 2002) said that they intended to have a new NHS complaints procedure in place by December 2002, but this new system has yet to be fully implemented and integrated across the NHS. At the time of writing (April 2006), the arrangements for 'local resolution' set out in the Complaints Regulations 2004 do not apply to primary care practitioners (GPs). The practice-based procedure booklets issued to primary care practitioners in 1996 continue to apply until the amended complaint regulations and guidance are issued in 2006. Following an approach by the Shipman Inquiry, ministers decided on a 'phased implementation' of the complaints system. The intention is to issue amended Complaints Regulations in 2006 once the Department of Health has been able to give proper consideration to any recommendations made by the Shipman Inquiry, which published its fifth report on 9 December 2004. The guidance will also be revised at that time. NHS Foundation Trusts have their own complaints procedures for dealing with internal complaints and these may differ from the 'local resolution' process that applies to other Trusts (Department of Health 2006a).

As far as 'local resolution' goes, the Complaints Regulations 1994 consolidate and rationalise the requirements set out in the various Department of Health directions since 1996. This means that 'local resolution' therefore remains broadly unchanged for NHS bodies and the new guidance updates information provided in existing guidance as well as expanding on the Regulations (Department of Health 2006a) (Table 3.1).

The Department of Health (2004) states that the most satisfactory outcome to complaints often comes when complaints are dealt with fully and effectively at 'local resolution'.

First steps

Initially a patient may approach a nurse or complaints manager to complain and they may feel able to deal with the matter on the spot or may refer it to a line manger (Department of Health 2006b). Alternatively, a patient may approach his/her local Patient Advice and Liaison Service (PALS). PALS have been established in every NHS Trust and primary care trust. PALS are not part of the complaints procedure itself but they might be able to resolve the patient's complaint informally or tell them more about the complaints procedure and the independent complaints advocacy services (ICAS). ICAS provides advice and support to people who want to complain about the NHS. Details of how to contact local ICAS services can be seen on the Department of Health complaints web page (Department of Health 2006b). Department of Health advice to patients on complaining also states that patients can contact NHS Direct.

If all these avenues fail then the patient can embark on making a formal complaint.

Table 3.1 Outline of changes to the complaints process		
	Old process (established 1996)	New process
Stage 1 Local resolution	Patient, or someone acting on their behalf, could complain to the organisation or practitioner concerned	(Unchanged) Patient, or someone acting on their behalf, complains to the organisation or practitioner concerned
Stage 2 Independent review	If the patient was unhappy with the response s/he got at stage 1, s/he could apply for an independent review, which was overseen by an NHS convener – usually a non-executive director of the Trust to which s/he complained	If the patient is unhappy with the response s/he got at stage 1, s/he can apply to the Healthcare Commission for an independent review. Trusts can also refer complaints to the Healthcare Commission with the patient's consent. Complaints managers, Independent Complaints Advocacy Service staff and PALS staff should notify patients of this option
	If the patient was unhappy with the convenor's initial response, a panel consisting of the convenor, a chair nominated by the strategic health authority and one other would form a panel to hear the complaint	If the individual is still unhappy after the initial review and investigation by the case manager, s/he has the option of having his/her case heard by an independent panel. See below for the timescales and phases the Healthcare Commission will be working to in handling these requests
Stage 3 Health Service Ombudsman	If a patient was unhappy, the complaint could be referred to the Health Service Ombudsman	(Unchanged) If a patient is unhappy, the complaint can be referred to the Health Service Ombudsman. In some circumstances the Healthcare Commission will refer complainants directly on to the Ombudsman
Source: Healthcare Commission 2004		

The complaints stages

Local resolution

The first stage for NHS complaints is local resolution. This stage seeks to provide prompt investigation and resolution of the complaint at local level, aiming to satisfy the complainant while also being fair to staff. The basis of the NHS local resolution stage can be found in the National Health Service (Complaints) Regulations 2004 SI No. 1768 and in the Department of Health guide (Department of Health 2004).

It is important for the nurse, as the person likely to spend the most time with patients and often their first NHS contact, to be aware of the complaints procedures. Currently these regulations are not applicable to primary care practitioners and new regulations are anticipated in 2006.

Patient safety, litigation and complaints in the National Health Service

The Department of Health (2004) states the importance of NHS staff knowledge about the complaints process:

❝ The complaints process will be more effective if all NHS staff understand the reformed procedure and the role played by the Healthcare Commission within that procedure. Training will enable all staff and non-executives of NHS trusts, primary care trusts and strategic health authorities to deal with someone wishing to make a complaint.... [1.6] It will be helpful also for staff to know how to deal with concerns informally, for example with the help of the Patient Advice and Liaison Services (PALS). PALS and Modern Matrons can each help to address people's concerns on the spot.

The key elements of local resolution (Department of Health 2004)
Handling and consideration of complaints by NHS bodies
Arrangements for the handling and consideration of complaints
Regulation 3

(1) Each NHS body must make arrangements in accordance with these Regulations for the handling and consideration of complaints.

(2) The arrangements must be accessible and such as to ensure that complaints are dealt with speedily and efficiently, and that complainants are treated courteously and sympathetically and as far as possible involved in decisions about how their complaints are handled and considered...

3.1 NHS bodies must have a well-defined procedure in place for investigating and resolving complaints. The procedure should be open, fair, flexible and conciliatory and should encourage communication on all sides. The primary objective is to resolve the complaint satisfactorily.

3.2 Complaints managers should involve the complainant from the outset and seek to determine what they are hoping to achieve from the process. The complainant should be given the opportunity to understand all possible options for pursuing the complaint, and the consequences of following these options. Throughout the process, the complaints manager should assess what further action might best resolve the complaint. The complainant should be kept informed.

3.3 Complaints managers will need to keep a complete documentary record of the handling and consideration of each complaint – these records will be particularly important if the complaint is referred to the Healthcare Commission or Ombudsman. Complaints records should be kept separate from health records, subject to the need to record information which is strictly relevant to their health in the patient's health records.

3.4 At all times NHS staff should treat patients, carers and visitors politely and with respect. However, violence, racial, sexual or verbal harassment should not be tolerated. Neither will NHS staff be expected to tolerate language that is of a personal, abusive or threatening nature.

Responsibility for complaints arrangements
Regulation 4
Each NHS body must designate one of its members, or in the case of an NHS trust a member of its board of directors, to take responsibility for ensuring compliance with

the arrangements made under these Regulations and that action is taken in the light of the outcome of any investigation.

Complaints manager
Regulation 5
(1) Each NHS body must designate a person, in these Regulations referred to as a complaints manager, to manage the procedures for handling and considering complaints and in particular – (a) to perform the functions of the complaints manager under this Part; and (b) to perform such other functions in relation to complaints as the NHS body may require.
(2) The functions of the complaints manger may be performed by him or by any person authorised by the NHS body to act on his behalf.

Complaints to NHS bodies
Regulation 6
Subject to regulation 7, a complaint to an NHS body may be about any matter reasonably connected with the exercise of its functions ….

Acknowledgement and record of complaint
Regulation 11
(1) The complaints manager must send to the complainant a written acknowledgement of the complaint within 2 working days of the date on which the complaint was made.
(2) Where a complaint was made orally, the acknowledgement must be accompanied by the written record mentioned in regulation 9(2)(a) with an invitation to the complainant to sign and return it.
3.39 Acknowledgements must be in writing and sent within two working days of the date on which the complaint was made (see Regulation 9(3)). It is good practice for the acknowledgement to be conciliatory, and indicate that the response will be provided by the Chief Executive within an agreed timeframe (see Regulation 13(2))….

Handling and consideration of complaints by the Healthcare Commission

Independent review (also applicable to primary care practitioners)
If the complainant is unhappy with the response to the informal stage, then the Healthcare Commission can be asked for an independent review (stage 2). They can only review the complaint if the complainant has already raised it with the organisation or practitioner concerned (first stage) and is dissatisfied with their formal written response, or if the complaint has been with the health-care provider for 6 months and has not been resolved. The Healthcare Commission (2006a) states:

" You may be dissatisfied because:

- you feel that the investigation by the local NHS organisation or practitioner was inadequate, incomplete or unsatisfactory
- you have reason to believe that the underlying issues, which led to the complaint, have not been fully uncovered or understood
- you feel that the healthcare provider's response did not address all the issues raised by your complaint.

Complaints that are forwarded to the Healthcare Commission are dealt with in the following way.

Initial review

A case manager will undertake an initial review of the case, with the help of expert advice if necessary, to determine whether there needs to be further investigation, and s/he will write a report. The Healthcare Commission states (2004a) that the investigation will be proportionate to both the substance of the complaint and the way in which it has been handled locally. If there are options for resolution at this stage, they will be explored. The report will be given to the complainant and also those complained against and will include any recommendations for improving services or actions to rectify the situation.

The case manager may decide to (Healthcare Commission 2004a, 2006a):

- take no further action
- refer the complaint back to the health-care provider or NHS body for further action
- refer the complaint to another body, e.g. the General Medical Council or the Health Service Ombudsman, for further action or investigation
- refer the complaint for action by another section of the Healthcare Commission
- carry out a full investigation of the complaint
- refer the complaint for a panel hearing
- decide that the complaint is not eligible because it does not meet the Healthcare Commission's criteria.

The criteria

There are also criteria for further investigation (Healthcare Commission 2004a):

" The Healthcare Commission may decide that investigation is necessary because:

- the investigation at local level was inadequate and there is uncertainty about the events that occurred, or
- the complaint covers more than one service and some issues were not properly answered locally, or
- there is reason to believe that the underlying circumstances that have led to the complaint have not yet been fully exposed, and additional information is likely to be exposed by the Healthcare Commission investigation, or
- the relationship between the complainant and complained against has broken down to the extent that resolution is not possible, or
- the response of the organisation to the complaint appears to be unreasonable or incomplete, or
- the events raise serious issues about local services or complaints handling that may be clarified by a Healthcare Commission investigation.

The letter
A letter outlining the outcome of the initial review and whether further investigation is required will be given to the complainant and the organisation or practitioner about whom s/he is complaining (Healthcare Commission 2004b).

Complainant not happy
If a complainant is unhappy with the outcome of the initial review, s/he will be able to complain about the decision to the Health Service Ombudsman.

If the Healthcare Commission investigates a complaint?

The Terms of Reference
If the Healthcare Commission decides to investigate, the case manager will first need to finalise the matters for investigation in what are termed 'terms of reference'. Both the complainant and complained against will be able to comment on the draft terms of reference. If the case manager decides not to investigate certain parts of the complaint, s/he will explain the reasons why. When the investigation is completed, a draft report will be prepared and sent out for comment on factual accuracy. The report will summarise the investigation and make recommendations. The report will then be finalised and distributed to the following parties (Healthcare Commission 2006b):

- the complainant
- the patient if different from the complainant
- the person complained against
- the chief executive of the relevant NHS organisation
- any experts consulted
- the strategic health authority.

Recommendations
The recommendations made at the end of an investigation will be similar to those possible at the end of initial review. An investigation will normally be completed within 6 months of the date the Healthcare Commission decided to undertake it (Healthcare Commission 2006b).

What can the Healthcare Commission do for the patient/person complaining?
The Healthcare Commission cannot direct that compensation be paid. It will, however, seek an explanation and acknowledgement of what went wrong, and corrective action. It will seek an apology for the patient in appropriate circumstances. Recommendations can also be made on changing work practices so that events are not repeated. The terms of reference drawn up in consultation with the health-care provider complained against and the patient will help focus the issues and outcomes wanted by the patient (Healthcare Commission 2006a). If the complainant is unhappy with the outcome of the investigation, s/he has the right to request an independent panel to hear and consider the issues.

The panel

The panel (Healthcare Commission 2004, 2006b) will consist of three members of the public who are not connected with the NHS but who have been specially trained to deal with NHS complaints. The panel will hear both sides of the complaint and may also make recommendations for resolution or for improving services where appropriate. The case manager and chair of the panel will agree the terms of reference for the panel following comments from the complainant and the complained against. A panel coordinator will then take over with organising the panel and producing the report of the outcomes. All parties involved with the panel will have a chance to check the draft report for factual accuracy before it is finalised and distributed. The panel process will normally be completed within 4 months of the date of the request. This includes the distribution of the panel report. If a complainant is unhappy with the outcome of the panel hearing, s/he will be able to complain about the Healthcare Commission's decision to the Health Service Ombudsman.

The Health Service Commissioner (Health Service Ombudsman)

The Health Service Commissioner – also known as the Health Service Ombudsman (Health Service Ombudsman 2006) – represents what could be regarded as the third stage of the NHS complaints process. Usually, the complainant should have already complained to the organisation or practitioner involved and to the Healthcare Commission before contacting the Health Service Ombudsman before sending in the complaint. The Health Service Ombudsman recognises, however, that this is not always possible and s/he has power to consider complaints that have not been put to the relevant NHS body where s/he considers that, in the circumstances of the particular case, it is not reasonable to expect this.

Examples of the types of complaint the Health Service Ombudsman can look at include:

" • Receiving the wrong or poor treatment
• Errors in diagnosis or treatment
• Communication problems within or between services
• Significant mistakes over appointments to see a doctor or go to hospital
• Failure by an organisation to provide or pay for a service, e.g. continuing care
• Delay that could have been avoided
• Faulty procedures, or failing to follow correct procedures
• Unfairness, bias or prejudice
• Giving advice which is misleading or inadequate
• Rudeness and not apologising for mistakes
• Not putting things right when something has gone wrong.

Health Service Ombudsman 2006

The powers of the Health Service Ombudsman

After completing an investigation the Health Service Ombudsman may uphold the complaint in full or in part or may not uphold the complaint at all. The findings, with reasons, will be set out in his/her report. If the complaint is upheld, recommendations may include appropriate redress, which might include an apology, an explanation, improvements to practices and systems or, where appropriate, financial redress. In addition in a situation in which s/he believes that it is in the interests of patient safety, s/he may decide to refer individual health-care practitioners to their regulatory bodies (Health Service Ombudsman 2006, para 6.12). There is an expectation that the recommendations will be implemented and the NHS provider will be contacted to find out how they have been implemented (Health Service Ombudsman 2006 para 6.13).

The HSO reports reveal a wide catalogue of errors and failures that generally speaking, could easily have been avoided. A large number involve communication failures; the HSO (Health Service Ombudsman 1992b) commented: 'some topics – such as record keeping, complaints handling and observation of patients – feature regularly in … annual reports'. Seven years on, the same problems still persist (Health Service Ombudsman 1999a):

" Communication difficulties lay at the heart of a significant number of complaints about clinical care. Sometimes the problem was poor communication between professionals, and sometimes between professionals and patients (or their relatives). In other cases, while I was satisfied that reasonable clinical care had been given, an opportunity to resolve the complainant's concerns had been missed because of poor communication and complaint handling.

Nurses do feature in a number of complaints to the HSO. In 1999 (Health Service Ombudsman 1999a), the HSO found that 'The service area with the largest number of complaints about clinical care (26) was, not unexpectedly, hospital inpatients: about 35% were upheld. About 13% of clinical grievances investigated primarily involved nurses and 19% hospital doctors.'

The following case investigation report provides a good illustration of the problems that the HSO investigates, in a nursing context, W.232/90/91 (Health Service Ombudsman 1992a). A woman was terminally ill with cancer and was also suffering from claustrophobia. She was nursed during the week in a surgical ward and for hospital financial reasons was moved at the weekend to other wards and sometimes to a small side room. A decision was eventually made to transfer her to a hospice, where she died 3 days after the transfer. Her husband complained that the weekend ward transfers caused his wife unacceptable distress and that nursing staff in these wards were unaware that his wife suffered from claustrophobia. He said that there had been inadequate nursing care in one ward. He claimed that his wife had not been given help with washing, that pressure sores had been allowed to develop, and her urostomy and ileostomy bags had not been changed regularly. He complained of insensitivity on the part of a ward sister, who he stated had asked his wife to cut up an incontinence roll when supplies had run out. The roll was inadequate for his wife's needs and he had to buy another one. The sister, he claimed, had also been unwilling to arrange for an ambulance to take his wife to the hospice. Some of the husband's complaints were upheld. The HSO found 'a deplorable lack of regard by management for patient's welfare'. The health authority apologised.

The investigation reports of the HSO provide a useful perspective from which to view the professional accountability of the nurse. The HSO Annual Report (Health Service Ombudsman 1995) contains the following case:

" A woman developed a pressure sore while in hospital and I considered that there had been an avoidable delay in taking preventative measures. I also criticised the poor standard of record keeping. I found that nursing staff had not communicated satisfactorily with the patient's daughter. Board to check that monitoring of pressure area care standards was operating effectively. (S.104/93–94, Tayside HB)

The HSO reported the following in Case No.E.189/97–98 (Health Service Ombudsman 1998), which involved failures in medical and nursing care, delay in transfer to an intensive care unit at another hospital and unsatisfactory complaint handling. Findings include the following:

" The evidence indicates that Mr B's drip was out for about two hours. My assessors have said that that would not have had an adverse effect on his condition. I accept that. However, it is not satisfactory that Mr B was left with blood stained pyjamas and bedding until the family asked for them to be changed.

Complaints to the HSO can cover a range of matters involving GPs, doctors, nurses, dentists and so on. The HSO investigates a wide range of matters and a recent trend is that more clinically complex matters are coming to the Office (HSO1999a). A typical contemporary case involving nurses can be seen in E.2775/02–03 (Health Service Ombudsman 2004):

" **Inadequate planning and implementation of nursing care – E.2775/02–03**

" Miss C, a teaching assistant, who lived independently, was admitted to hospital suffering from chest pain. She also suffered from severe spina bifida and congenital hydrocephalus. Accident and Emergency initially prescribed painkillers for her chest pain. After being examined by a consultant physician, she was subsequently prescribed antibiotics and transferred to the medical admissions unit. Her condition deteriorated significantly and she was admitted to intensive care, where sadly she died a few weeks later. The cause of her death was given as multiple organ failure secondary to septicaemia (blood poisoning). Miss C's parents complained that the standard of care was very poor. In particular, they complained about the assessment of her presenting symptoms, the prescription and administration of medication, the management of Miss C's fluid levels and the Trust's response to her deterioration. They also complained about the attitude of staff towards their daughter and the way that staff treated them. We found that the planning and implementation of nursing care and the level of nursing documentation were inadequate. The Trust therefore apologised to Miss C's parents. They also agreed to implement a number of recommendations relating to:

- improving documentation and audit;
- providing better patient care and communication;

and more effectively managing people with disabilities.

The reports and investigations of the HSO show that the office is providing a very valuable and important function. The HSO reports are always clear, thorough and incisive. The value of the HSO lies in the Office's independence from the NHS, the Ombudsman reports to Parliament. The role of the HSO does need to keep pace with the changes in the NHS and should not be seen as a static. Experience of the HSO shows that the role will change to meet new demands. The extension of the HSO's jurisdiction to cover clinical judgment is one example of how the HSO role has positively developed.

CONCLUSION

There does seem to be a groundswell of opinion developing that is saying that all is not right with the NHS complaints system. When the complaints system was introduced in 1996 the accompanying Department of Health documentation looked very promising, with clear advice on strategies to avoid and handle complaints being given. Experience with the system over time has revealed difficulties that the HSO has noted above (Health Service Ombudsman 2005), which do need to be resolved if meaningful reform to the complaints system is ever going to happen. The Department of Health and the government have enough expert literature to make informed and evidence-based decisions on the system. Such determinations are going to have to take account of other initiatives in the NHS such as clinical governance (integrated governance), clinical risk management, patient safety systems, the NHS Redress Scheme and organisations such as the Healthcare Commission, the HSO, the NPSA and the NHSLA.

A complaints system cannot exist in 'splendid isolation' from these dynamic and focused health-quality improvement initiatives. To operate effectively it must be comprehensive, joined up and manifestly transparent and simple. The links will have to be carefully thought through to avoid overlaps and inconsistencies.

The nurse as 'patient advocate' will be expected to know much about the NHS complaints system and s/he should also participate in and be aware of hospital and practice patient safety systems. If patient harm is avoided in the first place then there is unlikely to be a complaint or legal claim made.

REFERENCES

Beecham L 2000 Milburn sets up inquiry into Shipman case. *British Medical Journal* 320: 401. Available online at: http://www.bmj.com/cgi/content/full/320/7232/401/a (Accessed 10/7/06).

Berrington L, Barnwell R 1995 Britain's moaning minnies who know their rights. *The Times* 26 January

Department of Health 1995 The patient's charter. Department of Health, London

Department of Health 1997 The new NHS, modern, dependable. Cmnd 3807. Stationery Office, London

Department of Health 2000 The NHS plan. Cmnd 4818-1. The Stationery Office, London

Department of Health 2002 Learning from Bristol: the Department of Health's response to the Report of the Public Inquiry into children's heart surgery at the Bristol Royal Infirmary 1984–1995. Cmnd 5363. Stationery Office, London

Department of Health 2004 Guidance to support implementation of the National Health Service (Complaints) Regulations 2004. Department of Health, London

Department of Health 2006a NHS complaints procedure. Available online at: http://www.dh.gov.uk/PolicyAndGuidance/OrganisationPolicy/ComplaintsPolicy/NHSComplaintsProcedure/fs/en (Accessed 10/7/06). Department of Health, London

Department of Health 2006b How to complain about the NHS. Available online at: http://www.dh.gov.uk/PolicyAndGuidance/OrganisationPolicy/ComplaintsPolicy/NHSComplaintsProcedure/NHSComplaintsProcedureArticle/fs/en?CONTENT_ID=4080897&chk=%2Bwi3Mr (Accessed 10/7/06). Department of Health, London

Dyer C 1999 Bristol trust admits liability in baby heart surgery case. British Medical Journal 319: 213. Available online at: http://www.bmj.com/cgi/content/full/ 319/7204/213/a (Accessed 10/7/06).

Hawkes N, Charter D 2006 NHS chief says hospitals must spend less on drugs and staff. The Times 12 April: 8

Healthcare Commission 2004 Q&As – complaints briefing note. Healthcare Commission, London

Healthcare Commission 2004a Reforming the NHS complaints procedure. Healthcare Commission, London

Healthcare Commission 2004b New independent system to review NHS complaints. Press release, 26 July. Healthcare Commission, London

Healthcare Commission 2005 NHS sees doubling of number of people demanding their NHS complaint be independently reviewed. Press release, 31 October. Healthcare Commission, London

Healthcare Commission 2006a Unhappy with the way your complaint has been handled by the NHS? Contact the Healthcare Commission. Reference BH/CW/20T/0605. Available online at: http://www.healthcarecommission.org.uk/Homepage/fs/en. Healthcare Commission, London

Healthcare Commission 2006b How the Healthcare Commission will handle complaints. Available online at: http://www.healthcarecommission.org.uk/ContactUs/ComplainAboutNHS/Complain/(Accessed 26/04/06). Healthcare Commission, London

Health Service Ombudsman 1992a Selected investigations completed October 1991–March 1992. HMSO, London

Health Service Ombudsman 1992b Annual Report for 1991–92. HMSO, London

Health Service Ombudsman 1995 Annual Report for 1994–95. HMSO, London

Health Service Ombudsman 1998 Investigations completed April-September 1998, 1st Report – Session 1998–99. Stationery Office, London

Health Service Ombudsman 1999a Annual Report for 1998–99. Stationery Office, London

Health Service Ombudsman 2004 Annual Report 2003–04. Stationery Office, London

Health Service Ombudsman 2005 Making things better? A report on reform of the NHS complaints procedure in England. Stationery Office, London

Health Service Ombudsman 2006 What can we look at? Available online at: http://www.ombudsman.org.uk/make_a_complaint/health/what_can_we_look_at.hml. Health Service Ombudsman, London

Hill G 1991 Complaints about clinical care: correct management. Medical Defence Union, London. Available online at: http://www.publications.parliament.uk/pa/cm199899/cmselect/cmhealth/cmhealth.htm

Medical Defence Union 1993 Talking to patients. Medical Defence Union, London

National Audit Office 2001 Handling clinical negligence claims in England, HC 403. Stationery Office, London

National Audit Office 2005 A safer place for patients: learning to improve patient safety, HC 456. Stationery Office, London

National Health Service Litigation Authority 2006 About the NHS Litigation Authority. National Health Service Litigation Authority, London. Available online at: http://www.nhsla.com/home.htm

National Patient Safety Agency 2004 Seven steps to patient safety: an overview guide for NHS Staff, 2nd print. National Patient Safety Agency, London

National Patient Safety Agency 2005 Building a memory: preventing harm, reducing risks and improving patient safety. The first report of the National Reporting and Learning System and the Patient Safety Observatory. National Patient Safety Agency, London

Powers M 2004 The risk management of everything: rethinking the politics of uncertainty. Demos, London

Simanowitz A 1985 Standards, attitudes and accountability in the medical profession. Lancet 2: 546

Tingle JH 1990 Complaints and the law. Nursing Standard 5(2): 44

Truelove A 1985 On handling complaints. Hospital and Health Services Review September (i):229

Vincent C, Young M, Phillips A 1994 Why do people sue doctors? A study of patients and relatives taking legal action. Lancet 343: 1609

3

Patient safety, litigation and complaints in the National Health Service

Legal aspects of expanded role, clinical guidelines and protocols, and nurse prescribing

John Tingle and Jean McHale

This chapter focuses upon certain specific issues that have important ramifications regarding nursing accountability, such as expanded role, the operation of clinical care guidelines and protocols, and nurse prescribing. In part one, John Tingle considers the area of legal aspects of expanded role, clinical guidelines and protocols and in part two, Jean McHale considers the issue of nurse prescribing.

LEGAL ASPECTS OF EXPANDED ROLE

John Tingle

DEVELOPMENTS IN NURSING PRACTICE

Today the number of tasks undertaken by nurses has increased. This is related to a number of factors, ranging from resource issues such as the need to reduce junior doctors' hours to the fact that nurses are being entrusted with wider responsibility as recognition of their role as independent practitioners. The government's published strategy for nursing midwifery and health visiting contained in *Making a Difference* (Department of Health 1999b) is notable for its proactive stance on nurses taking on more advanced activities. The government would like nurses to extend their role and to make better use of their knowledge and skills. It also wants to make it easier for them to prescribe. The former Health Secretary Alan Milburn laid down a 10-point challenge on nursing skills to be implemented throughout the National Health Service (NHS). This included nurses being able to order diagnostic investigations, e.g. pathology tests and X-rays, make and receive referrals direct to, for example, therapists or pain consultants, run their own clinics, e.g. ophthalmology or dermatology, and take a lead in the way local health services are organised and run (Department of Health 2000a). The momentum for role expansion has been growing steadily for a number of years and it has been firmly taken forward and promoted by the government. The NHS Plan further promoted expanded roles (Department of Health 2000b) and *Liberating the Talents* (Department of Health 2003) described how 'nurses with special interests', i.e. with additional expertise, can be developed by primary care trusts to improve patient care and increase local primary care capacity. Advice for managers on developing key roles for nurses and midwives is provided by the Department of Health 2002.

Nurses now undertake activities such as electrocardiography, defibrillation after a heart attack, verification of death (not in cases of unexpected death), taking blood samples and performing male catheterisation (Eaton 1993). There are nurse-led minor injuries units (MIUs) where nurses carry out a variety of activities, which can include suturing, X-ray, plaster and refer (Carlisle 1995). There are also nurse endoscopists (United Kingdom Central Council 2000). The Department of Health and the Royal College of Nursing (2003) gave some further examples of expanded and advanced roles in their resource to nurses, therapists, health-care professionals, managers and directors to clarify what nurses and allied health professionals (AHPs) are allowed and able to do within their professional codes of conduct. It focuses on the patient journey, and brings together examples in practice that show how practitioners are working to speed up and improve the patient journey and experience by challenging myths.

The advice also provides practical factsheets about the legal and professional frameworks that support and develop professional practice and some good examples of expanded and advanced roles are given:

" • ...GP referrals direct to nurse consultants
• extending the boundaries of pre-hospital care and admission avoidance
• Pre-hospital care and thrombolysis by paramedic staff or nurses
• Walk-in Centres providing early access for patients
• patient assessment and advice through NHS Direct and online
• extended out of hours services
• treatment at home or at scene, carried out by nurses or paramedics.

" Nurses and AHPs have expanded their practice to carry out clinical assessment of adults, children and young people with a range of clinical conditions and symptoms...

• see and treat and discharge with advice
• nurse-led ambulatory care services
• nurse-initiated thrombolysis
• nurse-led assessment
• use of Patient Group Directions (PGDs) to enable nurses to administer medication such as analgesia, anti-emetics.

" Nurses and AHPs with appropriate competencies are able to refer patients for tests and investigations as part of the clinical assessment. This does not always necessitate an additional course.

" Nurses and AHPs who have appropriate competencies can interpret test results and initiate treatment.

• ... nurse-initiated X-rays
• nurse-initiated abdominal ultrasound, Doppler and ultrasound
• nurse-initiated computed tomography scan of head for head injuries
• nurses interpreting X-rays
• nurse-initiated interventions based on blood results.

A contemporary view of nurses working in advanced and extended roles is provided in *Department of Health and Royal College of Nursing 2005.* This publication reports the findings of a joint Royal College of Nursing (RCN) and Department of Health survey to find out more about nurses working in advanced and extended roles and how proactive they are in developing the roles and services. A total of 758 nurses were asked about what their role entailed, what gave them most satisfaction and how their job fitted in with other nursing roles. Nearly 70% returned completed questionnaires. Survey key findings included that a nursing background is essential to undertake these roles; they are maxi nurses and not mini doctors. Nurses were found to be very positive about these new roles and keen for further role expansion. Nurses are leading multidisciplinary teams, working across organisational boundaries and coordinating packages of care. The roles are having a positive impact on the care of patients and the level of job satisfaction was high among post-holders. The roles create important career development opportunities that allow nurses to retain significant patient contact.

EXPANDED ROLE: DEFINITIONAL ISSUES

The growth of the nurse's work has been termed 'expanded role' by some commentators. In the past the term 'extended role' was used when discussing the issue of nurses carrying out activities traditionally carried out by doctors (Tingle 1993). The position altered, however, in 1992 (Department of Health 1992). This change followed a report issued by the Standing Medical Advisory Committee and the Standing Nursing and Midwifery Advisory Committee (1989). The United Kingdom Central Council for Nursing, Midwifery and

The Nursing and Midwifery Council code (2004a) Clause 6 now covers role expansion and incorporates guidance on enlarging the scope of a nurse's practice previously published separately as the *Scope of Professional Practice* (United Kingdom Central Council 1992, p. 7), and provides:

6 As a registered nurse, midwife or specialist community public health nurse, you must maintain your professional knowledge and competence

6.1 You must keep your knowledge and skills up-to-date throughout your working life. In particular, you should take part regularly in learning activities that develop your competence and performance.

6.2 To practise competently, you must possess the knowledge, skills and abilities required for lawful, safe and effective practice without direct supervision. You must acknowledge the limits of your professional competence and only undertake practice and accept responsibilities for those activities in which you are competent.

6.3 If an aspect of practice is beyond your level of competence or outside your area of registration, you must obtain help and supervision from a competent practitioner until you and your employer consider that you have acquired the requisite knowledge and skill.

6.4 You have a duty to facilitate students of nursing, midwifery and specialist community public health nursing and others to develop their competence.

6.5 You have a responsibility to deliver care based on current evidence, best practice and, where applicable, validated research when it is available.

Health Visiting (UKCC) stated that the terms 'extended' or 'extending roles' are no longer favoured as they 'limit, rather than extend the parameters of practice' (United Kingdom Central Council 1992).

Many see role expansion as presenting an exciting opportunity to develop new specialisms. However, expanding the nursing role has been controversial and there has been disagreement within the nursing profession as to what approach should be taken. There is no national standard or catalogue of expanded roles. Practices differ from region to region and even within hospitals (Standing Medical Advisory Committee and Standing Nursing and Midwifery Advisory Committee 1989). Some nurses argue that nursing may as a result become too technical and less patient-centred (Giles 1993, Shepherd 1993, Healy 1996). Eaton (1993) quotes Derek Dean (formerly Director of Policy and Research at the RCN): 'The worry among nurses, many of whom welcome this additional responsibility, is that they are being asked to do extra work without anyone extra to take the load off them. A lot of members have expressed concern. They have said, 'We are being asked to do things and are rushed off our feet.'

Similarly, Waters (1996) quotes RCN community adviser Mark Jones, who presented at a conference a catalogue of cautionary tales illustrating the dangers of nurses overreaching themselves. The list included one case where a practice nurse with no formal midwifery training had taken over antenatal care and had missed a fetus dying in utero.

A report by Doyal and colleagues (1998) looked in detail at the development of four new nursing posts. Each post involved nurses taking over some part of the work previously done by junior doctors. This study explored the views of nurses themselves and was quite revealing. While the study revealed excitement at the professional challenges they faced, the study also indicated that practitioners received little support and there was considerable confusion surrounding their new roles. Some legal and accountability issues were also noted:

" there were many staff who admitted that they did not know about the arrangements for accountability. They included consultants, ward nurses and junior doctors who worked with the postholders. Certain factors seemed to contribute to the confusion about the understanding of the arrangements for the postholder's accountability. One of these was lack of clarity about the role. So for instance, at Site X, the doctors saw the postholder's role as a support worker for them and hence the postholders' accountability was described as being to the doctors. Senior nurses, however, interpreted the role as that of a nurse specialist with accountability identified within the nursing framework.

The authors make a number of recommendations for managers and postholders about the management of change which include:

" • Areas of work should be identified which the postholder can take over completely with maximum autonomy and minimum dependency on junior doctors for completion of the work
• Nurses and doctors should be equal partners in planning and managing such developments

- The GMC, UKCC and NHS Executive need to clarify and harmonise relevant regulations concerning the scope and standards of new clinical roles, influence legal process and educate the public about changing professional roles.

The authors of this report were also in a small working group that looked in further detail at the accountability of changing nurses' roles. The analyses were published in the *British Medical Journal* (Dowling et al 1996). They noted that the resulting uncertainties about appropriate management for clinical roles evolving between the professions, coupled with a public increasingly going to court, put nurses and consultants at risk. These health-care professionals faced a risk of complaints, litigation and possible disciplinary hearing. Recommendations to reduce risk included: doctors and nurses as equal partners in planning the new roles; patients should also be informed adequately of the postholder's role and relevant training. Staff should have access to legal advice and support.

This report should now be read alongside *Department of Health and Royal College of Nursing 2005*, which also looked at how extended and advanced roles are understood and utilised (Table 4.1). Two questions in the joint survey asked whether respondents had ever had a referral or investigation request refused because of being a nurse (not a doctor). Almost one in four (23%) of those who referred patients (*n* = 428) had had their referrals refused because they were a nurse rather than a doctor. The report also states that a third (33%) of the 315 respondents who ordered investigations had been refused on the same grounds. The likelihood of having referrals refused depends on both job title and sector. The report give more details:

" Those in nurse practitioner (37%) and advanced nurse practitioner (45%) posts are more likely to have had their referral refused, compared with specialist nurses/CNS (17%) and nurse consultants (24%). Some but not

Table 4.1 Views re roles being understood (%)

	Strongly agree	Agree	Neither	Disagree	Strongly disagree	*n*
My professional judgement is respected by nursing colleagues	46	49	5	1	0	506
My professional judgement is respected by other healthcare staff	38	56	6	1	0	507
Patients generally regard me as a nurse	33	52	9	6	0	505
My role is understood by other nurses	13	45	19	21	2	504
Patients have difficulty understanding my role	3	15	23	50	9	506
Other staff make appropriate use of the services in my role	12	63	15	9	1	506

Source: *Department of Health and Royal College of Nursing 2005*

all of this variation would seem to relate to the different distribution of posts between the sectors, and the fact that community/primary care based nurses were twice as likely to have had referrals refused compared with their hospital based colleagues (33% v. 16%). But even within the same sector, those in specialist nurses are least likely to have had refusals (13% in acute and 16% in community/primary). Nurses' views about the way in which their roles are understood sheds some light on this area.

It would be helpful if all these organisations could reach an understanding on expanded role.

Uniform guidance should also be drawn up and a consensus statement issued by the Department of Health with all the professional organisations together, the Nursing and Midwifery Council (NMC) and the General Medical Council (GMC), in conjunction with bodies such as the British Medical Association (BMA) and the RCN, regarding such practice.

The current advice, as will be shown, shows marked differences of approach. It seems from *Department of Health and Royal College of Nursing 2005* that whether a nurse who is performing an expanded or advanced role can get a referral appears to be just a matter of luck, which clearly should not be the case.

The emphasis today is upon the nurses themselves making the decision as to whether to undertake an expanded role. If the nurse believes that s/he has the necessary competence, then s/he may undertake the task him/herself. The UKCC was opposed to the use of certificates of competence, a view no doubt shared by its successor, the NMC. Such certificates state that the nurse has undergone a training programme and therefore may be competent to perform a particular task.

" In order to bring into proper focus the professional responsibility and consequent accountability of individual practitioners, it is the Council's principles for practice rather than certificates for tasks which should form the basis for adjustments to the scope of practice.

United Kingdom Central Council, 1992, p. 8

It was suggested that the fact that a nurse has been given a certificate might give the nurse a false sense of security and lead her/him to think that accountability for actions had shifted to his/her assessor. But at the same time, before a nurse undertakes an expanded role, appropriate training is essential and such knowledge needs to be sustained and updated.

Employers would need to ensure that a safe system of work is in operation for both staff and patients. As Giliker & Beckwith (2004) state: 'Employers are required to take reasonable steps to organise and supervise the work of their employees, and to give proper instructions and guidance to employees and check that it is adhered to.'

There is also the common law duty on the employer to provide competent staff. In addition, the nurse maintains a professional duty to act competently through the tort of negligence (*Crawford, Bolam,* etc., discussed in Ch. 3) and the contract of employment. The requirements of Post-registration Education and Practice (PREP) also imposes an obligation to keep up to date. The NMC (Nursing and Midwifery Council 2004b) states:

" **The PREP (CPD) standard**

" The PREP requirements include a commitment to undertake continuing professional development (CPD). This element of PREP is referred to as PREP (CPD). The PREP (CPD) standard is to:

- undertake at least five days or 35 hours of learning activity relevant to your practice during the three years prior to your renewal of registration
- maintain a personal professional profile (PPP) of your learning activity
- comply with any request from the NMC to audit how you have met these requirements.

" You must comply with the PREP (CPD) standard in order to maintain your NMC registration.

A key tool to ensure a safe environment of care may be through the use of guidelines for tasks that have been delegated by doctors to nurses, or where a new role has been developed. The issue of guideline development will be discussed later. In August 2006, the PREP practice will change to 450 hours over three years (NMC 2006).

DELEGATION

It is interesting to note that while the discourse in nursing practice is that of the nurse her- or himself undertaking an expanded role, difficult issues remain as to the boundaries of practice and where ultimate responsibility lies. Nurses may take on an increased role because they are acting as independent practitioners. Alternatively it may be because they have been delegated certain tasks to be performed by doctors. Guidance has been issued by the General Medical Council on the issue of delegation stating that (General Medical Council 2001):

> *Delegation and referral*
>
> 46. Delegation involves asking a nurse, doctor, or medical student or other health care worker to provide treatment or care on your behalf. When you delegate care or treatment you must be sure that the person to whom you delegate is competent to carry out the procedure or provide the therapy involved. You must always pass on enough information about the patient and the treatment needed. You will still be responsible for the overall management of the patient.
>
> 47. Referral involves transferring some or all of the responsibility for the patient's care, usually temporarily and for a particular purpose, such as additional investigation, care or treatment, which falls outside your competence. Usually you will refer patients to another registered medical practitioner. If this is not the case, you must be satisfied that such health care workers are accountable to a statutory regulatory body, and that a registered medical practitioner, usually a general practitioner, retains overall responsibility for the management of the patient.

There is recognition that doctors can refer cases to nurses as opposed to delegating care; however, overall responsibility still lies usually with the doctor.

Where tasks are delegated, the doctor delegating the task should follow appropriate guidelines. Should the doctor fail to do so and harm results to the patient, the doctor may be held liable in negligence for the harm caused. It may also be the case that, even where the delegation is properly undertaken, the doctor is held ultimately responsible in any event under what is known as the 'captain of the ship' approach (Montgomery 1992). It is interesting to note that both the GMC and the BMA assume that, where delegation takes place, the doctor retains ultimate accountability (British Medical Association, 1996, 2006). In discussing the competence and curriculum framework for the new NHS post of Medical Care Practitioner the BMA (British Medical Association 2006) state:

" 12. ...We believe that non medically qualified practitioners should operate within the limitations of pre-determined protocols for specific circumstances under the supervision of a doctor who will be ultimately responsible for the overall patient care. We seek assurance and independent evidence to show that all medical care practitioners are competent to provide safe and effective patient care in all instances of patient contact within their remit.

It may, however, be questioned to what extent such an approach is appropriate as the role of the nurse develops and s/he is recognised as having greater personal autonomy, and indeed whether the courts would be more likely to hold that the nurse was solely liable where tasks have been legitimately delegated.

The boundaries between activities that are undertaken as part of expanded role and those that follow from delegation are unclear. Darley & Rumsey (1996) note that the use of language such as 'delegation' is indicative of hierarchy. They suggest that it would be better to talk in terms of 'shared care' or 'referral'; this would have the advantage of emphasising the partnership and teamwork aspects. To avoid confusion a coordinated approach on these matters is urgently needed from both the GMC and UKCC and from other bodies such as the BMA and RCN (see further Dowling et al 1996).

THE PROBLEM WITH CODES

A key issue inherent with any code, protocol or guidance is the extent to which you can incorporate satisfactorily quite difficult concepts such as competence and accountability without trivialising them or making them too simplistic. Codes can spell out the conventional wisdom of a group of people or organisation, for example the NMC, but the enforceability and absorption of that wisdom are more difficult questions. The *Scope* document sought to change professional cultures, which is a hard thing to do, and therefore such change will be necessarily incremental and slow. Government initiatives such as the 10-point challenge on nursing skills and the NHS National Plan (Department of Health 2000a, 2000b) have, however, speeded up the pace of change to our present position where expanded role and advance nursing practice are essential to keep the NHS operating. Initiatives such as NHS Direct and walk-in centres would not be able to operate or exist without general acceptance of the extended and advanced roles of nurses. The whole NHS would probably grind to a halt without them.

Case study

A case involving a negligent practice nurse illustrates some difficulties regarding accountability (Parker & Wilson 1992):

A 34-year-old man attended his GP to have his right ear syringed. On examination the GP suspected that the patient had an abscess and prescribed penicillin, asking him to return a week later to see the nurse and have his ear syringed. When the patient returned, his ear was syringed by a locum practice nurse. (The patient later admitted that during the procedure he had felt excruciating pain and dizziness.) Two days later the patient said that his ear had been incompletely syringed and the same nurse repeated the procedure. The patient then returned to the surgery complaining of a sore ear and the nurse referred him to the GP. On examination, the patient was found to have a perforated eardrum and antibiotics were prescribed. Fortunately, he made a good recovery but sued, alleging negligence.

The Medical Defence Union sought expert opinion from a GP and a nurse and was advised that the GP had fallen below the acceptable standard of care in delegating the procedure to the nurse without first having established her competence to carry out the procedure. The nurse, who had not performed ear syringing for some 20 years, was also deemed liable for not declining to perform the procedure. The MDU settled the claim.

CLINICAL NEGLIGENCE AND PROFESSIONAL MISCONDUCT

The crucial issue for the employer, then, is to ensure that, first of all, the nurse is lawfully undertaking the task. The GP in the case above should have at least asked the nurse whether she had performed an ear syringe before and, if so, how long ago. On the facts of the case, the GP could be viewed as wrongfully assigning the procedure to the practice nurse. This may mean that the GP was acting negligently. Creating and stating job competencies and assessment sorts this problem out. Last et al (1992) raise the point:

" How can chief nurses, directors of nursing services and nurse managers be sure that all practitioners are safe to enlarge the scope of their practice? How can managers allow those who are able to fly to do so, yet provide a safety net to those who could never fly, or even worse, those who think they can but cannot, from falling down?

Managers, doctors and nurses have to be trusted to operate the system satisfactorily and in a way that does not compromise patient safety. Overloading the nurse may also have implications for the management should the nurse be unable to perform his/her role because s/he has developed some form of stress-related illness. A nurse who falls ill and claims that this was caused by unduly high stress levels in the workplace may bring legal proceedings claiming compensation for the harm suffered.

The fact that a contract of employment may stipulate stressful working conditions does not by itself mean that a nurse who suffers physical or psychological harm consequent upon that stress cannot bring a claim for damages. This was made clear by the case of *Johnston* v. *Bloomsbury AHA* ([1991] 2 All ER 293). Here, a junior hospital doctor brought an action claiming that his employer had broken an implied duty to take reasonable care for his safety and had broken his contract of employment. He was required by his contract to work a basic week of 40 hours and to be available for up to 48 hours per week overtime. In the Court of Appeal a majority of the judges held that he had an arguable case. Stuart Smith L.J. held that the health authority was under a duty to provide a safe system of work. While the obligation to work up to 88 hours per week was contained in a junior doctor's contract, this had to be set against an employer's duty to take reasonable care for the employee's safety.

One difficulty in bringing such actions is that of showing that stress-induced psychiatric injury is foreseeable. Much depends on the circumstances of the individual case. In some instances employers can justifiably argue that they were not aware that their employee had been subject to what were excessive stress levels. Where an employer is, however, put on notice that an employee is susceptible to such a breakdown and then that employee returns to work and suffers a second nervous breakdown due to stressful working conditions, an action consequent upon the second breakdown may meet with more success (*Walker* v. *Northumbria County Council* [1995] 1 All ER 737). A nurse would also have to establish that it was the stressful working conditions themselves that amounted to a material cause of his/her breakdown. This may itself be problematic; in many situations stress levels are influenced by factors external to the employment relationship itself, such as home and family life. It is also the case that the assessment of stress levels is a matter that would fall under the employee obligations under the Health and Safety at Work Act 1974.

LEGAL STANDARD OF CARE TO BE EXERCISED BY A NURSE PERFORMING AN EXPANDED ROLE

Where a nurse performs traditional nursing duties the standard of practice required is that of the ordinary skilled nurse in his/her speciality in the circumstances of the case – the *Bolam* principle. But what is the standard of care s/he must reach if performing an expanded role? Guidance can be taken from the case *Wilsher* v. *Essex Area Health Authority* ([1986] 3 All ER 801).

Wilsher case

The plaintiff, Martin Wilsher, was an infant child born about 3 months early. He was very ill. He was placed in a special care baby unit where a junior and inexperienced doctor monitoring the oxygen in the plaintiff's bloodstream made a mistake and mistakenly inserted a catheter into a vein rather than an artery. He asked a senior doctor to check what he had done. The registrar failed to notice the mistake and, when replacing the catheter himself some hours later, made the same mistake himself. The catheter monitor failed to register correctly the amount of oxygen in the baby's bloodstream. He was given excess oxygen. It was alleged that the excess oxygen in his bloodstream had caused an incurable condition of the retina, retrolental fibroplasia. Martin is now completely blind. A key issue discussed by the Court of Appeal was the standard of legal care to be exercised by the junior doctor in the case. Mustill L.J. stated:

" In a case such as the present, the standard is not just that of the averagely competent and well-informed junior houseman (or whatever the position of the doctor) but of such a person who fills a post in a unit offering a highly specialised service. (p. 813)

Glidewell L.J. stated:

" In my view, the law requires the trainee or learner to be judged by the same standard as his more experienced colleagues. If it did not, inexperience would frequently be urged as a defence to an action for professional negligence. (p. 831)

On the facts before the court the junior doctor was not found negligent. He had done the reasonable thing and asked his superior, but the registrar was found to be negligent. The case went on appeal to the House of Lords on the issue of causation and eventually was set down for retrial. The case was settled for £116 724.40 (Kerry 1991). The key point to be taken from the Wilsher case is that a nurse is liable to be judged by the professional standard of the post that s/he is performing at that time. This means that if the nurse is performing an expanded role, s/he is expected to operate at the level of skill and competence outlined in the expanded role. A further point is that, as Kloss (1988) argues:

" If a nurse undertakes a task for which she knows she has insufficient training, this in itself may constitute negligence, even if she is acting on the orders of a doctor…. If a nurse takes on the doctor's role she will be judged by the standard of the reasonable doctor.

There is much older legal authority (*Philips* v. *William Whitley Ltd* [1938] All ER 566) that could be used to argue against the *Wilsher* elevated legal standard of care proposition. It appears that the *Wilsher* approach is more likely to be followed. The case of *Djemal* v. *Bexley Health Authority* ([1995] 6 Med LR 269) supports the *Wilsher* approach.

The issue of the appropriate standard of legal care for nurses performing medical tasks to exercise has been brought into sharp focus by a number of recent initiatives where new health-care professional posts have been created that involve the performance of some medical activities, for example transplant clinician's assistants and cardiac surgeon's assistants. These posts can be occupied by nurses or other health-care professionals. If a negligence case involving one of these members of staff occurred, the court would have difficulty in assessing the appropriate standard of care for the professional to exercise. The posts are so new and there may only be one or two in existence. The court could look at the nature of the tasks performed and determine who normally performs those tasks. If doctors normally undertake them then a medical standard of care and skill will be expected (Caine 1993, Naish 1995, Peysner 1995). Dowling et al (1996) highlight some useful criteria that a court considering an expanded role case might take into account in determining the standard of care. These include the nature of the task and the way the nurse 'holds him/herself out' to patients. With regard to the second of these criteria, relevant factors would include dress, name badge, language, socialisation and the way the nurse is perceived by patients.

Conclusions

If the nurse undertakes a role previously undertaken by a medical practitioner then his/her competence to perform that role is that of the level of the medical practitioner. The courts may be looking for the nurse to exercise and maintain medical knowledge, and if the nurse cannot demonstrate this s/he could be found negligent and in breach of the NMC Code (Nursing and Midwifery Council 2004a). Inexperience is not a defence to a nursing negligence action. It is very important that nursing staff closely adhere to Clause 6 of the NMC Code, which concerns maintaining professional knowledge and competence.

ADVANCED PRACTICE SITUATIONS

Clinical guidelines, protocols and the law

The setting of guidelines or protocols is fast becoming an increasingly important aspect of nursing and health care as strategies to ensure quality and avoid risk take effect. The development of clinical guidelines is a government priority and an important aspect of its commitment to enhance the quality of patient care, and this is identified in the NHS National Plan (Department of Health 1999c, 2000b). A special health authority, the National Institute for Clinical Excellence (NICE) has been set up to promote best health-care practice. NICE has had its remit developed and is now known at the National Institute for Health and Clinical Excellence. It was set up on 1 April 1999 to provide the NHS, patients and the public with authoritative, robust and reliable guidance on current 'best practice' (National Institute for Clinical Excellence 1999).

NICE is now a key player in clinical guideline creation in the NHS in England and Wales (National Institute for Clinical Excellence 2004). The development of the Institute's clinical guidelines involves:

" • The Institute
• National Collaborating Centres (NCCs)

- Guideline Development Groups
- The Patient Involvement Unit
- Guideline Review Panels
- Stakeholders
- The Citizens Council.

The roles of these groups and individuals are described in the National Institute for Clinical Excellence 2004. A list of the information is available on the Institute's website.

The establishment of NICE and its clinical guidelines focus have created a momentum for guideline development. Clinical guidelines can now be clearly seen to be operating at a national, macro level and a local, micro level.

At the macro level NICE and other health-care organisations such as professional nursing, medical groups, university professional associations and the royal medical colleges create clinical guidelines. At the micro level, wards and care teams in hospitals, primary care groups and Trusts, GPs and individual care practitioners can also be seen to produce guidelines.

A nurse may be working with national and locally produced clinical guidelines. It is important to remember that clinical guidelines at the national and local level are advisory only: they should never be used automatically and without proper regard to the care of the patient.

NICE (National Institute for Clinical Excellence 2004) lists key features of good clinical guidelines:

" • The purpose and scope of the guideline are clear
- Stakeholders are involved in the process
- The development of guideline recommendations follows a rigorous process
- The guideline is clear and well presented
- The recommendations can be applied in practice
- Conflicts of interest have been recorded by the guideline developers.

Key principles underlying the Institute's clinical guidelines are stated (National Institute for Clinical Excellence 2004) as follows.

NICE clinical guidelines:

- aim to improve the quality of clinical care
- assess the clinical and cost effectiveness of treatments or management approaches
- are advisory, but are expected to be taken into account by clinicians when planning care for individual patients
- are developed through a process that takes account of the views of those who might be affected by the guideline (usually including health-care professionals, patients and their carers, service managers, NHS trusts, the wider public, government and the health-care industries)
- are based on the best possible research evidence and expert consensus
- are developed using methods that are sound and transparent and that command the respect of the NHS and NHS stakeholders, including patients
- set out the clinical care that might reasonably be suitable for the majority of patients using the NHS in England and Wales.

These principles underpin NICE clinical guideline development and appraisal. It is logical to suggest that they should also underpin local clinical guidelines development.

It is stated in the key principles that clinical guidelines are advisory. This is a common-sense principle and reflects the legal position of guidelines. Clinical guidelines do not suspend clinical autonomy. Nurses remain reflective and autonomous practitioners and a patient's condition may clearly contra-indicate the application of a clinical guideline. The patient's condition should always be assessed before applying a clinical guideline. However, if a clinical guideline is not followed, a proper reason should be advanced as an explanation. This principle will be explained further later in the chapter.

Clinical guidelines are care management tools that broadly set out the procedure to be followed by the nurse in an advanced practice situation, for example the MIU or the Well Woman Clinic. A GP may develop, with the practice nurse, a guideline or a protocol for the giving of inoculations.

The practice of setting guidelines or protocols raises important professional and legal issues, some of which have already been noted. It should be said at the outset, however, that the use of terminology by authors in the literature is not consistent or clear. As well as clinical guidelines or protocols, a variety of other terms such as practice parameters, clinical pathways and algorithms are used, often to describe the same tool.

Guidelines or protocols can be seen to be guidance statements based on sound practice. For ease of reference, the term 'clinical guidelines' will be used. Protocols are generally regarded as being more directive than guidelines. The law relating to guidelines applies equally to protocols.

The Department of Health (1996a) defines clinical guidelines as 'systemati-cally developed statements, which assist the individual clinician and patient in making decisions about appropriate health care for specific conditions'. NICE has a similar definition (National Institute for Clinical Excellence 2004).

Legal issues

Fundamentally, the existence of clinical guidelines may impact upon the operation of the *Bolam* test (Ch. 2). If a guideline is in existence and a nurse has failed to follow it, then this may be a factor that a court takes into consideration when discussing the legal duty of care and whether this has been breached. Nonetheless, the fact that a guideline exists does not mean that the court will accept the guideline. As noted in the previous chapter, the court may overrule the decision of a responsible body of professional practice.

Reasonable clinical guidelines

The *Bolam* principle will apply to the creation and use of clinical guidelines. The case of *Early* v. *Newham Health Authority* ([1994] 5 Med LR 214) illustrates the application of the case to clinical guidelines.

The plaintiff, aged 13 years, was having an appendectomy. The anaesthetist gave an intravenous injection of thiopentone (100 g fentanyl and 100 mg suxamethonium). Unfortunately, he was unable to successfully intubate the plaintiff. The effect of the thiopentone wore off before the effect of the short-term paralysing drug suxamethonium wore off and the plaintiff came to. She came to in a state of panic and distress as she was still partly paralysed by the drug. She alleged that the anaesthetist was negligent in failing to intubate her the first time and that the health authority's failed intubation guidelines were faulty. No negligence was found.

The judge considered the guidelines and found them reasonable. He was not satisfied that the guidelines were such that no reasonably competent authority would have adopted them. Before the hospital had adopted the guidelines they were put before the Division of Anaesthesia and the con-sultants discussed them. They decided that this was the proper procedure to adopt and minutes of the discussion were kept. The key point was that the judge found that a responsible body of medical opinion in the *Bolam* sense would have adopted the failed intubation guidelines that were used. The standard of legal care was therefore satisfied in the case.

In order to satisfy the legal standard of care under *Bolam*, nurses, in drafting and using clinical guidelines, have to act as ordinary skilled nurses in their speciality would have acted. There must be a responsible body of opinion, albeit minority opinion, that regards their practice as proper. The *Bolitho* case, *Bolitho* v. *City and Hackney Health Authority* ([1998] Lloyd's Rep. Med. 26), can be said to add a gloss to *Bolam* in that it is clear from the speech of Lord Browne-Wilkinson (at p. 33) that this opinion should be evidence-based, it must have a logical basis and a risk benefit analysis should have been done.

Foster (1998) advances an interesting view about the effect of *Bolitho*:

" Although *Bolitho* did not change the law, many people think it has, and so it is likely to alter in a few respects the way that litigation is conducted. Experts will have to appear not only respectable but also reasonable. The defendant will be judged not only by the cut of his expert's suit. Experts will have to be prepared to say not only that they do something a particular way, but why? Reports will have to be more carefully reasoned and referenced.... If the published evidence makes a wholly one-sided case against a particular medical practice, it will be difficult for any expert to say that its adoption by the defendant was reasonable, even though he or she is in august medical company in doing so.

Furthermore, the decision of the Court of Appeal in *Penney and Others* v. *East Kent Health Authority* (*The Times*, 25 November 1999 (CA); Tingle & Rodgers 1999) is notable. This case hints at the possible future for clinical negligence, with more reliance on clinical guidelines than on the clinicians themselves. A judge may disagree with the experts and prefer other expert evidence (see discussion in Ch. 2).

Inappropriate use of clinical guidelines

Situations change and a clinical guideline drafted some months previously may not now fit into the appropriate clinical care setting. Resource levels may have deteriorated or there may have been staffing changes affecting the ward skill mix. The conventional wisdom on a ward may be that a particular clinical guideline is no longer appropriate. If there are reasonable concerns about the effectiveness and safety of a clinical guideline then good practice dictates that it should be withdrawn and re-evaluated. It may be negligent not to do so as, as noted in Chapter 2, health-care professionals are required to keep up to date as to the scope of their professional practice.

Not a substitute for professional judgment

When considering the NICE clinical guidelines programme it was stated earlier, and it is worth emphasising again, that when using clinical guidelines nurses must always practice as reflective practitioners and responsibly exercise their clinical discretion. They must use their own professional judgment and skill and judge the appropriateness of the clinical guidelines for the particular care situation. If they decide to deviate from a clinical guideline then they should record on the notes their reasons for so doing. If they are unsure about the use of a clinical guideline, advice should be sought from more experienced colleagues.

Clinical guidelines should be reviewed systematically

If a particular clinical guideline became an issue in a nursing negligence case, a key issue would be the review system in operation in the hospital or surgery. The court would want to be satisfied that a clinical guideline was being used appropriately and updated where necessary. Concepts of risk management and quality assurance would also demand a systematic review system.

Clinical guidelines are legally disclosable

Clinical guidelines that were used in the care of a patient would be relevant documents for the purposes of a nursing negligence action. The clinical guideline would be subject to a fairly detailed examination in court. Having a clinical guideline based on reasonable criteria, good research and good practice would provide an indication that a reasonable and reflective care system was in operation. The key point would be to show that the clinical guideline was appropriate to the circumstances of the particular case and was followed by the staff involved. The fact that it was followed or not followed should always be recorded. A clinical guideline shows at the very least that there is a controlled environment of care.

Evidence-based clinical guidelines

The government pledge to improve the quality of health care in the NHS has seen a strong, centrally led policy adherence to the concept of evidence-based care. This concept underpins the work of NICE and can be seen as an underlying judicial philosophy in cases such as *Bolitho*.

While this is controversial, it is certainly the case that, if a particular approach was deemed to be appropriate after evidence-based evaluation had taken place, then this may be held to be accepted professional practice. Again, however, that does not mean that there would be automatic judicial acceptance.

A court examining a clinical guideline would be looking at the information that underpins the clinical guideline, quality of research and clinical practice. This was done in the Penney case. Unrealistic clinical guidelines that tried to do too much and those based on poor research, practice, etc. would be criticised by the NHS Executive (Department of Health, 1996b) and by NICE.

Conclusions

Clinical guidelines do raise a number of important legal issues. They are being used in legal proceedings and will be seen increasingly as an established quality improvement and clinical risk management tool in the health-care environment. Clinical guidelines must be used reflectively. They are not substitutes for professional judgment. Effectively used, they have the potential to reduce the level of complaints and litigation in health care by improving communication processes and the quality of care.

NURSE PRESCRIBING

Jean McHale

One notable example of the developing role of the nurse is through the role in prescribing drugs/medical appliances (Jones 1999). In 1986 the Cumberlege report stated that community nurses should have prescribing rights (Department of Health and Social Security 1986). This was followed by a Crown Report in 1989 that stated that health visitors and nurses should have the power to prescribe medication from a 'nurse's formulary' to benefit patients (Department of Health 1989). Legislation was introduced in 1992 in the form of the Medicinal Products (Prescription by Nurses) Act of that year.

A Midwives Supply Order allows midwives to possess and use certain controlled drugs. Powers also have been given to enable occupational health nurses to administer prescription-only drugs. This may be undertaken as long as they do so only in writing and under a doctor's supervision (Medicines (Products Other Than Veterinary Drugs) (Prescription Only) Order 1983 SI 1983 No. 1212 as amended; NHS Pharmaceutical Services (Amendment) Regulations SI 1996 No. 698 r8).

Nurses have also been administering medication in accordance with protocols produced by doctors, who themselves would actually prescribe the drug. Controversy arose in 1996 over this practice. Advice was given by union lawyers to the effect that this was illegal (Naish & Garbett 1996). In contrast, the Medical Defence Union (MDU) stated that nurses could administer such medication as long as they were working to a protocol. This, it is argued, was in accordance with section 58(2) (b) of the Medicines Act 1968, which provides that: 'No person shall administer (otherwise than to himself) any such medicinal product unless he is an appropriate practitioner or a person acting in accordance with the directions of an appropriate practitioner'.

The appropriate practitioner would be the doctor in this instance. The arguments advanced by the MDU are in accordance with the guidance which was issued by the UKCC to the effect that: 'Nurses can administer medicines according to the directions of a doctor and a detailed protocol would satisfy this requirement. However, nurses cannot supply medicines for the patient to take away unless there is a signed prescription.'

Nonetheless, there was a question mark regarding the status of administration under protocol (Mayor 1997). It appeared that the direction under the statute applies to a specified individual and it has been argued that this would not cover administration to groups of patients.

THE CROWN REVIEW

The whole issue of nurse prescribing was the subject of a review by the Department of Health chaired by Dr June Crown (Department of Health 1998, 1999a). Its purpose was to:

" develop a consistent framework to determine in what circumstances health professionals could undertake new roles with regard to the prescribing, administration or supply of medicines in the course of clinical practice; and to consider possible implications for legislation, and for professional training and standards.

The Review produced two reports. The first examined the supply and administration of medicines under protocol and the second the wider prescribing issues. On the legal issues regarding administration under protocol, Crown commented that:

" Advice to the Department of Health is that group protocols may not meet the requirements in sections 55(1) (b) and s58 (2) (b) Medicines Act 1968 for the supply and administration of medicines 'in accordance with the directions of a doctor' and that in order to meet the requirements of current legislation, protocols should leave the minimum of discretion to the health profession involved. Protocols which specify the patient by name (patient specific protocols) are more likely to be within the law than those which apply to groups of patients.

It recommended that the use of protocols should continue but that this should be subject to certain guidelines. The content should deal with the clinical condition to which the protocol applies and which patients can/cannot be included. Staff who are authorised to supply and administer medicines should be detailed, including qualifications and measures of competence. The treatment that was to be given under protocol should be included, along with details of drugs involved such as dose and methods of administration. The names of the professionals/professional advisory group involved in drawing up the protocol should be given.

The Report recommended that protocols should be drawn up on a local basis by an interdisciplinary committee – doctor/pharmacist/named representative of each professional likely to contribute care under protocol. The protocol would require approval of those professional managers using it, with all participants in care under protocol signing a copy. Group protocols are not only to be used in the context of nurses but should also cover persons who are not professionally trained but who have been suitably trained and approved as competent in relation to the protocol. The Report emphasised the need for safety and that in all situations group protocols should ensure that patient safety is not compromised or put at risk. Those using a protocol should be professionally trained, although in some situations those not so trained could be included if they were acting under the directions of those who were professionally trained.

PATIENT GROUP DIRECTIONS

This recommendation was taken forward subsequently. First steps were taken to formalise the operation of group protocols. Group protocols are now referred to as 'patient group directions' (PGDs) (Health Service Circular 2000/026. Prescription Only Medicines (Human Use) Amendment Order 2000; Medicines (Pharmacy and Sale) Exemptions Order 2000; Medicine (Sale and Supply; Miscellaneous Provisions (Amendment) Regulations 2000). It should be emphasised that PGDs are not prescribing powers: instead, the nurse is acting under circumscribed discretion regarding the supply and administration of drugs.

PGDs are defined as 'written instructions for the supply and administration of medicines to groups of patients who may not be individually identified for presentation for treatment'. They are not 'patient-specific directions'. Patient-specific directions are traditional written instructions from doctors, dentists and nurse prescribers for medicines to be supplied and administered to a named patient. This covers most medicines.

Guidance states that PGDs must be drawn up by a 'multidisciplinary group' a doctor, dentist, pharmacist, representative of any professional group that is expected to supply medicines under a PGD (HSC 2000/026). The guidance also suggests that it is good practice to involve the local Drug and Therapeutic Committee, Area Prescribing Committee and similar advisory bodies.

Who can supply/administer under patient group directions?

In contrast to independent and supplementary prescribing, no specific training is required for those supplying/administering medicines under PGDs. They may be used by a range of health-care professionals acting as named individuals.

- Nurses
- Midwives
- Health visitors
- Optometrists
- Pharmacists
- Dietitians
- Chiropodists
- Radiographers

This applies in the NHS and also in some non-NHS situations such as independent hospitals, clinics registered under the Care Standards Act, prison health care and the police.

What must a patient group direction contain?

There are a number of legal requirements for PGDs. They must contain the following information:

- Name of the organisation to which it applies
- When it comes into force and when it expires
- Description of the medicine to which it applies
- Which health professionals can supply/administer the medicine
- Signature of a doctor/dentist and also of a pharmacist
- Must be signed by an appropriate health organisation
- Must state the clinical condition to which it applies
- Description of those patients excluded from treatment under the direction
- Situations in which further advice should be sought from doctor/dentist and arrangements for referral
- Details of appropriate dosage/quantity/pharmaceutical form and strength/frequency of administration
- Maximum and minimum period over which it should be administered
- Relevant warnings, including potential adverse reactions
- Details of any necessary follow-up action and circumstances
- Statement of records to be kept for audit purposes

What drugs are included under the scope of patient group directions?

- Most licensed medicines
- Black triangle drugs – which are recently licensed and subject to special reporting arrangements – where this is an exceptional use that is justified by reference to best clinical practice and a direction that clearly describes the status of the product
- Black triangle vaccines (if in accordance with the schedule recommended by the Joint Committee on Vaccination)
- Schedule 4 and 5 controlled drugs, with the exception of anabolic steroids

The guidance does suggest caution in relation to the prescription of antibiotics because of public health concerns and the fact that overuse may give rise to an increase in drug-resistant conditions.

There are some potential problems with such PGDs. For example, the localised nature of group protocols works against the policy concerning centralisation and quality through the establishment of bodies such as NICE and the Healthcare Commission, although admittedly some decisions such as those made by research ethics committees are predominantly made on a local basis. Nurses need also to be aware that undertaking an enhanced role involves increased responsibilities, with the prospect of liability in negligence if a patient who is being treated under protocol suffers harm.

INDEPENDENT AND SUPPLEMENTARY PRESCRIBING

The second Crown report was much broader in scope and had the effect of removing the dominance of the medical profession sanctioning prescribing on a far broader basis. The report recommended that legal authority in the UK to prescribe should be extended. This should include those specific therapeutic areas that were related to the particular competence and expertise of the prescribing group. There would be independent prescribers who were to be those responsible for the assessment of patients with undiagnosed conditions and for decisions about the clinical management required, including prescribing. Examples of such independent prescribers included

- family planning nurses
- tissue viability nurses (who assess viability of patients' skin – particularly in their own homes)
- chiropodists and podiatrists (who undertake some forms of foot surgery)
- specialist physiotherapists.

There was also to be a category called 'dependent prescribers'. These would include groups such as:

- specialist diabetes nurses, who already give advice to patients, training them in the use of insulin, and who, as dependent prescribers, could take over from doctors once the initial diagnosis of diabetes was established
- specialist asthma nurses, who could vary diagnosis and prescribe further medication as was required
- specialist palliative care nurses, who could review and revise medication as necessary.

Certain groups of medicines would not be available for certain new groups of prescribers (para 6.53), for instance controlled drugs (subject to the Misuse of Drugs Act 1971) or drugs over which there was continuing professional concern, for instance drugs used to treat children and young people with mental health problems.

The dependent prescriber would be someone who was involved in continuing care of patients who had been clinically assessed by an independent prescriber. This could include prescribing, which will usually be informed by clinical guidelines and usually within designated treatment plans. They would have discretion to vary some aspects of repeat prescription, for example dose/frequency/presentation/active ingredient group. There was provision for regular clinical review by assessing clinician. The dependent prescriber would be different from the nurse administering drugs under group protocol because:

- the dependent prescriber would be working under a care plan drawn up for an individual patient following full assessment by the clinician
- supply and administration, in contrast, was used in the case of patients who were not individually identified for presentation for treatment
- dependent prescribers would have greater discretion over choice of treatment regime.

The Report suggested that:

" Administration or supply within a group protocol may be a suitable model where patient's clinical needs are broadly similar and individual prescriptions would be unwieldy or impracticable (as in mass vaccination campaigns), or where there is a need for urgent treatment (as in relief of acute asthma attacks by ambulance paramedics). Dependent or independent prescribing will be preferable where more detailed clinical assessment is needed and the range of treatment options required to meet the clinical needs of the patients is wider (as in family planning clinics).

The new scheme would be administered by a new prescribing authority, which would have the task of assessing existing prescribing rights for different groups of nurses and ensuring that the training was of a sufficiently high standard. The body would be drawn from current prescribers, other relevant health-care professions, professional regulatory bodies, education and training accrediting bodies, NHS commissioners and provider units, and patient groups.

TAKING PRESCRIBING FORWARD

In 2001 the government took forward the proposals in the second Crown Report. Section 63 of the Health and Social Care Act 2001 provided that new groups of health-care professionals could be designated to prescribe medicines for human use. There are today three categories of prescribers. First, those district nurses, midwives and health visitors who are able to pre-scribe under the provisions set out above. Second, 'independent prescribers', and third, 'supplementary prescribers' – the term now used to describe 'dependent' prescribers.

Who can prescribe?

District nurses and health visitors

As before, district nurses and health visitors can prescribe under the provisions set out in the Medicinal Products Prescription by Nurses Act 1992 discussed above. They can prescribe from the Nurse Prescribers Formulary, which is set out in Part XVII B(i) of the Drug Tariff. This training is today incorporated into university-based specialist programmes for new district nurses and health visitors.

In addition, from 1 May 2006 a new category of independent prescribers can prescribe any licensed medicine within their competence, including some prescribed drugs (this is a change to the previous position, where nurses prescribed from the extended prescribers formulary). The law requires that these must be first-level registered nurses or registered midwives and that the name must be held on the nurses and midwives professional register with annotations saying that they have successfully completed the training. In addition, nurses must also comply with their own professional practice guidelines.

Additional requirements have also been imposed by the Department of Health. The nurse will need the ability to study at level 3 and at least 3 years post-registration clinical experience or part-time equivalent. A medical prac-titioner must be willing to contribute to/supervise the nurse's 12-day 'learning in practice' element. The nurse's employer must also confirm that the post is one in which they will have the need/opportunity to prescribe from the extended formulary. Where the nurse is in primary care, the employer must confirm that they have access to a prescribing budget on completion of the course.

The Department of Health guidance states that the principles used to prioritise applications are

- patient safety
- better use of nurses' skills.

Sensitive to the concerns that this expansion of role could be seen as being 'forced' on nurses the Department of Health guidance states that 'No nurse should be required to undertake training unless he/she wishes to do so'.

Who can prescribe for whom?

- Practice nurses – can only prescribe for patients registered for their practice
- Nurses in a primary care trust – can only issue prescriptions for patients of the GP practices within the primary care trust
- The nurse can prescribe for visiting relatives of patients if they are temporarily resident with the GP practice
- Travelling families – nurses may prescribe for travelling families if the necessary application forms have been completed

Nurses should also only write a prescription for a patient for whom they have personal responsibility. In addition, they should only write a prescription on a pad bearing their unique number.

Who are the nurse independent prescribers?

There are a number of legal requirements for such practitioners (Medicines and Human Use (Prescribing) (Miscellaneous Amendments) Order May 2006):

- Must be first-level registered nurse/registered midwife/registered specialist community public health nurse
- Name must be held on the nurses and midwives professional register along with an annotation that they have successfully completed the training

In addition the Department of Health guidance provides that the nurse must have:

- Ability to study at level 3 (degree level)
- Normally at least 3 years post-registration clinical nursing experience; 1 year of this should be in the clinical area in which they intend to prescribe
- Assessed as competent to take a history/undertake a clinical assessment/make a diagnosis
- Medical practitioner must be willing/able to contribute and supervise the 12-day learning in practice part of training

- Employer must identify this as being a post where they will have 'need and opportunity' to act as an independent prescriber
- There must be a local need for the prescriber
- Access to budget to meet the cost of prescriptions
- Access to continuing professional development
- Will work within a robust clinical governance framework

(Department of Health 2006; para 19)

The NMC validates prescribing training and a nurse will only be registered as an independent prescriber if s/he completes such an approved course (Department of Health 2006, para 32). While training will be undertaken at the outset, nurses are expected to maintain their professional practice skills (Department of Health 2006, para 45).

What can they prescribe?

'Any licensed medicine, which includes certain controlled drugs, for any medical condition which is within their clinical competence'

Nurses are required to act within Clause 6 of their professional code and prescribe only where this is within their level of skill and competence (Department of Health 2006, para 14). Medicines that are outside their UK licensed indications may be prescribed but only where it is accepted clinical practice, and nurses cannot prescribe unlicensed medicines (Department of Health 2006, para 54).

Conflicts of interest

It is important to ensure that, when prescribing, the nurse is not subject to conflicts of interest in relation to pharmaceutical companies (Department of Health 2006, para 26). Section 7.2 of the NMC Code of Professional Conduct provides that the nurse must:

" ensure that your registration status is not used in the promotion of commercial products or services, declare any financial or other interests in relevant organisations providing such goods or services and ensure that your professional judgment is not influenced by any commercial considerations.

SUPPLEMENTARY PRESCRIBING

Following Crown, the government also indicated that it intended to take forward the 'dependent prescriber' recommendations, which were renamed 'supplementary prescribing'. This has been defined as being 'a voluntary partnership between an independent prescriber and a supplementary prescriber to implement a patient-specific clinical management plan with the patient's agreement'. This was introduced consequent upon s63 of the Health and Social Care Act 2001 and amended Prescription Only Medicines Order in force 4 April 2003. The control of the supplementary prescriber process is ultimately with the independent prescriber. The independent prescriber needs to ascertain whether the patient will benefit from supplementary prescribing.

Who are the supplementary prescribers?

Initially this was rolled out from April 2003 to:

- first-level registered nurses
- registered midwives
- registered pharmacists.

It was then subsequently, from April 2005, extended to cover:

- chiropodists
- physiotherapists
- radiographers (Medicines for Human Use (Prescribing Order) 2005, SI 2005, No. 765).

Nurses who are at level 3 degree level are to have 26 taught days followed by 12 learning in practice days.

The essence of the supplementary prescriber is that of the 'partnership' but it is a partnership in which the independent prescriber is the dominant figure. The initial assessment has to be undertaken by the independent prescriber. The independent prescriber determines:

- which patients may benefit
- which nurses may be prescribers.

It is the independent prescriber who will also undertake the initial diagnosis.

What types of medicines are included?

" • General sales list
- Pharmacy
- Various prescription-only medicines (including antimicrobials/black triangle drugs/some controlled drugs/products outside UK licensed indications, i.e. off-label/unlicensed drugs – with the agreement of both independent and supplementary prescriber.

Clinical management plan

Crucial to supplementary prescribing is the 'clinical management plan'. The regulations provide that the clinical management plan must be in place before prescribing can go ahead. It can be written or in electronic form. It must relate to a named patient and to that patient's specific condition. The regulations provide that it must contain:

- The name of the patient
- The illness/condition to be treated
- The date when the clinical management plan is due to come into effect
- Reference to the type of medicine which must be administered
- Any restriction/limit of strength/dosage
- Any known sensitivities of the patient and any difficulties which they may have with particular medicines and appliances
- Any suspected/known adverse reactions/ circumstances which may lead to death or to deterioration in the patient's health

The nature of the prescribing partnership must be explained to the patient and the patient must agree to it. In addition, the agreement of the patient must be included in the clinical management plan and the patient's prescribing record, and without this agreement supplementary prescribing cannot go ahead (Department of Health 2002, para 28). While the patient does not have to sign, nonetheless his/her agreement should be recorded.

Where the independent prescriber changes, the supplementary prescriber cannot continue without negotiating a new prescribing partnership. Ongoing control is in the hands of the independent prescriber (Department of Health 2002, para 19).

Regular clinical review

The Department of Health guidance states that ideally there should be a regular clinical review within 12 months of the start of the clinical management plan (Department of Health 2002, para 17). There is provision, however, for the review to be undertaken at an interval longer than 12 months 'occasionally' and where 'the patient's condition has been shown to be stable and deterioration of the condition is not expected during a period longer than 12 months'. The supplementary prescriber must at all times work within his/her clinical competence. The Department of Health guidance states that the supplementary prescriber must '[pass] prescribing responsibility back to the independent prescriber, if the agreed clinical reviews are not carried out within the specified interval ... or if they feel that the patient's condition no longer falls within their competence ...' (Department of Health 2002, para 20).

Record keeping

Nurses are required to keep contemporaneous records that are 'unambiguous and legible' (Department of Health 2006, para 73) and moreover these should be completed immediately or 'as soon as possible after a consultation' (Department of Health 2006, para 74). The Department of Health guidance goes on to state that 'Only in very exceptional circumstances (e.g. the intervention of a weekend or a public holiday) should this period exceed 48 hours from the writing of the prescription'.

Adverse reaction reporting

If there is an adverse reaction this must be reported immediately through national reporting procedures. Suspected adverse drug reactions should be reported through the 'Yellow card scheme' (Department of Health 2006, para 78). In addition, harm or a 'near miss' due to an adverse incident involving drugs should be reported to the National Patient Safety Agency (Department of Health 2006, para 80).

LIABILITY AND EXPANDED ROLE PRESCRIBING

When prescribing drugs the nurse will be judged by the standard of the experienced nurse undertaking such a role. There is the prospect that s/he will be held personally accountable in the courts should harm result to a patient. The Department of Health guidance provides that:

" Prescribers are accountable for all aspects of their prescribing decisions. They should therefore only prescribe those medicines they know are safe and effective for the patient and the condition being treated. They must be able to recognise and deal with pressures (e.g. from the pharmaceutical industry, patients or colleagues) that might result in inappropriate prescribing.

Department of Health 2006, para 85

If nurses are involved in prescribing drugs, they must check the dose given; negligent prescription of an overdose may lead to an action in negligence (*Dwyer* v. *Roderick* (1983) 127 SJ 806), as may writing an illegible prescription (*Prendergast* v. *Sam and Dee* [1989] 1 Med LR 36). Given that expanded accountability may give rise to expanded liability, it is particularly important that nurses have requisite protection in the form of indemnity insurance, as is recognised in Clause 9 of the NMC Code (Nursing and Midwifery Council 2004a). The Department of Health comment in their 2006 guidance that 'All prescribers should ensure that they have sufficient professional indemnity insurance, for instance by means of membership of a professional organisation or trade union which provides this cover' (Department of Health 2006, para 86).

Enhanced prescribing powers are illustrative of the increasing autonomy given to nurses exercising an expanded role. However it does also provide another illustration of an area where, through expansion of responsibility, there is a risk of expansion of liability.

REFERENCES

British Medical Association 1996 Protecting patient safety. Joint Consultants Committee. BMA, London.

British Medical Association 2006 Competence and curriculum framework for the medical care practitioner. BMA, London

Caine N 1993 Heart to heart. Health Service Journal 103: 22

Carlisle D 1995 Nurse-led unity. Nursing Times 91(47): 14

Darley M, Rumsey M 1996 The scope of professional practice: work to date. Nursing Times 11(4): 32

Department of Health 1989 Report of the Advisory Group on Nurse Prescribing. HMSO, London

Department of Health 1992 The extended role of the nurse. Scope of professional practice. PL/CNO (92)4. Department of Health, London.

Department of Health 1996a Promoting clinical effectiveness: a framework for action in and through the NHS. Department of Health, London

Department of Health 1996b Delivering the future. Department of Health, London

Department of Health 1998 Report on the supply and administration of medicines under group protocols (Crown Part I). HMSO, London

Department of Health 1999a Review of prescribing, supply and administration of medicines: final report (Crown Part II). HMSO, London

Department of Health 1999b Making a difference. PL/CNO (99) (6). HMSO, London

Department of Health 1999c Faster access to modern treatment: how NICE appraisal will work: a discussion paper. Department of Health, London

Department of Health 2000a Health Secretary lays out plans to liberate nurse talents. Press release, 2000/0209. Department of Health, London

Department of Health 2000b The NHS plan. Cmnd 4818-1. Stationery Office, London

Department of Health 2002 Developing key roles for nurses and midwives-a guide for managers. Department of Health, London

Department of Health 2003 Practitioners with special interests in primary care. Implementing a scheme for nurses with special interests in primary care: liberating the talents. Department of Health, London

Department of Health 2006 Improving patients' access to medicines : a guide to implementing nurse and pharmacist independent prescribing within the NHS in England. Department of Health, London

Department of Health and Royal College of Nursing 2003 Freedom to practise: dispelling the myths. Department of Health/Royal College of Nursing, London

Department of Health and Royal College of Nursing 2005 Maxi nurses: advanced and specialist nursing roles. Department of Health/Royal College of Nursing, London. Available online at: www.rcn. org.uk/publications

Department of Health and Social Security 1986 Neighbourhood nursing: a focus for care. HMSO, London

Dowling S, Martin R, Skidmore P et al 1996 Nurses taking on junior doctor's work: a confusion of accountability. British Medical Journal 312: 1211–1214

Doyal L, Dowling S, Cameron A 1998 Challenging practice: an evaluation of four innovatory nursing posts in the south west. Policy Press, University of Bristol, Bristol

Eaton L 1993 Vein hopes. Nursing Times 89(36): 18

Foster C 1998 Bolam: consolidation and clarification. Health Care Risk Reports 4(5): 5–7

General Medical Council 2001 Good medical practice. GMC, London

Giles S 1993 Passing the buck. Nursing Times 89(28): 42

Giliker P, Beckwith S 2004 Tort, 2nd edn. Sweet & Maxwell, London

Healy P 1996 Nurses doing junior doctor's work are safe claims unions. Nursing Standard 10(34): 5

Jones M 1999 Nurse prescribing. Baillière Tindall, Edinburgh

Kerry DG 1991 Lawyers comment, *Martin Wilsher* v. *Essex Area Health Authority* and causation. AVMA Medical Legal Journal 12

Kloss DK 1988 Demarcation in medical practice: the extended role of the nurse. Professional Negligence 4: 41

Last T, Seld N, Kassat J, Rawan A 1992 Extended role of the nurse in ICU. British Journal of Nursing 1: 675

Mayor S 1997 Working to protocol. Practice Nurse 13: 187

Montgomery J 1992 Doctors handmaidens: the legal contribution. In: McVeigh S, Wheeler S (eds) Law health and medical regulation. Dartmouth, Aldershot

Naish J 1995 The extended role of the nurse: risk management implications. Health Care Risk Report 1: 22–24

Naish J, Garbett R 1996 Don't administer drugs, says union. Nursing Times 92(47): 5

National Institute for Clinical Excellence 1999 A guide to our work. NICE, London

National Institute for Clinical Excellence 2004 The guideline development process, an overview for stakeholders, the public and the NHS. NICE, London

Nursing and Midwifery Council 2004a The NMC code of professional conduct: standards for conduct, performance and ethics. Standards 07.04. NMC, London

Nursing and Midwifery Council 2004b The PREP handbook. NMC, London

Nursing and Midwifery Council 2006 NMC News May 15: 7

Parker S, Wilson C 1992 An introduction to medico-legal aspects of practice nursing. Medical Defence Union, London

Peysner J 1995 The captain on the bridge. Health Care Risk Report 1: 8

Shepherd J 1993 Nurses are changing not extending their roles. British Journal of Nursing 2: 447

Standing Medical Advisory Committee and Standing Nursing and Midwifery Advisory Committee Joint Working Party on Extended Role 1989 DHSS professional letter. PL/CMO (89) 7. HMSO, London

Tingle JH 1993 The extended role of the nurse; legal implications. Care of the Critically Ill 9: 30–34

Tingle JH, Rodgers ME 1999 Clinical guidelines, NICE and the Court of Appeal. Nottingham Law Journal 8: 95–100

United Kingdom Central Council 1992 The scope of professional practice. UKCC, London

United Kingdom Central Council 2000 The scope of professional practice – a study of its implementation. (Dr Sandra Jowett, Mark Peters, Professor Jennifer Wilson-Barnett, Heidi Reynolds). UKCC, London

Waters J 1996 Horror stories warn of need for training. Nursing Times 92(16): 9

Legal aspects of expanded role, clinical guidelines and protocols, and nurse prescribing

Consent to treatment I: General principles

5

Jean McHale

One of the most fundamental principles of health-care law and ethics is that treatment should be given only with the patient's consent. The nurse is frequently the person who has to obtain the patient's consent to treatment, whether on the wards or in the community. Even if the doctor has the task of obtaining the patient's consent, the patient may turn to the nurse for clarification or further information regarding the proposed treatment. The importance of obtaining consent is inherent in law and also in professional practice. The Nursing and Midwifery Code provides that

> 3.1 All patients and clients have a right to receive information about their condition. You must be sensitive to their needs and respect the wishes of those who refuse or are unable to receive information about their condition. Information should be accurate, truthful and presented in such a way as to make it easily understood. You may need to seek legal or professional advice or guidance from your employer in relation to the giving or withholding of consent.
>
> *Nursing and Midwifery Council 2004*

This chapter begins by considering the types of consent: express and implied, written and oral. Second, it examines when a patient is legally capable of giving consent and the basis on which treatment may be given to an incompetent patient. Third, liability in criminal and civil law is discussed where treatment is given without consent.

TYPES OF CONSENT

Consent forms

Nurses are familiar with the consent forms given to patients to sign before they go in for an operation. The Department of Health (2001a) has published model consent forms that provide guidance to health professionals.

In law, while a consent form may provide evidence that the patient has consented, the act of signing a form does not itself make the consent obtained legally valid. What is important is that the consent that is given is 'real', that is to say it has been obtained freely, without pressure being placed upon the patient and that the patient understands the implications of what s/he is consenting to. There may be situations in which consent may be implied through the patient's actions. But considered consent is necessary in relation to all serious medical procedures, and failure to obtain that consent may leave a nurse in danger of being held liable in the criminal courts or of being sued for damages in the civil courts.

Express and implied consent

Consent may be either express or implied. Consent may be expressly given in writing or orally. Alternatively, a patient may through his/her actions signify consent, for example the patient proffering her wrist to be bandaged. There are risks in assuming that a patient, in seeking treatment, is consenting to any medical procedure being undertaken. What is important is to ensure that the decision making process is appropriately documented (Nursing and Midwifery Council 2004, para 3.5).

CAPACITY

Generally, patients are presumed to be capable of making their own treatment decisions. But in some situations capacity may be called into question. A patient may not appear to understand what s/he has been told or may appear confused. The nurse may need to assess whether this patient is capable of making a particular treatment decision. This task may prove to be particularly difficult if a person has a learning disability or suffers from fluctuating mental capacity. In *Re C* the court upheld the right of a 68-year-old paranoid schizophrenic who had developed gangrene in his foot to prevent amputation in the future without his express written consent (*Re C* [1994] All ER 819). Thorpe J. suggested a three-part test to determine whether a patient possessed capacity. Did the patient comprehend the information given to her/him? Did s/he believe it? Had s/he weighed up the information balancing needs and risks before reaching a decision? At the hearing it was claimed that C was not competent because of his delusions that he was a doctor and that whatever treatment was given to him was calculated to destroy his body. But despite these claims Thorpe J. held that he was satisfied that C was capable of giving consent because he understood and had retained the relevant treatment information and believed it and had arrived at a clear choice.

One difficulty with the test laid down in *Re C* is that it makes capacity dependent upon the information that the patient is actually given (Grubb 1994). If the nurse provides a patient with a great deal of complex information, the patient may not understand it and so it may not fall within the definition of capacity set out in *Re C*, whereas had the patient been given a very simple basic explanation about the same treatment procedure s/he would have possessed the necessary capacity to consent.

The approach taken in *Re C* was confirmed by the Court of Appeal in *Re MB*, a case discussed more fully in Chapter 9 in the context of enforced caesarean sections. In this case the Court of Appeal adopted a version of the test of capacity stated in earlier cases. They held that a person is not capable of making a decision where:

" (a) the person is unable to comprehend and retain the information which is material to the decision, especially as to the likely consequences of having or not having the treatment in question: and

(b) the patient is unable to use the information and weigh it in the balance as of the process of arriving at a decision.

Should capacity include the right to make an 'irrational' decision?

> If a patient refuses treatment on what the nurse treating him or her regards as an irrational basis, can treatment still be given?

As Brazier (1991) comments, an elderly woman with a diseased tooth may have sufficient capacity to understand the suggestion made to her that it should be removed but she may nevertheless allow her fear of dentists and of the pain of treatment to overcome her wish to have the tooth extracted. One approach to problem patients such as this elderly lady would be to categorise her decision as 'irrational' and to override it. A variation on this approach suggested by Kennedy (1991) is that an irrational decision should be respected where it derives from long-held beliefs and values on the basis of which a patient has run his/her life but not if it is the result of a temporary delusion. Nevertheless, attempting to distinguish between different 'irrational' decisions may be difficult practically. Furthermore, there is also a real risk that those refusals that are found to be 'irrational' will be those of the mentally handicapped and the demented patient (Brazier 1991).

In *Re MB*, in which MB refused a caesarean section because of her needle phobia, the Court of Appeal discussed the cases in which a caesarean section was authorised, noting that, in all those cases save *Re S*, the court had decided that the woman in question lacked capacity. After again stressing the right of the competent adult to consent or to refuse treatment, Butler Sloss L.J. commented that:

" A competent woman who has the capacity to decide may, for religious reasons, other reasons, for rational or irrational reasons or for no reason at all, choose not to have medical intervention, even though the consequence may be the death or serious handicap of the child she bears, or her own death. In that event the courts do not have the jurisdiction to declare medical intervention lawful and the question of her own best interests objectively considered, does not arise.

(Re MB [1997] FLR 426, pp 436–437)

She went on to state that:

" Irrationality is here used to connote a decision which is so outrageous in its defiance of logic or of accepted moral standards that no sensible person who has applied his mind to the question to be decided could have arrived at it.... Although it might be thought that irrationality sits uneasily with competence to decide, panic, indecisiveness and irrationality in themselves do not as such amount to incompetence, but they may be symptoms or evidence of incompetence. The graver the consequences of the decision the commensurately greater the level of competence is required to take the decision.

(Ibid. p. 437)

The Court of Appeal noted that, in *Re C*, Thorpe J. had suggested that a compulsive disorder/phobia may have the effect that the decision is not 'a true one'. Temporary incompetence, as the Court of Appeal commented, may erode capacity. This may be due to such factors as were mentioned by Lord Donaldson in the earlier case of *Re T* – 'confusion, shock, pain and drugs'.

Thus a patient has, as in *Re C* itself, the ability to make a decision which some may regard as being irrational even though this may have serious consequences for their health while in other situations a decision which may be irrational may be linked to a lack of competence. This is a fine line and is a matter which is likely to come before the courts again in the future. The law in this area is also reflected in the Nursing and Midwifery Council Professional Code which (Nursing and Midwifery Council 2004) states that

" 3.2 You must respect patients' and clients autonomy – their right to decide whether or not to undergo any health care intervention – even where a refusal may result in harm or death to themselves or a fetus, unless a court of law orders to the contrary. This right is protected in law, although in circumstances where the health of the fetus would be severely compromised by any refusal to give consent, it would be appropriate to discuss this matter fully within the team and with a supervisor of midwives and possibly to seek external advice or guidance.

Fluctuating capacity

> An elderly lady is cared for in a nursing home. She has good days and bad days. She can throw tantrums and yet later appear totally lucid. How far do the nurses caring for her need to respect her wishes?

Where a patient has a fluctuating mental state it may be acutely difficult to assess capacity, which creates real difficulties for the nurses treating the patient. In such a situation it is tempting to say that s/he lacks capacity, because English law allows a mentally incompetent patient to be given such treatment as those treating her/him believe to be in his/her best interests (*Re F* [1990] 1 AC 1). In *Re T* ([1992] 4 All ER 649) the Court of Appeal held that the capacity of an adult patient is to be judged by reference to the particular decision to be made. This approach was at variance with an earlier Court of Appeal decision, in which it was held that a child with fluctuating mental capacity was to be regarded as totally incapable (*Re R* [1991] 4 All ER 177). The approach in *Re T* is surely right, reinforced by the decision in *Re C*, which states that the test for capacity is decision-specific.

In assessing capacity, in practice much will depend upon the discretion of the individual practitioner. Good practice would suggest that as far as possible patients should be left to make their own decisions.

The adult lacking mental capacity

Best interest test

Take a situation in which a nurse is asked to care for a patient who has a profound mental handicap or severe brain damage: on what basis can s/he lawfully treat that patient? Until 1990, the legal position as to treating adults lacking mental capacity was uncertain. Prior to the Mental Health Act 1983 the court had had an 'inherent jurisdiction' to act for the benefit of adult patients lacking mental capacity, as they have today with regard to child patients (Ch. 6). The basis for such treatment was discussed by the House of Lords in 1990. In *Re F* ([1990] AC 1), the court was asked to authorise the sterilisation of a 36-year-old woman with severe learning disabilities. The House of Lords held that the operation could be undertaken; it held that the court had no power to authorise treatment of an adult lacking mental capacity through the use of inherent jurisdiction, as it had regarding a child patient (Ch. 6). Prior to *Re F* it was common practice to get the relatives to sign the consent form. In *Re F* the court said that such consent had no legal effect. No one had a legal right to give consent on behalf of an adult lacking mental capacity. However, that did not mean that treatment could not be given. The House of Lords said treatment could be given on the grounds of necessity where this was in the patient's best interests.

'Best interests' was originally assessed by reference to what a responsible body of professional practice would regard as being in this patient's best interests (the *Bolam* test discussed in Ch. 2). However in later cases a more expansive approach has been taken. Over time the courts have moved away from a totally medically based approach to 'best interests'. In *Re S* ([2000] 3 WLR 1288), a case that concerned an application to sterilise a 28-year-old woman with severe learning disabilities, Thorpe J. held that:

" In deciding what is best for the disabled patient the judge must have regard to the patient's welfare as the paramount consideration. That embraces issues far wider than the medical. Indeed it would be undesirable and possibly impossible to set bounds to what is relevant to a welfare determination.

He suggested that while *Bolam* may assist in ascertaining what treatment alternatives are available this is only one part of the assessment. Butler Sloss P also held in that case that *Bolam* was 'irrelevant to the judicial decision once the judge is satisfied that the range of options was within the range of acceptable opinion among competent and responsible practitioners'.

In *Re F* the court said that there was no legal duty to refer all cases concerning treatment of an adult lacking mental capacity to the court for approval. Nevertheless in certain situations, for example before major surgery is performed, it believed that referral of the issue to the court would be desirable. This raises the question of whether it is appropriate to leave this assessment to the health professional at all.

The nurse acting as the patient's advocate may take the view that what a doctor believes to be medically expedient is not actually in that patient's best interests. The nurse should be able to raise concerns and to take the matter further should s/he believe that the patient's interests are being disregarded.

What medical procedures are capable of being authorised under the 'best interests' principle was left uncertain after *Re F*. While it appears that generally therapeutic procedures would clearly fall within 'best interests', the legality of many non-therapeutic procedures such as non-therapeutic clinical trials is questionable. This issue is returned to below.

Mental Capacity Act 2005

The law in this area will be soon subject to change due to the enactment of new legislation in the form of the Mental Capacity Act 2005. This legislation followed an extensive examination of this area undertaken by the Law Commission, a body established by the government to examine areas of law and make recommendations for reform. In its report *Mental Incapacity* (Law Commission 1995), the Law Commission recommended creating a statutory decision-making structure for adults lacking mental capacity. It took a decade from the Law Commission Report for the final legislation to be enacted. The Law Commission Report proved extremely controversial, in particular those recommendations that concerned end-of-life decision-making, which certain pro-life groups believed constituted the promotion of euthanasia (see Ch. 10).

In the years that followed, the government consulted upon the reforms. Finally a Bill was introduced in 2003 and this subsequently led to the legislation being enacted in May 2005.

The Mental Capacity Act 2005 builds upon the common law in the area, structuring decision-making concerning adults lacking mental capacity within a statutory framework. The Act is due to come into force in 2007. Here we consider the main provisions concerning assessment of capacity. Other specific issues that have arisen as a result of the legislation in relation to clinical research and end-of-life decision making are examined in Chapters 8 and 10 respectively.

In the test for capacity the Mental Capacity Act 2005 builds upon and develops the common law test in *Re C*. Section 1 of the Act sets out a series of 'principles' that are to underpin decision-making. These are to include a presumption in favour of capacity; the requirement that all reasonable steps are to be taken to ensure that the individual makes the decision; and that decisions must be reached on the basis of the 'best interests' of the individual. Section 2(1) states that a person will lack capacity where they are unable to make the decision because of 'an impairment of or a disturbance in the functioning of the mind or brain'. As with the test suggested by Thorpe J. in *Re C*, any test for capacity is decision-specific; this emphasises the fact that a person may be capable of making one decision while at the same time being incapable of making another decision. Section 3(1) provides that a person is unable to understand the information that is necessary in relation to this decision; unable to retain it; unable to use or weigh the information up as part of the decision-making process or unable to communicate the decision by any means. Information here includes information regarding the foreseeable consequences of the necessary decision (s.3(4)). If a person acts on the best interests of an adult lacking capacity they will not be subject to legal liability if they have undertaken reasonable steps to ascertain that the adult lacks capacity and if they reasonably believe that the person lacks decision-making capacity and that the decision is in the person's best interests (s.5).

Decisions concerning the adult lacking mental capacity will be as at common law made on the basis of the 'best interests' of the individual. Guidance is given in the legislation, in section 4, as to what constitutes an individual's best interests. Factors that should be taken into account 'as far as is reasonably practicable' include an individual's past and present wishes and feelings, any beliefs and values that would have been taken into account if they had capacity; and any 'other factors that he would be likely to consider if he were able to do so' (s.4(6)). The Mental Capacity Act Draft Code of Practice 2006 states that, where certain decisions arise that concern 'serious medical treatment', these should be referred for judicial determination. These include withholding or withdrawing artificial nutrition or hydration, non-therapeutic sterilisation of a person lacking capacity to consent, some termination of pregnancy cases and 'other cases where there is a doubt or dispute about whether a particular treatment will be in a person's best interests' (Department of Constitutional Affairs 2006, para 7.17.)

INFORMATION PROVISION

Criminal law liability

Bringing a criminal law prosecution against a nurse or doctor where a medical procedure has been undertaken without consent may seem only a remote possibility, but such a prosecution is not totally unforeseeable. In November 1992, a press report appeared concerning a 51-year-old journalist who woke up in hospital after a 'deep scrape' operation to find that during the operation her womb and ovaries had been removed (*Sunday Times* Nov 1992). The surgeon found a swelling in her abdomen, although it was not a life-threatening condition, and had gone on to cut out her ovaries. He said that 'I thought at her age it was the wiser thing to remove them'. The woman took her case to the Director of Public Prosecutions, who considered prosecution, although ultimately this was not proceeded with.

Failure to obtain consent to treatment may amount to the crime of battery, a common law offence. Some types of battery cannot be consented to, such as prize fighting or beatings for sexual gratification (*R* v. *Donovan* [1934] QB 638 and *R* v. *Brown* [1994] 1 AC 212). However, it appears to be the case that reasonable surgical interference does not constitute an inherently unlawful action and that no crime will be committed as long as the patient has consented to the operation being undertaken (*AG Ref (No. 6 of 1980)* [1981] QB 715). There is the possibility that serious surgical procedures may also constitute an offence under section 18 of the Offences Against the Person Act 1861. This section makes it an offence to cause grievous bodily harm 'unlawfully and maliciously' to a person with the intention of causing grievous bodily harm. A court is unlikely to find that an operation to improve the patient's health has been undertaken unlawfully.

Finally, there is the chance that an operation might be held to be unlawful regardless of consent because it constituted the crime of maim. This is an ancient crime that makes it an offence to perform an operation or give an injury that has the effect of permanently disabling/weakening a man. Skegg (1984) suggests that such a prosecution is unlikely to be successful even if it were to be brought. First, most medical treatment does not have the effect of permanently disabling a man and rendering him less useful for fighting. Second, even if an operation did have that effect it might still be lawful if undertaken for therapeutic purposes. In a consultation paper that examines the scope of criminal liability in relation to consent to treatment, the Law Commission (1996) recommended reform of the law to recognise the legality of the performance of medical procedures such as surgical operations.

Civil law liability

Battery

While a criminal prosecution may be brought it is far more likely that failure to obtain consent will lead to the patient suing for damages in the civil courts. This may be on the basis either that the treatment amounted to a battery or that the nurse or doctor was negligent in providing the patient with inadequate information. A battery refers to any unlawful touching. Consent is a defence to battery. But what amounts to consent? In *Chatterson* v. *Gerson* ([1981] QB 432), Bristow J. said:

> " In my judgment once the patient is informed in broad terms of the nature of the procedure which is intended and has given her consent then that consent is real and the cause of action on which to base the claim is negligence not trespass.

It is sufficient that the patient understands the type of operation that is to be performed. The patient doesn't have to be informed of all the potential risks and implications of the clinical procedure.

Treating on the basis of temporary incapacity

Consent is not required if treatment is necessary in an emergency. The patient brought in bleeding and unconscious to Accident & Emergency can be treated without his/her consent. If it was claimed that treatment was unlawful then the nurse could claim the defence that the treatment was 'necessary'.

If, during an operation, it is found that a patient is suffering from, for example, a life-threatening tumour then this tumour may be removed if it is necessary to save the patient's life, even though the medical team do not have the patient's express consent to removal. But, while it is lawful to undertake treatment without consent where it is necessary to do so, how far does this principle extend? Guidance can be taken from two notable decisions in Canada. In *Marshall* v. *Curry* ([1933] 3 DLR 260) the plaintiff sought damages against a surgeon for battery. During a hernia operation the surgeon had removed a testicle. He claimed that the removal was necessary because otherwise the patient's life would have been in danger. The court held that the surgeon was correct to go ahead and that it would have been unreasonable to have delayed removal by waiting to obtain the patient's consent, then undertaking a second operation.

But 'reasonableness' is a question of degree and dependent upon the urgency with which the operation should be undertaken. This was illustrated in the later case of *Murray* v. *McMurchy* ([1942] 2 DLR 442). A woman underwent a caesarean section. While operating, the doctor found that the woman's uterus was in such a state that it would have been exceedingly dangerous for her to undergo another pregnancy. He decided to sterilise her there and then and tied her fallopian tubes. On recovering from the operation and discovering what had happened, the woman brought an action for battery. The court upheld her claim. They were of the view that the doctor should have postponed the sterilisation operation until after the patient's consent had been obtained. In view of the uncertainty as to what constitutes necessary treatment, nurses should be exceedingly careful before proceeding with treatment in the absence of consent, save in an emergency situation where it is required to preserve the patient's life.

The patient who refuses treatment

> A woman who is lying in Accident & Emergency critically ill after a car accident refuses treatment because she says that she is opposed to conventional medical therapies and in particular will not receive blood products. Can she be treated?

If the nurse goes ahead and gives treatment against the patient's wishes this may well amount to a battery. Take, for example, the Canadian case of *Malette* v. *Schumann* ([1990] 67 DLR (4th) 321). The plaintiff was brought into hospital after a road accident. A nurse found a card in her pocket identifying her as a Jehovah's Witness and requesting that she never be given a blood transfusion. Despite this the doctor went ahead and administered the transfusion. On recovering her health the patient brought an action for battery and was awarded some $20 000 damages.

But while this is the general rule the English courts have indicated that there may be situations in which treating a patient against his/her express wishes may be lawful. In *Re T* ([1992] 4 All ER 649), T, a woman 34 weeks pregnant, was taken to hospital after she had been involved in a road accident. She developed pneumonia and her condition deteriorated. While in hospital she was visited by her mother. Although T was not a Jehovah's Witness, her mother was. There was some discussion between T and the medical team treating her as to whether she should be given a caesarean section. After some time alone with her mother T stated clearly that she did not want a blood transfusion. T then gave birth to a stillborn child. T's condition subsequently deteriorated. The hospital went to the court and asked for a declaration stating whether it would be lawful for T to be given a transfusion should it prove necessary. The court granted the declaration.

The Master of the Rolls, Sir John Donaldson, stressed that a patient's refusal to consent should lead those treating the patient to ask: was the patient capable of refusing consent to that treatment? He emphasised that refusals varied in their degree of seriousness and the scope of the refusal must be considered: did it apply to all situations?; was it based upon assumptions that had not been realised? He recommended that consent forms should be redesigned so that the consequences of refusal were brought forcibly to the patient's attention. This is a very controversial judgment. Were it to be followed, nurses and other members of the health-care team would have to scrutinise very carefully any decision to refuse treatment. The other judges in this case did not go so far as Lord Donaldson, preferring to base their decision upon the fact that T had made her decision under pressure from her mother. Where there is doubt as to the patient's capacity to refuse treatment,

Lord Donaldson stressed that the health-care team should seek a declaration from the court.

Subsequently, the courts have confirmed the right of a competent patient to refuse treatment regardless of the consequences, as we noted above in relation to *Re MB*. In 2002 the court upheld the decision of Ms B, a former social worker, to have artificial ventilation withdrawn even though the consequence of withdrawal of the ventilation was that she would die (*Re B (Adult: Refusal of Medical Treatment)* [2002] 2 All ER 449). This case is discussed further in Chapter 10. Here the Court awarded nominal damages reflecting the fact than the hospital had continued to treat her against her will.

What is clear is that the law does not allow nurses or other health-care professionals to force a competent patient to receive treatment simply because they believe that the patient has made a totally irrational decision. If there is real doubt as to whether to proceed against the patient's wishes and the patient's life is in danger, advice should be sought from the court as to the legality of proceeding with treatment. This issue is discussed in the context of decisions relating to the end of life in Chapter 10.

Using compulsion in health care – public health powers

Generally speaking, in order for clinical procedures to be lawful a patient must give consent freely. However, in some situations compulsion may be sought. In the next chapter, the operation of the Mental Health Act 1983 is examined. In addition, there are a number of powers relating to compulsory care in the context of public health. If a patient is suffering from a notifiable disease, then the Public Health (Control of Disease) Act 1984 s.37 allows such a patient to be forcibly removed to hospital. The order must be made by a magistrate. The statute applies to those persons suffering from notifiable diseases such as cholera or typhoid. While human immunodeficiency virus (HIV) and acquired immunodeficiency syndrome (AIDS) are not notifiable conditions, special regulations have extended the power to make an order to persons who are HIV-positive or who have AIDS (Public Health (Control of Infectious Diseases) Act 1984). There are also provisions under the National Assistance Act 1948 section 48 that allow the removal of persons who are aged, infirm, suffering from chronic disease, who are incapacitated, from their homes to hospital. Removal can only be undertaken after a magistrate's order has been obtained. This order allows removal for a period of up to 3 months. There is also a special provision allowing a person to be removed in an emergency for a period of up to 3 weeks (National Assistance (Amendment) Act 1951 s1(1)). This may be undertaken on the recommendation of the community physician if supported by another practitioner.

Negligence

Once the patient has been told in general terms what is involved in medical procedures then there will no longer be liability in battery. But the patient may claim that while s/he has been given a general explanation s/he has not been told of the risks of the treatment and that this amounts to negligence. In establishing negligence for failure to inform, the legal principles are the same as in any other negligence claim (Ch. 2). The claimant must show that s/he was owed a duty, that there was a breach of duty and that damage resulted from that breach.

In English law there is no doctrine of 'informed consent'; no requirement to inform the patient of all risks. This was made clear by the courts in the case of *Sidaway* v. *Bethlem Royal Hospital Governors* ([1985] 1 All ER 643). Mrs Sidaway underwent an operation after having suffered for some time from a recurring pain in her neck, right shoulder and arm. The operation was performed by a senior neurosurgeon at the Bethlem Royal Hospital. Even if carried out with all due care and skill there was a 1–2% risk of damage to nerve root and spinal column. While the risk of damage to the spinal column was less than to the nerve root, the consequences were more severe.

The plaintiff was left severely disabled after the operation. She claimed that she had not been given adequate warning as to the risks of the operation and she sought damages for negligence. During the proceedings it was found that, while the surgeon had told the patient of the risks of damage to the nerve root, he had not told her of the risks of damage to the spinal column. In doing this, he had conformed with what in 1974 would have been accepted as standard medical practice by a responsible and skilled body of neuro-surgeons. The House of Lords rejected the claim that the surgeon had acted negligently. The majority held that the test that the courts should use in deciding whether the advice given was negligent was the same as that used in deciding whether medical treatment was negligent – the *Bolam* test. This test provides that a doctor: 'is not guilty of negligence if he has acted in accordance with a practice accepted as proper by a responsible body of medical men'.

That does not mean, however, that the court will always accept the word of the health-care professional as to which risks should and which should not be disclosed. Only one member of the court in *Sidaway*, Lord Diplock, unreservedly accepted the *Bolam* test. Lord Bridge said that a judge could disagree with the evidence given to him:

  ❝ I am of the opinion that the judge might in certain circumstances come to the conclusion that disclosure of a particular risk was so obviously necessary to an informed choice on the part of the patient that no reasonably prudent medical man would fail to make it.

Lord Templeman stressed that it was for the court to decide whether the doctor had acted negligently or not.

The requirement that the standard of disclosure should be that which would be recognised by a competent body of health-care professionals can be contrasted with the approach taken in certain other countries that have recognised the doctrine of 'informed consent'. In the US case of *Canterbury* v. *Spence* ([1972] 464 F 2d 772), the court declared that:

  ❝ respect for the patient's right of self-determination on particular therapy demands a standard set by law for the physician rather than one which physicians may or may not impose on themselves.

Several states adopted a standard of disclosure based upon the information that a 'prudent patient' would expect to receive In *Sidaway* one member of the House of Lords, Lord Scarman, favoured the informed consent approach, but he was very much in the minority. Whether such a test would make a radical difference to the amount of information a patient receives is open to question. It is interesting to note that, in the USA, some courts have used the notion of therapeutic privilege to restrict the requirement to disclose (see also the discussion of therapeutic privilege, below). A broader duty of disclosure has also been recognised in the Australian case of *Rogers* v. *Whittaker* ([1993] 4 Med LR 79).

Overriding the responsible body of professional practice

However, while the court has the ultimate power to overrule the view of the responsible body of professional practice as to what risks should be disclosed, the courts have been traditionally unwilling to do so. In *Maynard* v. *West Midlands Health Authority* ([1984] 1 WLR 643), for example, the trial judge preferred one body of professional medical opinion to another and was held to have been wrong to do so. Even if the body of professional practice is very small in number, four or five out of 250 specialists, for example, the court will still be prepared to accept its opinion (*De Freitas* v. *O'Brien* [1995] 6 Med LR 108).

Nonetheless the fact that a responsible body of medical practice does support the actions of the clinician is not by itself necessarily conclusive. In *Smith* v. *Tunbridge Wells Health Authority* ([1994] 5 Med LR 334), the failure to warn a 28-year-old man of the risks of impotence subsequent to surgery upon a rectal prolapse was found to constitute negligence. It was held that, while some surgeons were not providing warnings of that risk at that time, nonetheless the omission to inform in this particular case was 'neither reasonable nor responsible'.

The House of Lords in *Bolitho* subsequently illustrated the fact that there is greater judicial willingness to scrutinise the opinion expressed by the body of professional practice (*Bolitho* v. *City and Hackney Health Authority* [1998]AC 232). Lord Browne Wilkinson stated that:

" In particular where there are questions of assessment of the relative risks and benefits of adopting a particular medical practice, a reasonable view necessarily presupposes that the relative risks and benefits have been weighed by the experts in forming their opinions. But if, in a rare case, it can be demonstrated that the professional opinion is not capable of withstanding logical analysis, the judge is entitled to hold that the body of opinion is not reasonable or responsible. I emphasis that in my view it will be very seldom right for a judge to reach the conclusion that views genuinely held by a competent medical expert are unreasonable.

In this case Lord Brown Wilkinson excluded from his discussion the issue of disclosure of risk. He stated (at p. 243) that:

" in cases of diagnosis and treatment there are cases where, despite a body of professional opinion sanctioning the defendant's conduct, the defendant can be properly held liable in negligence (I am not here considering questions of disclosure of risk).

However the application of *Bolitho* to diagnosis and treatment was considered recently in the decision of *Pearce* v. *United Bristol NHS Trust* ([1999] PIQR P53

(CA)). Here the Court of Appeal looked at both the decisions in *Bolitho* and the earlier House of Lords judgment in *Sidaway*. Lord Woolf held that:

> " if there is a significant risk which would affect the judgment of a reasonable patient then in the normal course it is the responsibility of a doctor to inform the patient of that significant risk, if the information is needed so that the patient can determine for him or herself as to what course that she should adopt.

On the facts of that particular case the plaintiffs failed to establish negligence, in that had the risk of the stillbirth been disclosed the evidence suggested that she would still have gone ahead with a natural delivery. Nonetheless the approach taken by the Court of Appeal in this case indicates that this decision may again be regarded as a further step towards a broader duty of disclosure upon clinicians (Grubb 1999). Jones (1999) has argued that the effect of the judgments is that of a combination of the 'prudent patient' standard with the reasonable doctor standard and that in the light of this case it could be argued that 'no reasonable doctor would fail to disclose a risk regarded as significant by a reasonable patient'. Moreover, it appears to be the case that the risk does not necessarily have to be such that the patient would have changed his/her mind had s/he known about this particular risk, but rather that it could be sufficient if this risk is one which is relevant, alongside other factors, in reaching a decision.

The movement towards enhanced disclosure was confirmed in the subsequent case of *Chester* v. *Afshar* ([2005] 1 AC 234). This case concerned a patient with back pain who on consulting a rheumatologist was found to have a significant deterioration of the spinal disks. She saw Mr Afshar, a consultant neurosurgeon. He advised her that surgery was needed to remove three disks. Miss Chester asked Mr Afshar about the 'horror stories' of such operations. There was a conflict of evidence between Mr Afshar and Miss Chester as to what information had actually been given. Mr Afshar stated that he had informed her that there was a small risk of lower spinal cord nerve root disturbance, haemorrhage and infection. Miss Chester stated that she had not been given this information, rather that she had been told by the consultant that he 'hadn't crippled anybody yet'. She said that, had she been given that information, she would not have gone ahead with the information at the time and would have then sought further opinions as to the best course of treatment.

At trial Miss Chester's evidence was preferred. The trial judge held that 'the defendant's failure to advise the claimant adequately was negligent'. The House of Lords held that failure to inform about the risks constituted negligence. This case is fundamentally rooted in the issue of whether, if there has been a breach of duty in failure to disclose, it 'caused' the harm that resulted. This issue is considered below.

Following *Pearce* and *Chester* v. *Afshar* the prospect of such enhanced judicial scrutiny of information provision to patients may suggest that in the future it will become increasingly difficult to justify withholding information from patients regarding the risks of treatment. This may also be reflective of the fact that there is a tendency today in health care towards enhanced disclosure on a routine basis and that in many cases the responsible body of professional practice is likely to favour broader disclosure.

Consent after Bristol

The duty of disclosure required under the *Sidaway* test is not fixed: it changes as the approach taken in professional practice changes. The approach taken by health-care professionals to information disclosure was subject to considerable criticism by Professor Sir Ian Kennedy at the Bristol Inquiry (Department of Health 2001b and see Ch. 1). This report dealt specifically with the issue of consent in a section entitled 'Respect and honesty'. The report suggested that consent should be best regarded as being a 'process'. It provided that:

" 24. The process of informing the patient and obtaining consent on a course of treatment should be regarded as a process and not a one-off event consisting of obtaining a patient's signature on a form.

25. The process of consent should apply not only to surgical procedures but all clinical procedures and examinations which involve any form of touching. This must not mean more forms; it means more communication.

26. As part of the process of obtaining consent, except when they have indicated otherwise, patients should be given sufficient information about what is to take place, the risks, the uncertainties and possible negative consequences of the proposed treatment, about any alternatives and about the likely outcome, to enable them to make a choice about how to proceed.

The Report suggested that information should be tailored to the needs, circumstances and wishes of the individual. This approach reflects very much the approach taken by Lord Woolf in the Court of Appeal in *Pearce.*

The guidelines of the General Medical Council *Seeking patients' consent: the ethical considerations* (General Medical Council 1998), which slightly predate the Bristol Report, are illustrative of the changing approach in health-care practice. This document giving guidance to doctors regarding the provision of information states that:

" 6. When providing information you must do your best to find out about patients' individual needs and priorities. For example, patients' beliefs, culture, occupation or other factors may have a bearing on the information they need in order to reach a decision. You should not make assumptions about patients' views, but discuss these matters with them, and ask them whether they have any concerns about the treatment or the risks it may involve. You should provide patients with appropriate information, which should include an explanation of any risks to which they may attach particular significance. Ask patients whether they have understood the information and whether they would like more before making a decision.

As patient expectations change regarding their involvement in decisions concerning their treatment, so the levels of disclosure required of practitioners are likely to change.

This is a very patient-based test. Similarly the government, in their response to Bristol confirmed the importance of informed consent, and this led to revised Department of Health guidelines in relation to examination and treatment. So, for example, the Department of Health document *Good practice in consent; implementation guidance* (Department of Health 2001a) provides that:

" Patients and those close to them will vary in how much information they want; from those who want as much detail as possible including details of rare risks, to those who ask health professionals to make decisions for them. There will always be an element of clinical judgment in determining what information should be given. However the presumption must be that the patient wishes to be well-informed about the risks and benefits of the various options. Where the patient makes it clear (verbally or non-verbally) that they do not wish to be given this level of information, this should be documented.

Therapeutic privilege

There may be some situations in which it is thought that the patient would be unable to cope if told all the details of the prognosis. In *Sidaway*, Lord Scarman indicated that in such a situation information may be withheld on therapeutic grounds, the so-called 'therapeutic privilege'. This must of course be exercised sensitively. Generally, nurses should be cautious today before withholding information from patients, particularly in the light of the trend towards greater information disclosure.

The questioning patient

A patient is provided with information about the proposed treatment but then asks questions as to the risks of the treatment and any complications that may arise. To what extent is the nurse obliged to give a full answer?

In *Sidaway*, it was suggested that there might be a duty to respond fully if the patient asked specific questions. For example, Lord Bridge said that:

" when questioned specifically by a patient of apparently sound mind about the risks involved in a particular procedure proposed, the doctor's duty must, in my opinion, be to answer both truthfully and as fully as the questioner requires.

However, the statements made were only judicial opinions, which did not relate to the decision in that case and so were obitur not binding on later courts.

In the later case of *Blyth* v. *Bloomsbury AHA* ([1987] (1993) 4 Med LR 151 CA) the court indicated that the *Bolam* test should also apply to this situation. The plaintiff, Mrs Blyth, was a qualified nurse. She went into hospital to give birth. After the birth she was given a vaccination against rubella and an injection of the contraceptive Depo-Provera. Mrs Blyth said that she did not want to be given Depo-Provera until she had been told about the side effects. At the trial her claims as to what information she had been given were disputed. Expert evidence put forward at the trial indicated that at that time it was the practice to inform the patient that Depo-Provera led to irregular bleeding but not to inform about the other side effects. Kerr L.J. said that there was no obligation to disclose all information when a question was asked; it was sufficient if the information given was that which would be given by a responsible body of clinical practitioners (the *Bolam* test). In responding to questions he stressed that the answer given should depend upon the circumstances, the nature of the information, its reliability and relevance, the condition of the patient, etc. In deciding what information should be given initially, the nurse would need to examine the patient to see if s/he is capable of comprehending the information. However this approach was criticised in later cases. In *Pearce* v. *United Bristol NHS Trust* ([1999] PIQR P53 (CA)), Lord Woolf stated – obitur that 'it is clear that, if a patient asks a doctor about the risk, then the doctor is required to give an honest answer'. Failure to answer questions did arise in the case of *Chester* v. *Afshar*, although this point was not considered as part of the decision of the House of Lords in that case.

Given the trend of judicial decisions in this area and the movement towards increased information provision in clinical practice, it is clear that the nurse would be well advised to ensure that the questioning patient is treated with respect and his/her questions are given a serious response.

Therapeutic v. non-therapeutic treatment

While the general obligation regarding disclosure of information relates to the standard of the responsible body of clinical practice, should that standard apply to all types of medical procedure? This question came before the courts in the case of *Gold* v. *Haringey Health Authority* ([1987] 2 All ER 888). Mrs Gold underwent a sterilisation operation. The operation was unsuccessful. She brought an action claiming that the surgeon was negligent because she was not told of the risk that the sterilisation operation might be reversed naturally, nor the fact that a vasectomy operation upon her husband would have carried less risk of reversal. At the time she underwent her operation there was a body of medical opinion that supported giving further information, but also a body of medical opinion that supported what her surgeon had done.

At first instance, Schiemmann J. drew a distinction between the level of information that had to be given in cases involving therapeutic as opposed to non-therapeutic treatment. He said that a sterilisation operation was non-therapeutic treatment and as such the approach taken in *Sidaway* was not applicable. It was for the court to decide whether or not the person giving advice should mention the chance that the operation would not achieve the desired result. However, on appeal, this approach was rejected. In the Court of Appeal, Lloyd L.J. said that the *Bolam* test applied. He saw problems in trying to draw a line between advice given in relation to therapeutic treatment and non-therapeutic treatment. For example, a plastic surgeon carrying out a skin graft might be acting therapeutically, but he might not be if he were carrying out a facelift or some other cosmetic operation.

Causation

As with any negligence claim, if the patient can show that s/he was given inadequate information by the nurse treating him/her, the patient must still go on to show that the failure to provide such information as to the risks of a particular clinical procedures caused the harm that s/he suffered. The court will ask, 'If this patient here had been given the information which she should have been given then would she have decided to go ahead with the treatment?' (*Chatterson* v. *Gerson* [1981] QB 432). This test for causation can prove problematic in relation to informed consent. What if, had the risk been disclosed, the person would still have gone ahead with the operation? This issue arose in the case of *Chester* v. *Afshar* ([2005] 1 AC 234) discussed above. Here, if Miss Chester had this operation there was a risk consequent upon the surgery. However, even though Miss Chester might still have gone ahead and had the operation if she had been told, the House of Lords still held that the failure to inform was actionable. In a departure from the traditional approach to causation, and following the approach taken in the Australian case of *Chappel* v. *Hart* ([1998] HCA 55), the House of Lords held that disclosure here was necessary in order to safeguard Miss Chester's autonomy and rooted their final decision in concern for individual autonomy. This was even though the breach of duty would not have necessarily 'caused' the harm. Lord Hope took the view that, unless such an approach was taken, this 'would render the duty useless in the cases where it is needed the most'. Unless the claim was allowed this would have the effect that those who admitted that they would still have gone ahead with the surgery were placed in a worse position than those persons who concealed that fact.

Providing information: professional conflicts over disclosure

> In some situations the nurse may be of the view that a doctor or another nurse treating the patient has not provided the patient with adequate information or that the patient has not understood the information given. What should the nurse do?

The nurse should first make this clear to the doctor/other nurse. It may be that they have simply not appreciated the degree of information necessary for that particular patient to make informed consent. But what if the nurse draws the doctor's/other nurse's attention to the perceived problem but they disagree with her/him? What should s/he do?

The standard of disclosure laid down by the courts is that of the responsible body of professional clinical practice. If, for example, a doctor had given a patient the amount of information that a body of professional opinion would believe was sufficient, then s/he would have acted lawfully even though the nurse might disagree with the amount of information which has been given. It is very unlikely that the court would go against the approach that the doctor has taken.

Should the nurse inform the patient him/herself? If s/he does then s/he may be put at risk of being disciplined for overstepping authority and disobeying the doctor. It is also possible that the doctor may be withholding the information for a specific reason, such as on therapeutic grounds, and the patient may not be able to cope with the information once given and may actually suffer harm. In such a situation, the nurse is at risk of an action subsequently being brought against her/him in negligence. The court would examine the nurse's actions and determine whether his/her conduct was such as would be supported by a responsible body of professional nursing practice.

If the nurse fails to act and the patient suffers harm, then the nurse may also be at risk of legal proceedings. However, were proceedings to be brought against the nurse, s/he could claim to be simply following the doctor's orders. In earlier cases the courts have been willing to find that a nurse was not negligent because s/he had been following the orders of the doctor (*Gold* v. *Essex CC* [1942] 2 All ER 237). However, with the increasing autonomy of the nurse and the growth of professional practice, whether this approach would be given unreserved acceptance may be questioned.

In practice, should this situation arise it is suggested that the nurse should not go ahead and disclose immediately. S/he should ask the doctor why more information is not being given. If the doctor gives what the nurse regards to be an inadequate reason, then the matter should be referred to his/her line manager.

CONCLUDING COMMENTS

The principles of consent to treatment outlined in this chapter underpin much of health-care law. Matters of consent are considered in the chapters on reproductive choice, medical research and end of life. In the following chapter, consent in relation to two particular groups of patient – child patients and the mentally ill – are considered.

REFERENCES

Brazier M 1991 Competence, consent and proxy consents. In: Brazier M, Lobjoit M (eds) Protecting the vulnerable. Routledge, London

Department of Constitutional Affairs 2006 Draft Mental Capacity Act Code of Practice. The Stationery Office, London

Department of Health 2001a Reference guide to consent for examination and treatment. Department of Health, London

Department of Health 2001b Learning from Bristol: the report of the Public Inquiry into children's heart surgery at the Bristol Royal Infirmary 1984–1995. Stationery Office, London

General Medical Council 1998 Seeking patients' consent: the ethical considerations. GMC, London

Grubb A 1994 Treatment without consent: adult. Medical Law Review 2: 92

Grubb A 1999 Refusal of treatment (child): competence – *Re L* (Medical treatment: Gillick competency). Medical Law Review 7: 61

Jones M 1999 Informed consent and other fairy stories. Medical Law Review 7: 103

Kennedy I 1991 Consent to treatment. In: Dyer C (ed.) Doctors, patients and the law. Blackwell Scientific, Oxford

Law Commission 1995 Mental incapacity. Report No. 231. HMSO, London

Law Commission 1996 Consent in the criminal law: a consultation paper. No. 139. HMSO, London

Nursing and Midwifery Council 2004 NMC Code of professional conduct: standards for conduct, performance and ethics. NMC London

Skegg PDG 1984 Law medicine and ethics. Oxford University Press, Oxford

Consent to treatment II: Children and the mentally ill

6

Jean McHale

In Chapter 5 the basic principles of the law as it relates to consent to treatment were examined. This chapter focuses on the treatment of two particular groups of patients, children and the mentally ill. The basis on which treatment may be given and from whom consent to treatment should be obtained is examined in relation to the child patient. Particular difficult treatment issues arise with the child patient, as with the adult counterpart, in the context of treatment refusal. These issues are further complicated in the context of the child patient in a situation in which conflicts arise between child and parent. The second part of the chapter considers legal regulation of treatment of the mentally ill patient in hospital and the community. Here, a statutory regime exists which regulates treatment procedures in the form of the Mental Health Act 1983.

TREATING THE CHILD PATIENT

Where the nurse is treating a child patient s/he must take care to ensure that the appropriate consent has been obtained. Where a child is very young, consent must be obtained from the person with 'parental responsibility'. This may be the child's mother, married father and unmarried father (s2 and s4 Children Act 1989) (with agreement with the mother or where a court order has been made giving him that power), a person holding a residence order (s12) or a local authority (s33). But there may be situations in which there is not sufficient time to consult a person with parental responsibility. For example, a child on her way to school is injured by a hit and run driver. She is taken to hospital bleeding profusely, in a critical condition. In an emergency, such treatment may be given as is immediately necessary, without parental consent being obtained. In addition, a child minder or a teacher has the right to do what is 'reasonable in all the circumstances' of the case for the purpose of safeguarding or promoting the child's welfare. This would include authorising medical treatment (s3 (5) Children Act 1989). The Family Law Reform Act 1969 gives children who are 16 years and over the right to give consent themselves to surgical, medical or dental treatment (s8 Family Law Reform Act 1969).

Many uncertainties remain, however, as to what exactly constitutes 'treatment' for these purposes. It is obvious that the plaster on the wound, the surgery on the car accident victim are covered. What is less clear is the extent to which procedures ancillary to treatment are lawful. A difficult issue

117

concerns the use of constraints upon young children, e.g. holding down a child to give treatment. It is submitted that wherever possible treatment should be given with the cooperation of the child and that the use of compulsion should be contemplated only in highly exceptional circumstances. Generally the performance of non-therapeutic procedures on a child creates difficulties because often they cannot be said to be in the child's best interests. One approach is to say that certain procedures are justifiable as long as they are not *against* the child's best interests (*S* v. *McC, W* v. *W* [1972] AC 24). Whether parents can consent to involvement in certain non-therapeutic procedures such as organ donation or involvement in clinical research are discussed further in later chapters.

The parental power of consent does not cover whatever treatment they believe to be in the child's best interests. Any treatment given is ultimately dependent upon the health professional's assessment of whether that treatment is appropriate for the child. Second, certain procedures are unlawful per se. For example, a mother cannot consent to her daughter being circumcised, because this practice was made illegal by the Prohibition of Female Circumcision Act 1985.

When is the child competent to consent to medical treatment?

A young girl approaches a school nurse and wants advice because she intends obtaining the contraceptive pill. What is the legal position? Can such a girl be given such medication without parental consent?

As seen above, there is a statutory right for children aged 16 years and over to consent to medical or dental treatment. However, some children reach maturity earlier than others – 16 years is an arbitrary point. In *Gillick* v. *West Norfolk and Wisbech AHA* ([1985] 3 All ER 402), the House of Lords clearly stated that, even if a child was under 16 years of age s/he might be able to give consent to medical treatment. In this case Mrs Victoria Gillick sought a declaration that the Department of Health and Social Security had been wrong to issue a direction indicating that a doctor might give contraceptive advice/treatment to a child under 16 years without parental consent. The House of Lords, by a narrow majority, dismissed her claim. Lord Fraser held that a doctor would be justified in giving a girl contraceptive advice without her parent's knowledge and/or consent. He suggested a number of factors to be taken into account in making such an assessment. These included that:

- the doctor is satisfied that the girl would understand his advice
- he has been unable to persuade her to tell her parents or to let him tell her parents
- the girl is likely to begin having intercourse with/without contraceptive treatment
- without contraceptive advice/treatment her physical or mental health could suffer
- it would be in the girl's best interests to receive contraceptive assistance without her parent's consent.

Another member of the House of Lords, Lord Scarman, saw the issue in terms of the rights of the child:

❝ as a matter of law the parental right to determine whether or not a minor child below the age of 16 will have medical treatment terminates if and when the child achieves a sufficient understanding and intelligence to enable him to understand fully what is proposed. It will be a question of fact whether a child seeking advice has sufficient understanding of what is involved to give a consent valid in law. (p. 423)

Two members of the House of Lords, Lords Brandon and Templeman, dissented. Lord Templeman said that there are many things that a girl under 16 years needs to practice but sex is not one of them.

After the *Gillick* decision it is clear that a child under 16 years may consent to medical treatment if s/he is judged to be competent to give that consent. The difficulty with the test laid down in *Gillick* is that it means that a nurse treating a child patient has the task of assessing whether this particular child is competent to consent to this particular treatment. A child may have sufficient maturity to consent to one type of treatment, such as treatment for cuts and bruises, while at the same time not being competent to decide about another type of treatment, such as an operation. It must be emphasised that, even if a child is under 16 years, good practice would dictate that, wherever possible, an effort should be made to involve the child in any decisions regarding care and treatment.

The *Gillick* decision was confirmed recently in the *Axon* case (discussed further in Ch. 8).

Court orders

The vast majority of treatment decisions are straightforward and will present no legal difficulties as long as the nurse complies with the general legal principles in relation to disclosure of information set out in the previous chapter, and if s/he obtains consent from the appropriate person. There are, however, some situations in which difficult dilemmas arise. The health-care professionals may be uncertain as to what action to take. There are three main routes through which an application may be made to the court. The case may be referred under what is known as the court's 'inherent jurisdiction'; the court has a power to make orders regarding medical treatment. The child may be made a ward of court. This power was limited by the Children Act 1989 and today a local authority cannot apply for wardship, although other interested bodies such as a health authority may do so. In addition, wardship cannot be sought if the child is in local authority care. The third option is to ask the court to make one of two orders created by the Children Act 1989. The first of these is a 'prohibited steps' order; this has the effect of stopping a parent exercising his/her parental responsibility without the consent of the court. Second, an application could be made for a 'specific issue order'. This involves asking the court to give directions on a specific question before it, for example, giving consent to treatment (s8). In making an order the court considers whether the child's welfare dictates that the treatment be undertaken. The importance of making an application to the court where there is a dispute with the parents as to what treatment should be undertaken is considered in the next section.

Refusal of treatment by those with parental responsibility

What if a course of treatment is proposed for a critically ill child but the parents refuse to give their consent? Can treatment be given? The parents may be refusing treatment for a particular reason, such as their own ethical or religious beliefs. In such circumstances health-care professionals should hesitate before treating. The impact upon the child, were treatment to be authorised in the face of parental opposition, requires some consideration. Were treatment to be given in such a situation, this might have the effect that the child is alienated from his/her own family. The action taken is likely to relate to the urgency with which treatment is required. If a child is literally bleeding to death then, it is suggested, it is justifiable to treat, even in the face of parental opposition.

But if, while a child's life is in grave danger, death is not imminent, then the matter may be referred to the court by the hospital or by the local authority under the court's inherent jurisdiction, or through a specific issue order asking for clarification of their legal position in undertaking treatment.

Such an issue came before the courts in the case of *Re S (a minor)* ([1993] 1 FLR 376). A $4^1/2$-year-old child was suffering from T-cell leukaemia with a high risk that death would occur. Chemotherapy was offered but this required a blood transfusion. S's parents, who were dedicated Jehovah's Witnesses, refused to consent to the treatment. The local authority went to court and asked for an order under its inherent jurisdiction and the parents asked for a prohibited steps order. In authorising treatment, Thorpe J. noted that the parents' refusal of treatment would deny their son the 50% chance of survival that was offered by the therapy. It had been suggested that one reason why treatment should not be given was that the child would have to live for years to come with parents who 'believed that his life was prolonged through an ungodly act'. Thorpe J. recognised that by providing the child with a transfusion there was a further risk of conflict between child and parent. However, as the judge said: 'The reality seems to me that family reactions will recognise that the responsibility of consent was taken from them, and as a judicial act, absolved their conscience of responsibility.'

In the case of *Re O (a minor) (Medical Treatment)* ([1993] 2 FLR 149), a baby was born prematurely. The child suffered from a respiratory distress syndrome, which meant that she would require a blood transfusion. The parents were Jehovah's Witnesses and were opposed to the transfusion. Other options were tried but it was realised that a blood transfusion was inevitable. The inherent jurisdiction of the High Court was invoked. Johnson J. gave directions to the effect that if medical advice deemed it necessary the child should be given a blood transfusion.

A contrasting case provides an illustration of judicial willingness to support a parent's decision to refuse treatment. In *Re T* ([1997] 1WLR 242), a child was born with a liver defect that was life-threatening. An operation had initially been carried out on the child at the age of $3^1/2$ months that had been unsuccessful and had resulted in the child suffering a great deal of pain. The child then needed a liver transplant. At the time of the hearing both child and parents were in a foreign country. The parents, who were health-care professionals, were opposed to the treatment being undertaken. The mother did not want the child to undergo the suffering that this procedure would involve. The operation was not available in the Commonwealth country where the treatment was being given and, had an order been made, the parents would have had to bring the child back to this country for treatment.

At first instance, the judge held that leave should be given to the health professionals to perform the operation despite parental opposition. In the Court of Appeal this order was reversed. Butler Sloss L.J. examined a number of cases involving the decision to treat the incompetent minor. She noted the exceptional nature of this case and stated that:

> " This mother and child are one for the purpose of this unusual case and the decision of the court to consent to the operation jointly affects the mother and son and it also affects the father. The welfare of this child depends upon his mother.

The decision of the Court of Appeal in *Re T* has proved controversial. The court placed great weight on the views of the parents. This case may appear to run contrary to a number of cases concerning refusal of treatment by parents on religious grounds, where the views of the parents have been overridden by the courts. Emphasis was placed upon the fact that the parents were health professionals. Does this place the opinions of such parents in a special category apart from those of parents generally – even where the parents possess deep religious convictions? While the decision of the Court of Appeal in *Re T* has attracted considerable public attention its wider implications remain to be assessed. In *Re T* the court stressed the unusual nature of this case and the close emotional attachment that existed between the mother and baby. It may be speculated as to whether the location of the parties may have had some influence on the ultimate decision reached, as the parents were abroad at the time. There are a number of cases in which the court has granted orders allowing active treatment to be withheld from newly born infants and these cases are explored in Chapter 12 below.

An illustration of some of the difficult issues which may arise in the context of parental treatment refusal was provided by the case of. *Re C (HIV Test)* ([1999] 2 FLR 1004). Here the parents of a 4-month-old baby refused to have the child tested for HIV. The mother was HIV-positive, although the father had tested negative. The parents were opposed to the testing. They said that the child was healthy and they wanted to they decide what was in her best interests.. They were both alternative health practitioners and were sceptical regarding conventional medical treatment. The mother was breast-feeding the baby. The judge held that he was prepared to sanction the test and that here there was an 'overwhelming case' for the baby to be tested. The order applied only to testing and the local authority would be required to return for a further order in relation to treatment. The Council had not sought an order preventing the mother from breast-feeding. Mr Justice Wilson was of the view that had such an order been sought it would have been unenforceable. As he stated: 'My belief is that the law cannot come between the baby and the breast'. The parents sought leave to appeal but their application was dismissed. They had argued that the judge should have evaluated why they were critical of the use of orthodox clinical approaches to HIV, that parents in a developing area of medicine such as this should be given certain clinical autonomy and that the court should not intervene with this. The Court of Appeal rejected the appeal. They held that there was strong medical evidence that the child was at risk of harm unless the test was undertaken. Moreover the court could overrule the decision of a parent even though this decision might be reasonable.

Article 8 of the European Convention of Human Rights, which concerns the right to privacy of home and family life and includes a right to autonomy, may be used in such cases under the Human Rights Act 1998. The extent to which this provision will be successfully used to alter the judicial approach in cases such as *Re C (HIV Test)* has been questioned. (Grubb 2000). Grubb has suggested that 'it would, however, require a substantial "U-turn" in judicial behaviour and inclination and would contradict the philosophy of the Children Act which sees the child's welfare as paramount' (s.1(1)). It is submitted that this is the better view and that, unless there is a radical recon-ception of the role of parent's rights in treatment decision making, successful use of Article 8 is somewhat unlikely.

Parental conflict and the conjoined twins case

A notable case concerning the issue of parental decision making and children is that of *Re A* in 2000 4 All ER 961. Here conjoined twins were born in St Mary's Hospital Manchester to parents who came from the island of Gozo, Malta. The surgeons sought to separate the twins. The consequence of the separation operation was that the weaker twin, 'Mary', would die but it would be likely that the stronger twin, 'Jodie', would survive and have a good quality of life. The parents, who were devout Roman Catholics, were opposed to the surgery going ahead. Ultimately the Court of Appeal sanctioned the surgery. The judgments are complex to interpret as different approaches were taken by different members of the Court of Appeal. The case was determined by reference to principles of family law, health-care law and criminal law.

The Court of Appeal considered whether the operation could be seen as being in the best interests of Mary, the weaker twin. Two members of the Court of Appeal were of the view that separation would not be in Mary's best interests, although one member, Robert Walker L.J., supported the view that the operation would be in her best interests because to continue her life for 'a few months' would not be to confer any advantage. One difficulty facing them was that the result of ordering the surgery would be for Mary to die – would that then contravene criminal law? The Court of Appeal held that the operation to separate the twins could not be classed withdrawal of treatment amounting to an omission – the approach that had been taken by the House of Lords in the *Bland* case (discussed in Ch. 10). This meant that the surgery would constitute murder unless there was some defence. Brooke L.J. held that the surgery was supported under the doctrine of necessity;

Walker L.J. agreed but also suggested that it could be supported under the doctrine of double effect. Ward L.J. rather saw this in terms of 'quasi' self-defence. He commented that there was:

" no difference in essence between that resort to legitimate self-defence and the doctors coming to Jodie's defence and removing the threat of fatal harm to her presented by Mary's draining her life blood.

Although this case is obviously an emotive one, and one that at the time gave rise to considerable discussion both in the media and in the academic literature, it is suggested that in the future the impact of this decision is likely to be limited, because of the exceptional nature of the facts in this case, to further cases concerning separation of conjoined twins.

Compelling treatment

What if the parents and the health-care professionals disagree as to a particular course of treatment in a situation in which the parents want the treatment carried out but the professionals are opposed? This issue has arisen in relation to end-of-life decision making and is discussed more extensively in Chapter 10. However here we should note the case of *Glass* v. *UK* [2004] 1 FLR 1019. This case arose as a result of a dispute of treatment of a child who, at the time of the incidents that led to the litigation, was 12 years old. Following a respiratory tract infection David Glass, who has severe disabilities, was being treated in hospital. The doctors treating him were of the view that further treatment was hopeless, issued a Do Not Resuscitate order without informing his mother and sought to administer diamorphine without parental consent. This led to violent incidents in the hospital that led subsequently to litigation. The Trust informed the parents that they would not further pursue life-sustaining treatment and advised them to seek treatment in another local hospital. This led to litigation in the English courts where the family were not successful (see discussion in Chapter 10); however, their action before the European Court of Human Rights (ECHR) succeeded. The ECHR held that treatment here in the face of parental opposition without having obtained judicial sanction constituted a violation of Article 8 of the European Convention on Human Rights. It is interesting to note that in 2004, the year of the ECHR judgment, David Glass turned 18. Thus, if there is a dispute between parents and medical staff as to the legitimacy of a particular course of treatment which has life-threatening consequences, and it is proposed to treat or not continue to treat in the face of parental opposition, then a court order should be sought. In practice, application can be made very swiftly to a judge sitting in chambers.

Disagreement between the parents

Tom wants his 18-month-old son Jack to be given the MMR injection; his wife Lisa refuses. She says that she is frightened of the risk of autism. Can Tom compel Jack to have the injection?

This is a situation concerning married parents and thus both have decision-making authority in law – but what should happen if they disagree? This issue arose in the case of *Re C* ([2003] 2 FLR 678). Here a dispute arose between parents in two couples over the administration of the MMR vaccine. The court was prepared to order that the children should be given the vaccine.

In contrast, in *Re J* ([2000] FLR 571), the father, who was a Muslim, wanted his 5-year-old son circumcised, while the mother, who was a Christian, was opposed. The father did not actively observe many of the religious practices of his faith and the mother was a non-practising Christian. Here the Court of Appeal refused to order the surgery. In delivering judgment the President, Dame Elizabeth Butler–Sloss, held that there were a number of decisions that, where there are two persons with parental responsibility, should not be arranged by a one-parent carer. She gave as an example sterilisation and stated that the decision to circumcise a child on religious grounds also came within this category. Again, should a dispute arise in such a situation the matter should be referred to the court for resolution prior to the treatment going ahead.

When can treatment be given in the face of a child's refusal?

> Parents bring their son to be vaccinated. The boy goes into the treatment room but then begins to scream and refuses to let the nurse touch him. Can he be compelled to have the injection?

In the case of a very young child, while actually giving this injection may not be very easy, in strict law the parent may consent to treatment despite the child's refusal. However, in practice, the nurse may suggest to the parents that s/he does not go ahead at that time but that they bring the child back another day. Difficult issues arise in relation to older children who are assessed as *Gillick*-competent. Such a child may be able to consent to medical treatment but what if s/he refuses? Can treatment be given and if so on what basis? In the professional role as patient advocate the nurse is required to respect the autonomy of his/her patient, which includes providing support for a patient who decides to refuse treatment or decides that treatment should be withdrawn. Nonetheless it has been noted that in law the power of the adult patient to refuse treatment is not unlimited (Ch. 5). As far as the child patient is concerned, it is clearly the case that the right to refuse treatment is again not absolute. It is also likely that where a child refuses treatment this will mean that, as with the adult patient, a more rigorous assessment is made of that child's competence.

The Court of Appeal has indicated that, if a competent child refuses treatment, his/her parents may override this refusal. In *Re R* ([1991] 4 All ER 177 CA) Lord Donaldson said that the fact that a child was competent to consent to treatment did not mean that all parental rights were removed. Once a child reaches maturity s/he receives a key to the door of treatment. However, the child's parents have keys and they keep the key once the child gains maturity. A parent can authorise treatment even though the child refuses. Lord Donaldson's words in that case were obiter and the other members of the Court of Appeal did not agree with his approach.

However, in the later case of *Re W* ([1992] 3 WLR 758) the Court of Appeal confirmed that the parents could lawfully override the refusal of a competent child. This case concerned an anorexic 16-year-old girl who opposed removal to a treatment centre where it was likely that an active treatment regime would be imposed. The court held that, although she was competent to consent to treatment, her refusal could be overridden. Lord Donaldson moved away from the keyholder analogy and instead said that a doctor acquires a legal 'flak jacket' as protection from being sued when he receives consent from a child over 16, a *Gillick*-competent child or a person with parental responsibility. He went on to say:

    " No minor of whatever age has power by refusing consent to treatment to override a consent to treatment by someone who has parental responsibility for the minor. Nevertheless such a refusal was a very important consideration in making clinical judgments and for parents and the court in deciding themselves whether to give consent.

The judgment in this case was contrary to general opinion as to the interpretation of the *Gillick* case and the Family Law Reform Act 1969. However, at present, even if a *Gillick*-competent child refuses medical treatment it appears that his/her parents may override the refusal. However, the court in *Re W* suggested that before a major surgical procedure is undertaken on a child against his/her will it is desirable for the issue to be referred to the court. The court would then determine what is in the child's best interests, taking into account the child's expressed wishes and the strength of the child's beliefs. It may be, for example, that while a child has strong convictions at present, this may be only a passing phase. The urgency of the treatment is also a relevant factor.

In *Re W* Nolan L.J. suggested that the court could intervene where the child's welfare was 'threatened by serious and imminent risk that the child will suffer grave and irreversible mental or physical harm', while Balcombe L.J. stated that the court should only intervene where refusal would lead to the child's death.

Children were given certain statutory rights to refuse court-ordered assessment and treatment under the Children Act 1989. This may seem rather at odds with the approach of the courts in *Re R* and *Re W*. However, in the case of *South Glamorgan CC v. W and B* ([1993] 1 FLR 574) the court confirmed that a court still possessed certain residual powers under its inherent jurisdiction to override a child's refusal. The decision in this case has been criticised on the basis that it goes against clear words of statute.

Authorisation of treatment in the face of a child's opposition may also give rise to problems as to the relationship between the powers to compulsorily treat under the Mental Health Act 1983 (which will be considered later) and the powers at common law. In *Re K, W and H (minors) (Medical Treatment)* ([1993] FLR 584), advance parental consent was required before children were admitted for treatment in a specialist psychiatric institution. Three children were admitted. They later complained as to their treatment, including the administration of emergency medication. An action was brought before the court under section 8 of the Children Act 1989 to clarify the legality of the treatment of these three children. Two were 15 years old and were suffering from unsocialised adolescent conduct disorder; the other child, who was almost 15 years, was suffering from bipolar affective disorder. Thorpe J. said that none of the children was *Gillick*-competent but that, even if they were, the doctor had received parental authorisation of treatment in the form of the advance consents before they had entered the psychiatric institution and thus was justified in law in going ahead and providing treatment. He commented that a specific issue order to authorise treatment under section 8 of the Children Act 1989 was not required where parental consent existed. The difficulty with such an approach is that it denies children the safeguards in the form of the statutory provisions limiting provision of treatment contained in the Mental Health Act 1983 (Bate 1994).

In *Re M* ([1999] 2 FLR 1097), a 15-year-old girl required a heart transplant without which she was likely to die within the week. M refused consent and claimed that she did not want to follow the long postoperative course of therapy with a daily course of tablets for the rest of her life and that she would rather die than live on with the heart of another person inside her. Johnson J. in the Family Division held that M was in effect incompetent. He commented, 'events have overtaken M so swiftly that she has not been able to come to terms with her situation'. While there were consequent risks in the heart transplant operation itself being undertaken, as Johnson J. noted these were overridden by what was otherwise the certainty that in this situation M would die.

Refusal of treatment – the 'competent' minor and the Human Rights Act 1998

Does the Human Rights Act 1998 have the potential to change the situation here (Garwood-Gowers 2001, McHale & Gallagher 2004)? Three rights under the European Convention on Human Rights may be potentially relevant. First, it could be argued that enforced treatment would violate Article 3, the prohibition on torture and inhuman and degrading treatment. Second, it can be argued that ordering an adolescent to be treated against his/her will would contravene Article 8, the right to privacy and autonomy of the person. Third, if the reason why the adolescent was proposing to reject the treatment was on the basis of religious or cultural beliefs, this could be seen as violating Article 9, the right to respect for religious and cultural beliefs. It remains to be seen how successful such a claim would be, and indeed it should be noted that Articles 8 and 9 are qualified rights and subject to other public interest considerations.

While certain powers are given to courts and parents to override the decisions of competent children, these powers should be used only in exceptional circumstances. Generally it is not clinically beneficial to treat a child where s/he is objecting, particularly where this involves detention against his/her will.

Refusal of treatment by both children and parents

What if both parents and child patient are in agreement in their opposition to treatment and emphasise that this is on religious grounds? In such a situation the consequences of refusal of treatment should be clearly explained to the child. Dilemmas may arise, however, where that refusal is likely to result in the patient's death. It may be the case that the child's will is being overborne, but equally the child may have a fundamental religious belief and have reached his/her own decision to refuse treatment on the basis of that belief. In such a situation where refusal of treatment would have the consequence that death would result, an application to the court would be appropriate, to ask for the authorisation of treatment.

This issue came before the courts in the case of *Re E (minor) (Wardship: Medical Treatment)* ([1993] 1 FLR 386). A was $15^3/_4$ years old and was suffering from leukaemia. A's parents were devout Jehovah's Witnesses, and both A and his parents were opposed to a blood transfusion. Consent was given to therapy that avoided a blood transfusion but only had a 40–50% chance of full remission, as opposed to 80–90% had treatment that involved a blood transfusion been given. The health authority made an application to the court when it became apparent that within a matter of hours blood platelet levels would fall to unacceptable levels and A was at risk of a stroke or heart attack. The judge, Ward J., stated that, although A was a calm and intelligent person, in his view he did not really understand the implications of his decision.

" I am quite satisfied that A does not have any sufficient comprehension of the pain he has yet to suffer, of the fear that he will be undergoing, of the distress not only occasioned by that fear but also – and more importantly – the distress he will inevitably suffer as he, a loving son, helplessly watches his parents' and his family's distress. They are a close family and a brave family, but I find that he has no realisation of the full implications that lie before him as to the process of dying.

While noting A's religious convictions he stated:

" I respect this boy's profession of faith but I cannot discount at least the possibility that he may in later years suffer some diminution in his convictions. There is no settled certainty about matters of this kind.

In *Re L (Medical Treatment: Gillick Competency)* ([1998] 2 FLR 810), L was a Jehovah's witness who was 14 years of age. She refused a blood transfusion, both orally and also by having executed a blood transfusion card. L fell into a bath of hot water and suffered severe scalds. 54% of her body surface was covered with severe burns. 40% were third-degree burns. Surgery was necessary to save her life – she required a blood transfusion. The hospital authority obtained an application under the inherent jurisdiction to administer blood and blood products as necessary during treatment without L's consent. Sir Stephen Brown stated that L lacked *Gillick* competence. She had not been informed by her family or by the doctors as to the distressing nature of her death. He held that here:

" It may be that because of her belief she is willing to say, and to mean it, 'I am willing to accept death rather than to have a blood transfusion', but it is clear that she has not been able to be given all the details which it would be right and appropriate to have in mind when making a decision.

This type of case poses difficult questions. In *Re L* the patient had not been appraised of all the circumstances when making the decision and the court's decision in that case reflects that fact. It is also the case that the patient's perception of the situation may alter consequent upon treatment. However while the patient's views may very well change, equally they may not. The minor in *Re E* died subsequently when, on reaching the age of 18 years, he refused treatment.

Seeking treatment and care when a child is being neglected or put at risk

A health visitor believes that a child is being neglected by his parents or that he is being abused. What can the health visitor do? His/her actions will obviously depend upon the gravity of the situation and the child's need for immediate care. If a child is suffering from a particular medical condition and it is believed that the child still needs care, what can be done? In this situation the matter should be referred to Social Services. All local authorities and county councils have child protection policies, which should be consulted by health-care professionals. The local authority may decide to instigate an investigation. The health visitor would be consulted while any investigation was being undertaken. Measures may be taken to bring the child under the care or supervision of the local authority. These are matters that go beyond the scope of this book and readers are referred to specialist texts on the subject.

TREATING THE MENTALLY ILL PATIENT

In Chapter 5 the question of treatment of mentally incompetent patients was examined. Here, the question of treatment of the mentally ill patient is considered. Mental illness and mental incompetence should not be equated. A mentally ill person may be perfectly competent to consent to involvement in some clinical procedures, for example involvement in clinical research, even though s/he has diminished competence in relation to other matters.

It is important for the nurse to be aware of the operation of the Mental Health Act 1983, not only if s/he intends to specialise in mental health nursing but also because issues involving treatment of the mentally ill arise in a wide variety of nursing situations. The nurse should also be aware of the Mental Health Act Code of Practice. This is not legally binding but provides an indication of good practice. For fuller discussion of this area the reader is referred to specialist texts dealing with mental health law (Gostin, 1985; Dimond & Barker, 1996; Hogget 1996; Bartlett & Sandland 2003). We are focusing on treatment given after detention under civil law power. Powers of detention are also available in the context of the criminal law.

Admission into hospital for treatment

A mentally disordered patient may be informally admitted to a hospital for psychiatric treatment in the same way as a patient may consent to enter hospital for any operation (*R* v. *Kirklees MBC ex parte C* [1993] 2 FLR 187). Such a patient may refuse any treatment and may leave hospital freely at any time (s131 Mental Health Act 1983). Any attempt to detain the patient may lead to a civil law claim for damages for false imprisonment. It appears that the use of 'constraints' such as special locks on doors to prevent patients wandering out on to the street is lawful (Hoggett 1996). However, as Hoggett notes 'consideration should be given to "sectioning" people who persistently and purposefully try to leave' (p. 143).

The scope of this section was considered further by the House of Lords in *R v. Bournewood NHS Trust ex parte L* ([1998] 3 All ER 289). L was a 48-year-old man with learning disabilities. He was living with paid carers in a 'family' situation. He attended a day centre. One day L was in a seriously agitated state. The carers could not be contacted and a local doctor gave him a sedative; he was taken to the Accident and Emergency unit at the local hospital. There he was assessed by a psychiatrist as requiring detention. He was admitted informally. The issue that arose was whether this informal admission was lawful. The House of Lords rejected the argument that he was unlawfully detained. Admission here did not amount to a deprivation of his liberty. His treatment in hospital was also held to be justified under the common law doctrine of necessity. This decision was challenged before the ECHR in *HL v. UK* ((2004) Application No. 45508/99). The ECHR confirmed that the decision was in violation of Article 5(1) of the European Convention on Human Rights – the right to liberty and security of the person – and constituted unlawful deprivation of his liberty. They were concerned at the lack of formal protection where detention was sanctioned under the common law doctrine of necessity in contrast to the detailed procedures and safeguards that existed under the Mental Health Act 1983. This absence of procedural safeguards failed to protect against arbitrary deprivation of liberty and thus amounted to a violation of Article 5(1). Although it was possible to challenge the detention through judicial review/habeas corpus – as discussed below – this would simply give the courts a power of review and that was not sufficient to ensure that the applicant had a procedure to challenge the detention that complied with Article 5(4) of the European Convention on Human Rights. Following the ECHR decision the government indicated that it would bring forward proposals to deal with this issue (Department of Health 2005).

Although wherever possible, preference should be given to informal admission in some situations it is necessary to compulsorily admit a patient. Considered first below is the basis on which a patient can be brought from the community into hospital and given treatment and second, the grounds for detaining a patient who is presently in a hospital on an informal basis.

Emergency removal under the Mental Health Act 1983

The Mental Health Act 1983 contains emergency powers enabling a person to be removed to hospital for treatment. Section 135 of the Act provides that a magistrate may authorise a warrant allowing a police officer to gain entry to premises and remove a person to a 'place of safety'. The warrant will be granted if a magistrate is satisfied that the person is suffering from mental disorder and 'has been or is being ill-treated, neglected or kept otherwise than under proper control, or is living alone and is unable to care for themselves'. When entering premises the Act requires a police officer to be accompanied by an approved social worker and a doctor. A person may only be detained under section 135 for up to 72 hours. After this point any continued detention must be authorised under one of the other powers contained in the Mental Health Act 1983.

Power of police to remove a person found in a public place

A man is found wandering in the street showing clear signs of mental disorder. If a policeman believes that the man is in immediate need of care/control, he may remove him to a 'place of safety', such as a hospital, for up to 72 hours (s136 Mental Health Act 1983). The powers under section 136 apply to 'any place to which the public has access'. They enable an individual to be examined by a doctor and interviewed by an approved social worker as a preliminary to providing care or admission to hospital for treatment under the Mental Health Act 1983. The operation of this section has come under considerable criticism, with claims that the section has been inadequately supervised, with details of patients admitted under the section being inadequately recorded.

At present, if a person opposes removal from his/her home and treatment is needed, there is no alternative but forcible removal to hospital under the Mental Health Act 1983.

Admission for assessment

Section 2 of the Mental Health Act 1983 allows a patient to be admitted for 'assessment'. Section 2 applies to patients suffering from a mental disorder justifying detention in hospital at least for a limited period. It must also be shown that detention is needed in the interests of the patient's own health and safety or to protect others. The application must be made by the patient's 'nearest relative' or by an approved social worker. The approved social worker should inform the nearest relative that an application is being made (s11(3)). The application must be supported by two doctors, one of whom must have been approved by the Secretary of State as having special experience in the treatment of mental disorder. The 'nearest relative' is defined in the Act as being the relative who usually lives with that patient or the person with the closest connection as determined in relation to a long list of relatives – in order of priority. The approved social worker is a social worker appointed to work under the Mental Health Act. Section 2 is intended to provide a short-term detention with the limited purpose of determining suitability for continued assessment (*R* v. *Wilson and Williamson* [1995] *The Independent* 19 April). Admission under this section is for a period of up to 28 days. This is a one-off admission, as the period cannot be renewed.

'Mental disorder' under this section is defined as 'mental illness, arrested or incomplete development of mind, psychopathic disorder and any other disability of mind' (s1(2)). The Act does not define mental illness but the courts have indicated that it should be given its ordinary meaning (*W* v. *L* [1974] QB 711). This is commonly known as 'the man must be mad' test (Hoggett, 1996). The definition of mental disorder expressly excludes sexual deviations and alcoholism (s1(3) Mental Health Act 1983). 'Psychopathic disorder' refers to a disorder/disability of mind (whether or not including significant impairment of intelligence) resulting in abnormally aggressive or seriously irresponsible conduct.

Admission for treatment

A person may be admitted for treatment for longer periods under section 3 of the Mental Health Act 1983. Application for admission under this section may be made by the same persons as under section 2. It must be shown that the patient is suffering from 'mental illness, severe mental impairment, psychopathic disorder or mental impairment' (s 3(2)). Mental impairment refers to arrested/incomplete mental development, including significant impairment of intelligence/social functioning and associated with abnormally aggressive/seriously irresponsible conduct. The condition must be of a nature such that it is appropriate for the patient to receive treatment in a hospital.

Where treatment is sought for psychopathic disorder or mental impairment it must be shown that the treatment is likely to alleviate or prevent deterioration in the patient's condition, although it is not necessary to show that it would provide a guaranteed cure. Treatment may include nursing and rehabilitation, including group therapy, which could result in the patient being rendered more cooperative (*R* v. *Canons Park Mental Health Review Tribunal Ex parte A* ([1994] 1 All ER 481). In addition, treatment may also include that which alleviates the symptoms of a disorder rather than alleviating the disorder itself (*Reid* v. *Secretary of State for Scotland* [1999] 1 All ER 481). Finally, it must be shown that admission is necessary for the patient's health and safety or for the protection of other persons and that necessary treatment cannot be given unless the patient is detained under this section. Admission under section 3 allows the patient to be detained for up to 6 months. This period can be renewed, initially for 6 months, then on an annual basis.

Emergency power – section 4

In an emergency a patient can be admitted under section 4 of the Mental Health Act 1983 if one doctor certifies that s/he is suffering from 'mental disorder'. The doctor should, if possible, already know the patient. A doctor who certifies admission under section 4 does not have to be a specialist in mental illness. The person making the application should have examined the patient in the previous 24 hours. Section 4 allows detention for up to a maximum of 72 hours. This period can be extended by conversion into 'admission for assessment' under section 2.

Detaining a patient in hospital

In some situations it becomes obvious that a patient receiving care in hospital on a voluntary basis requires compulsory detention. The Mental Health Act 1983 contains powers to allow a patient to be detained to enable assessment of whether prolonged detention is necessary. One of these powers applies expressly to the nurse. Section 5(4) of the Mental Health Act 1983 gives the nurse power to detain an inpatient if the nurse is of the view that the patient is suffering from a mental disorder to such a degree that it is necessary for the patient to be immediately restrained from leaving hospital, and a doctor is unable to examine the patient at that time.

The power applies to nurses on part 3 or part 5 or parts 13 or 14 of the statutory Register (part 3 includes first-level nurses trained in nursing people suffering from mental illness; part 5 first-level nurses trained in nursing those with learning disabilities; part 13 nurses who have obtained qualifications after following a course of mental health nursing; and part 14 those qualified from a course of learning disabilities nursing (Mental Health Nurses Order 1998, SI 1998/265)). If the nurse decides to exercise this power s/he must record this fact in writing. Detention under section 5(4) is limited to 6 hours or to the point at which the doctor can see the patient. This is an important power – and one the nurse should use with discretion. There is a danger that, as Unsworth notes, the nurse may be seen as 'gaoler' rather than carer (Unsworth 1987).

The Mental Health Act Code of Practice sets out a number of criteria which a nurse should take into account before exercising power under section 5(4) (para 9.2). The nurse should consider:

a. the likely arrival time of the doctor as against the likely intention of the patient to leave. Most patients who express a wish to leave hospital can be persuaded to wait until a doctor arrives to discuss it further. Where this is not possible, the nurse must try to predict the impact of any delay upon the patient.

b. the consequences of a patient leaving hospital immediately – the harm that might occur to the patient or others – taking into account:

- the patient's expressed intentions including the likelihood of the patient committing self-harm or suicide
- any evidence of disordered thinking
- the patient's current behaviour and in particular any changes in usual behaviour
- likelihood of the patient behaving in a violent manner
- any recently received messages from relatives or friends
- any recent disturbance on the ward
- any relevant involvement of other patients.

c. the patient's known unpredictability and any other relevant information from other members of the multidisciplinary team.

Code of Practice, para 9.2

The wording of section 5(4) appears to assume that a nurse should complete the forms before detaining the patient. But does this mean that the patient cannot be detained until the forms have been completed? The question is not expressly dealt with in the 1983 Act. At common law there were powers allowing the insane to be arrested. It is uncertain how far these powers still exist, though (*Black* v. *Forsey* (1988) *The Times*, 21 May). Although, as we saw above, the House of Lords in *R* v. *Bournewood NHS Trust ex parte L* ([1998] 3 All ER) confirmed that informal powers of detention may be used, a different approach was taken in *HL* v. *UK* in the ECHR. This issue thus still requires resolution.

The section requires that detention must be authorised by a suitably qualified nurse – a RMN or a RNMH. But what if there are no suitably qualified nurses on the ward? The Code of Practice provides, that if it is likely that section 5(4) might be used, then 'they should ensure that suitable arrangements are in place for a suitably qualified nurse to be available should the power need to be invoked'.

The holding power under section 5(4) applies for a maximum of 6 hours.

Detention may be authorised under section 5(2) by a doctor. The doctor must provide the hospital managers with a report as to why s/he believes that the patient's detention is required. Once the managers have obtained a copy of the report then detention can be authorised for a period of up to 72 hours. It should be noted that this power applies to inpatients as opposed to patients simply visiting the hospital for treatment. It should be noted that, while section 5(2) powers can be applied to any inpatient as long as the relevant criteria are satisfied, section 5(4) can be used by a nurse only in relation to a patient receiving treatment as an inpatient for a mental disorder.

It should be emphasised that sections 5(4) and 5(2) are holding powers to allow detention and assessment prior to possible authorisation of longer detention under one of the other provisions of the 1983 Act.

Providing the patient with information

A detained patient must be given information enabling her/him to understand the grounds for and conditions for detention (s132 Mental Health Act 1983). This duty is one that is likely to be delegated to the nurse. The patient must be informed of what provisions of the Mental Health Act 1983 s/he is being detained under, the right to apply to a mental health tribunal for discharge and how certain provisions of the Mental Health Act 1983, such as those relating to consent to treatment, affect her/him (s132 Mental Health Act 1983). This information must be given as soon as it is reasonably practicable to do so after detention has begun. Good practice dictates that the information should be given both orally and in writing. There should be a procedure in existence stating who should give the information to the patient.

Treatment of the detained patient

The Mental Health Act 1983 only regulates treatment given for the patient's mental disorder (s63); a mentally disordered person may still have capacity to give consent or refusal to other types of treatment. 'Treatment' includes medication and nursing care but may also extend to, for instance, feeding if the patient's mental illness leads to the refusal of food (*B* v. *Croyden HA* [1995] 1 All ER 683; *R* v. *Collins ex parte Brady* [2000] Lloyds Rep Med 355). It has been suggested that the definition of mental illness includes anorexia nervosa (*Riverside Mental Health Trust* v. *Fox* [1994] 2 *Med Law Review* 95). The section also applies to any mental disorder and is not restricted to the disorder in relation to which the patient has been initially detained (*R (on the application of B)* v. *Ashworth Hospital Authority* [2005] UKHL 20). There has been judicial criticism of the use of this section in relation to the authorisation of a caesarean section upon a protesting patient (*St George's NHS Trust v. S* [1998] 3 All ER 673 and see Ch. 9). It should be noted that, even where a patient may be compelled to receive medication within 3 months under section 63, every attempt must be made to obtain his/her consent.

Psychosurgery/surgical implantation of hormones

Section 57 sets out a special procedure for psychosurgery and for other procedures governed by regulations, including the surgical implantation of hormones. The patient must consent to the administration of this treatment. In addition, a second-opinion-approved doctor appointed by the Secretary of State and two other persons appointed by the Mental Health Act Commission must have 'certified in writing that the patient is capable of understanding the nature, purpose and likely effects of the treatment in question and has consented to it' (s57(2)(a)). One of these persons must be a nurse and the other should be neither a nurse or doctor.

The second-opinion-approved doctor is appointed for these purposes by the body which regulates the conduct of the Mental Health Act, the Mental Health Commission. The doctor must also certify that 'having regard to the likelihood of the treatment alleviating or preventing a deterioration of the patient's condition the treatment should be given' (s57(2)(b)). These safeguards apply both to patients detained under the Mental Health Act 1983 and to informal patients.

Electroconvulsive therapy and administration of medicines after 3 months

The administration of medicines and electroconvulsive therapy (ECT) is governed by section 58 of the 1983 Act. ECT may be appropriate, for instance, if a patient suffers from severe depression. As far as the administration of medicines is concerned, once 3 months have passed from the point when the patient was first admitted and given treatment for his/her mental disorder, special authorisation is required before the nurse may continue to administer any medicines. Before ECT is given or medicines are administered after 3 months, one of two additional criteria must be satisfied. Either the patient must consent, with this consent being verified by the practitioner treating the patient, or, if the patient refuses consent, treatment may still be given if authorised by a second-opinion-approved doctor but only if it is a 'medical or therapeutic necessity'. Unless that is shown then the treatment may constitute a violation of Article 3 of the European Convention on Human Rights – the prohibition on torture and inhuman and degrading treatment (*R (Wilkinson)* v. *Broadmoor Special Hospital Authority* [2002] 1 WLR 419). To comply with the Human Rights Act the standard is that it must be 'convincingly shown that it is a medical or therapeutic necessity' (*R (N)* v. *M and others* [2003] 1 WLR 562.)

The doctor must state that either the patient is not competent because s/he cannot understand the nature, purpose or likely effects of treatment or that, although the patient is competent and is refusing treatment, in view of the likelihood of it alleviating or preventing a deterioration in the patient's condition treatment should be given (s58(3)(b)). In forming his or her opinion, the second-opinion-approved doctor should also consult two other persons professionally involved in that person's care. The statute requires that at least one of these persons is a nurse (s58(4)). The grade of nurse is not specified. Again, the other person must be neither nurse nor doctor (s58(4)).

Treatment under sections 57 and 58 should be the subject of regular review. It should be noted that consents here are not always required on each separate occasion: it is sufficient that the consents relate to the overall plan of care (s.59).

Treating in an emergency

In an emergency the safeguards contained in section 57 and section 58 may be bypassed under section 62 of the Act. Treatment may be given, first, if it is immediately necessary to save the patient's life. Second, treatment that is not irreversible may be given to alleviate serious suffering by the patient. Third, treatment that is immediately necessary and represents the minimum interference necessary to prevent the patient from behaving violently or being a danger to him/herself or others may be given if it is not irreversible or hazardous in nature. 'Irreversible' is defined as treatment entailing unfavourable physical or psychological consequences. 'Hazardous' refers to treatment that entails significant physical hazard. Gunn & Rodgers (2000) have suggested that those situations in which treatment may be given lawfully under this section are likely to be exceedingly limited. It is difficult to see how the performance of psychosurgery or surgical implantation of hormones can be justified in an emergency. Medication can, in any case, be given in the absence of the patient's consent within 3 months of a person first receiving medication for mental disorder during any continuous period of detention within 3 months of a person being sectioned. The only situation in which Gunn & Rodgers (2000) envisage use of section 62 is in an emergency to give ECT to a patient who is in a catatonic stupor and who might otherwise die.

It has been claimed that in some instances treatment given under section 62 has extended beyond what is justifiable within the provisions of the section. For example, there have been three reported cases in Broadmoor special hospital where patients have died following doses of antipsychotic medication in excess of the guide produced jointly by the British Medical Association and the Royal Pharmaceutical Society of Great Britain (Fennell 1994). A nurse who believes that the criteria laid down in the Mental Health Act 1983 are not being followed should make his/her concerns known to those who authorised this treatment. If necessary, the nurse should inform the line manager. Where an abuse has occurred, the line manager should inform the hospital authorities and make the Mental Health Act Commission aware of the situation. (See also the discussion on whistleblowing in Ch. 7.)

Use of seclusion

The use of seclusion in mental hospitals came under scrutiny in the report into the abuses of mentally ill patients at Ashworth special hospital. Seclusion is defined in the Mental Health Code of Practice as: 'the supervised confinement of a patient in a room which may be locked for the protection of others from significant harm' (para 19.16). The Code of Practice emphasises that it must be used as a last resort and for the shortest time possible. It should also not be used as punishment/threat or as part of a treatment programme, as a measure because of staff shortages or where there is any risk of suicide or of self-harm.

The precise legality of seclusion is unclear. It may be lawful because it is the application of reasonable force which amounts to self-defence.

The Code of Practice provides that the nurse in charge of the ward may impose seclusion on a patient but where this is done a doctor should be immediately called. A number of criteria must be fulfilled. First, a nurse should be within sight and sound of the place where the patient is being held and should be present if the patient has been sedated (para 19.19). Second, the patient should be observed and a documented report should be made every 15 minutes as to whether seclusion is necessary (para 19.20). Third, if seclusion is continued then two nurses in the seclusion room should undertake a review every 2 hours and a doctor should review every 4 hours. Where the seclusion has continued for more than 8 hours consecutively or for more than 12 hours intermittently over 48 hours an independent review is required. This should be undertaken by a consultant 'or other doctor of suitable seniority' and a team of nurses and other health professionals, none of whom had been involved in the care of the patient when the original seclusion was undertaken (para 19;22).

Transfer

A patient detained under the Mental Health Act 1983 may be transferred to another unit managed by a different NHS trust or to a registered mental nursing home registered to take detained patients.

Discharging the patient

The period of detention may come to an end or the patient may leave as a result of being discharged. A trust or authority can discharge any patient who has been admitted for assessment or treatment at any time (s.23). The decision to discharge is to be taken by a committee of three persons (s24(4)(5)). The nearest relative may also apply to the hospital for the patient's discharge (s23(2)(a)) and must give notice in writing (s.25). The patient has the right to apply for discharge to a mental health review tribunal (s.66). In addition, an automatic reference will be made to a tribunal if the patient has not exercised the right to apply during the first 6 months of detention. Under section 68, automatic referral must be made if the patient has not been before the tribunal for 3 years. A Mental Health review tribunal (of which there are eight nationally) is a body comprised of three members, one legal, one medical and one lay. It is required to discharge patients if they are no longer suffering from mental disorder/illness or further detention is not required for the purposes of the patient's health or safety or to protect other persons. It is for those who are arguing for continued detention to show that the patient does meet the criteria for detention (Mental Health Act 1983, Remedial Order 2001 SI 2001/3712). It may also exercise a discretion to discharge even if these criteria have not been satisfied. If a responsible medical officer is of the view that the Tribunal's decision is wrong they still should not try to get round this by immediately re-admitting the patient under the Mental Health Act (*R* v. *East London and the City Mental Health NHS Trust, ex parte Von Brandenberg* [2003] UKHL 58).

Liability of the nurse under the Mental Health Act 1983

As long as a nurse acts in accordance with her or his statutory powers under the Mental Health Act 1983 then section 139 provides that:

" No person shall be liable… to any civil or criminal proceedings… in respect of any act purporting to be done in pursuance of this Act… unless the act was done in bad faith or without reasonable care.

This limits the possibility of a civil action against the nurse (*Poutney* v. *Griffiths* [1975] 2 All ER 881). A patient may still bring an action challenging his or her detention under judicial review on the basis the health-care professionals have acted outside their powers.

Treating in the community

Some patients suffering from a mental disorder may benefit from treatment in the community rather than in hospital. The 1983 Act allows such patients to be made the subject of what are known as 'guardianship' orders (s7(2) Mental Health Act 1983). A person of 16 years or over may be received into guardianship if s/he is suffering from mental disorder, i.e. mental illness, severe mental impairment, psychopathic disorder or mental impairment and the disorder is of a nature or degree warranting the use of guardianship and that it is in the interests of the patient or for the protection of others that guardianship powers be used. The guardian may be the local social services authority or other named person. An application for admission to guardianship may be made by an approved social worker or by the patient's nearest relative (s11(1)) and must contain the recommendation of two doctors. A clinical description of the patient's mental condition must be given and it must be explained why the patient cannot be appropriately cared for without the powers of guardianship.

One criticism made of the powers of guardianship has been that they are limited in scope. A patient may be required to live at a place specified by the guardian and required to attend for treatment, occupation, education or training (s8). In addition, the order may require that a doctor or approved social worker be given access to the patient at his or her residence (s.8). But a patient cannot be compelled to receive treatment. It appears that in practice these powers were rarely used (Gunn 1986).

If a patient detained under section 3 is then released into the community s/he may be required, as a condition of discharge, to continue taking medication. But section 3 cannot be used to admit a patient with the aim of requiring him/her to receive medication and then releasing that patient into the community (*R* v. *Hallstrom ex parte W* [1986] QB 1090). However as long as a 'significant component' of treatment is being provided in hospital, then the courts have been prepared to uphold a treatment plan in the case of a person detained under section 3 but who had leave of absence and lived in the community and attended hospital on certain days during the week (*R (on the application of DR)* v. *Merseycare NHS Trust* [2002] All ER D 28; *R* v. *BHB Community Healthcare NHS Trust ex parte B* [1999] 1 FLR 106; *R (on the application of CS)* v. *MHRT* [2004] EWCA 2958).

Some argued that patients were being released into the community but that there were inadequate powers for regulating their care, and thus patients would enter into a cycle of admission treatment and discharge followed by readmission. Concern as to this 'revolving door' led to the issue being considered by a House of Lords Select Committee in their 5th report (1992/93) and this was followed by a Department of Health Inquiry (Department of Health 1993b). The results of many of the recommendations for reform are to be found in the Mental Health (Patients in the Community) Act 1995. This legislation provides a new regime for supervision in the community of persons who have been released from detention (Mental Health Act 1983 s25A–H). The patient's responsible medical officer makes an application for supervision to the health authority which is to have responsibility for providing the patient with aftercare facilities (s25(A)s). The responsible medical officer (RMO) must be satisfied that supervision is justified on the basis of risk of harm to the patient or risk to the safety of others. In making this assessment the RMO should take into account the patient's views and those of persons who will be professionally concerned with the after care and others such as relatives who may be caring for the patient in the community (s25B). Once in the community the patient is under the care of a supervisor. As with guardianship the patient can be required to live in a particular place. The patient can be compelled to attend for treatment but cannot be compelled to receive treatment (s25D). However, unlike guardianship, if the patient refuses treatment this may lead to his/her condition being reviewed to see whether readmission is necessary. Supervision under this power is for an initial period of 6 months with the possibility of renewal for a further 6 months. It may be ended at any time by the responsible medical officer after undertaking consultation (s25H(1)–(3)). This measure considerably strengthens the power to treat in the community.

Monitoring care – the role of the Mental Health Act Commission

The Mental Health Act Commission was established under the Mental Health Act 1983 (s120(1)) (Bingley 1995). The Commissioners are drawn from medical practitioners and others, such as social workers, academics, psychologists and lawyers. The Commission has the task of monitoring care given under the Act. The special hospitals are visited by the commissioners on a regular basis. They also visit other NHS hospitals and mental nursing homes, which are registered to receive detained patients. They undertake periodic reviews of situations in which treatments have been authorised by the second-opinion-approved doctor. Where a nurse becomes concerned as to the regime at a mental health hospital and believes that his/her concerns have not been adequately addressed within the complaints structure available for hospital staff, then the Mental Health Act Commissioners provide one avenue through which s/he can address concerns as to standards of patient care (Department of Health 1993a) and they can also investigate complaints from patients (s120(1)(b) Mental Health Act 1983). They have the power to visit and interview detained patients. They can require the production of and inspection of records relating to detained patients.

The Commissioners may also make visits without giving advance warning if there is particular concern regarding patients. An example of this was a 'dawn raid' undertaken on 21 November 1996 on 31 acute psychiatric hospitals in England and Wales by the Mental Health Act Commission and the Sainsbury Centre for Mental Health. These raids led to a report that noted difficulties facing staff nursing and the mentally ill and the fact that staff appeared to be demotivated and that there were breakdowns in communication between staff and patients. The report noted that there were on average 80 patients for every 100 beds, which left little room for manoeuvre. The Commission monitors the implementation of the Mental Health Act Code of Practice.

The Commission publishes a biennial report which is laid before Parliament. It also publishes Practice Notes. Other functions include the appointment of second opinion doctors. The Mental Health Act Commission is itself accountable to the Secretary of State and to Parliament as a Special Health Authority.

Reforming the Mental Health Act

Over the last 7 years, reform of mental health law has been under the spotlight. A major report of a government appointed Expert Committee (the Richardson Committee) into the system of treatment and care for the mentally ill was published in 1999 (Richardson 1999). Chaired by Professor Genevra Richardson, the committee recommended a total reform of the system. It recommended a 'principle-based approach' with legislation setting out a list of rights-based care principles. The Richardson committee emphasised a capacity based test in relation to care and treatment decisions. It recommended that in authorising compulsory care and treatment the tribunal would apply differential criteria in a case in which the patient did or did not possess capacity. It proposed a higher threshold which would have to be established in a situation in which the patient did possess capacity. In contrast with the existing position it recommended that there should be power to make a compulsory treatment order in the community. The same criteria would apply whether the order was to take effect in hospital or in the community.

The Richardson Review proposed that the existing tribunal system should be reformed. It recommended that there should be an application to an independent tribunal for the imposition of care and of treatment over 28 days. It would go further than the existing powers to consider whether detention criteria are met on that day to looking at the basis for continued use of compulsory powers. It would consider evidence such as information from the formal assessment process and involve scrutiny of the proposed plan for continuing care and treatment.

The Richardson proposals were not taken forward. The government was unhappy regarding the emphasis the Committee had placed on capacity (Department of Health 1999). They saw the crucial issue in many cases as rather that of 'risk', influenced by concerns regarding the dangers of individuals with severe personality disorders who were not susceptible to further detention as they were not 'treatable' and who could harm others (Department of Health/Home Office 1999). Attention was directed at the case of Michael Stone, who had attacked and killed Lin Russell and her young daughter in 1996. The government stated that issues relating to the safety of the individual patient and of the public are of key importance in determining the question of whether compulsory powers should be imposed. Although assessment of capacity would still be integral to assessment of needs and risk, it would not be a primary factor in determining whether a compulsory order should be made.

The Government introduced a draft Mental Health Bill into Parliament in 2002. It included a broad definition of mental illness to include personality disorders. It proposed detention of those who were mentally ill even if not treatable and also included provisions for compulsory treatment in the community. The draft Bill met a storm of controversy. It was ultimately withdrawn. A revised draft Bill was published and given to a Joint Scrutiny Committee of Commons and Lords in 2004 (Joint Committee 2004). Some amendments were made. So, for example, individuals with personality disorders would be able to be treated but only if the treatment was 'clinically sound' and otherwise if treatment was not considered 'justified' but they were a risk to others they should be referred to other organisations such as the police, as appropriate. The controversy however did not diminish and the Bill was widely criticised. The definition of treatment was very broad. The Joint Scrutiny Committee commented that it was concerned that the Bill could be used as in effect a mental health Antisocial Behaviour Order (ASBO) (Joint Committee 2004). It could have the effect of imposing treatment on persons who constituted a nuisance as opposed to a genuine threat. Further concerns surrounded the size and complexity of the proposed legislation. There were proposals to abolish the Mental Health Commission and to transfer its functions to the Healthcare Commission. This met with some opposition as there were concerns in transferring such a role from a recognised body with specialised expertise and whether there was a risk that it may result in a diminution of the effectiveness of the scrutiny of mental health providers.

Ultimately in spring 2006 the government announced that it was abandoning the Mental Health Bill. Instead it has indicated that certain specific new powers would be introduced. First, they are intending to extend powers of compulsory detention to those patients who are deemed a risk to themselves or to others. Such persons would not have to satisfy the 'treatability test'. Second, new powers are to enable enforced community treatment to be given. If people fail to comply with community treatment orders then new powers will enable them to be taken to a clinical setting and treated against their will.

Reform is to be welcomed, but the present proposals have considerable limitations. The balance too is very much on the axis of risk and of public safety rather than that of patient autonomy. It is likely that these are issues which will be almost certainly need to be revisited in the light of the Human Rights Act 1998.

REFERENCES

Bartlett P, Sandland R 2003 Mental health law policy and practice, 2nd edn. Oxford University Press, London

Bate P 1994 Children on secure psychiatric units: out of sight out of mind. Journal of Child Law 6: 131

Bingley W 1995 The Mental Health Act Commission. Health Director, 14

Department of Health 1993a Guidance for staff on relations with the public and the media. Department of Health, London

Department of Health 1993b Legal powers of the care of mentally ill people in the community. Department of Health, London.

Department of Health 1999 Reform of the Mental Health Act 1983: proposals for consultation. Department of Health, London

Department of Health 2005 Government response to the report of the Joint Committee on the draft Mental Health Bill 2004. Cmd 6624. Stationery Office, London

Department of Health/Home Office 1999 Managing dangerous persons with severe personality disorder. Home Office, London

Dimond B, Barker F 1996 Mental health law for nurses. Blackwell Scientific, Oxford.

Fennell P 1994 Statutory authority to treat. Medical Law Review 2: 30

Garwood-Gowers A 2001 The autonomous patient after the Human Rights Act 1998. In: Garwood-Gowers A, Lewis T, Tingle J Healthcare law: the impact of the Human Rights Act 1998. Cavendish, London

Gostin LO 1985 Mental health services law and practice. Shaw & Sons, London

Gunn MJ 1986 Mental Health Act guardianship: where now? Journal of Social Welfare Law: 144

Gunn MJ, Rodgers L 2000 Mental health nursing law. In: Tingle J, Cribb A (eds) Nursing law and ethics, 2nd edn. Blackwell Scientific, Oxford

Grubb A 2000 Incompetent patient (child): HIV testing and best interest. *Re C (HIV test)*. Medical Law Review 8: 120–125

Hoggett B 1996 Mental health law, 4th edn. Sweet & Maxwell, London

Joint Committee on the Draft Mental Health Bill 2004 Draft Mental Health Bill session 2004–05. HL Paper 79-I. HC 95-I. Stationery Office, London

McHale J, Gallagher A 2004 Nursing and human rights. Butterworth Heinemann, Edinburgh

Richardson 1999 Report of the Expert Committee: review of the Mental Health Act 1983. Department of Health, London

Unsworth C 1987 The politics of mental health legislation. Clarendon Press, Oxford, p 332

FURTHER READING

Brazier M, Bridge C 1996 Coercion or caring: analysing adolescent autonomy. Legal Studies 16: 84

McHale J, Fox M 2006 Health care law text and materials. Sweet & Maxwell, London, Chs 7 and 9

Consent to treatment II: Children and the mentally ill

Privacy, confidentiality, and access to health-care records

Jean McHale

7

Confidentiality has long been emphasised in nursing practice. The Nightingale oath provided that:

> " every nurse should be one who is to be depended upon, in other words, capable of being a 'confidential' nurse… she must be no gossip; no vain talker; she should never answer questions about her sick except to those who have a right to ask them; she must, I need not say be strictly sober and honest; but more than this, she must be a religious and devoted woman; she must have a respect for her calling.
>
> *Nightingale 1859*

Confidentiality is still a fundamental part of nursing today. But as health care has grown in sophistication and complexity, so the boundaries of confidentiality have become increasingly difficult to define. Instead of receiving treatment all their life from one family doctor, today patients are usually cared for in a group practice. During their time with that practice they may be seen by many different doctors and nurses. If patients are cared for in hospital the number of persons treating them will be considerably larger. The difficulty in maintaining confidentiality was graphically illustrated by Marc Siegler, a US physician and academic (Siegler 1982). One of Siegler's patients threatened to leave hospital if he was not told just how many people did have access to his medical records. Siegler went away and came back with a figure of some 75 people – doctors, nurses, etc. – who had legitimate access to his medical records; that did not include, of course, those who might have obtained unauthorised access. This patient was receiving relatively straightforward treatment. It is perhaps no wonder that, after being told this, the patient retorted, 'Perhaps you could explain just what you mean by confidentiality?' Maintaining confidentiality may also be particularly problematic as health-care professionals may work caring for patients alongside other professionals drawn from, for example, social work, housing and education. Today, as will be seen below, confidentiality in health-care practice is increasingly rooted in human rights and in particular Article 8 of the European Convention on Human Rights (ECHR, McHale & Gallagher 2004). This safeguards the right to privacy of home and of family life. One aspect of privacy is that of 'informational privacy' – the ability of the individual to control access to his/her own personal health information.

This chapter examines the nurse's obligation to maintain his/her patient's confidence. (Difficulties relating to disclosure of the health-care professional's own medical information to patients are examined in a later chapter.) The first part examines the general obligation of patient confidentiality; the second considers those situations in which health-care information may be disclosed. Then are considered the problems facing nurses when there are conflicts between maintaining patient confidentiality and upholding standards of care. Finally, safeguards for the confidentiality of health-care records are discussed, and on what basis a patient may obtain access to such records.

GENERAL OBLIGATIONS

The nurse has an obligation to keep patient information confidential. This obligation covers both information disclosed to her/him directly and information that s/he obtains from other health-care professionals when treating the patient. The obligation of confidentiality is contained in the nurse's professional ethical code. The Nursing and Midwifery Code (Nursing and Midwifery Council 2004) provides that

     You must treat information about patients and clients as confidential and use it only for the purposes for which it was given. As it is impractical to obtain consent every time you need to share information with others, you should ensure that patients and clients understand that some information may be made available to other members of the team involved in the delivery of care. You must guard against breaches of confidentiality by protecting information from improper disclosure at all times. (para 5.1)

Second, the nurse's contract of employment requires her/him to keep patient information confidential. Unauthorised disclosure may lead the nurse to be disciplined by his/her professional body or to be dismissed by the employer. Guidance on confidentiality within the NHS has been provided by the Department of Health in their document *Confidentiality: NHS Code of Practice*, which was published in 2003 (Department of Health 2003). Third, where information has been disclosed in breach of an obligation of confidence, legal proceedings may follow, such as an injunction being obtained to stop further publication of the confidential information. For example, in *X* v. *Y* ([1988] 2 All ER 648) the medical records of two general practitioners who had developed AIDS were disclosed in a national newspaper. The court issued an injunction to stop further publication of the records. To bring legal proceedings for breach of confidence the patient must show that a duty of confidence, either express or implied, has arisen, that the information was given in confidence and that disclosure was made in breach of that duty (*Att. Gen* v. *Guardian Newspaper (No 2)* [1988] 3 All ER 545). A duty of confidence would be implied in a situation in which a patient discloses information to a nurse because of his/her status as a nurse.

Health-care confidentiality is today also reinforced through the application of the Human Rights Act 1998 and in particular Article 8 – the right to privacy of home and family life. The European Court of Human Rights has already confirmed that it protects health-care confidentiality. In *Z* v. *Finland*

((1997) 25 EHRR 371) a man was prosecuted for rape. At trial his wife's medical records, which revealed that she was human immunodeficiency virus (HIV)-positive, were disclosed. The European Court of Human Rights held that this was a breach of her right to privacy.

Although the English courts have rejected claims for a separate 'privacy tort' (*Wainwright* v. *Home Office* [2003] UKHL 53), nonetheless, the courts have been rooting protection for health-care confidentiality in the right to privacy. In *Campbell* v. *MGN* ([2004] 2 AC 457 (HL)) the model Naomi Campbell brought an action for damages regarding the publication of an article in the *Daily Mirror* that stated that she had been receiving treatment for drug addiction. Campbell claimed that, although there was justification in publication of information that corrected statements she had made in public about her drug addiction, which were false, the publication of an article that detailed information regarding her treatment for drug addiction and an additional photograph constituted an invasion of privacy. While this was not a health-professional–patient breach of confidence, the case does have important implications for the relationship between confidentiality and privacy. In the House of Lords their Lordships confirmed that the action for breach of confidence encompasses protection for personal privacy under Article 8 of the ECHR. The courts will consider whether a person has a reasonable expectation of personal privacy in all the circumstances. In addition, they will examine whether the issue is something that is obviously private or whether the disclosure could be seen as 'highly offensive to a reasonable person'.

The nurse is thus obliged in both law and professional practice to keep the patient's confidence. But this obligation is not regarded as absolute – in some situations the nurse may legitimately break confidence, as we shall see below. In addition, the nurse may be required to break confidentiality by court order or by specific statutory provision. These issues will be examined further below.

CHILDREN AND CONFIDENTIALITY

What right does a child patient have to confidentiality? It is ludicrous to suggest that a nurse shouldn't discuss a toddler's illness with the child's mother. But, children grow and begin to express the wish to control aspects of their own lives. If a 14-year-old girl approaches a school nurse and asks for advice regarding contraceptive treatment, what should the nurse do?

In *Gillick* v. *West Norfolk and Wisbech AHA* ([1986] AC 150) Mrs Victoria Gillick sought an assurance from her local health authority that her daughter would not be given advice concerning contraception/abortion or receive treatment without her consent. The authority refused to give the assurance and Mrs Gillick went to court and asked for a declaration that the authority's decision and the guidance of the Department of Health and Social Security on which the authority's refusal was based were unlawful. She was unsuccessful in her application. In the House of Lords it was said that the child is able to consent to medical treatment where s/he has sufficient maturity to do so. The *Gillick* decision was revisited recently in the context of the *Axon* case. In 2004 the Department of Health produced guidance called *Best practice guidance* for doctors and other health professionals on the provision of advice and treatment to young people under sixteen on contraception, sexual and reproductive health (Department of Health 2004). This guidance, which followed the decision in *Gillick*, provided that health professionals could provide such advice and treatment on sexual matters for persons under 16 years of age without parental knowledge or the consent of their parents subject to conditions.

Mrs Axon, a mother of teenage daughters, applied for judicial review challenging the Guidance. She argued that there was no duty to maintain confidentiality in this situation unless there were exceptional circumstances such that disclosure of the information would harm the health of the child. Her claim was unsuccessful. Silber J. followed the judgment in *Gillick* and upheld the guidelines. He noted the importance of safeguarding the human right of privacy under the ECHR and also noted the United Nations Convention on the Rights of the Child. He rejected the claim that the parental rights of privacy were infringed in this case but then went on to say that, even if they were, such infringement was justifiable under Article 8(2) on the public policy basis, ensuring that adolescents seeking advice and treatment regarding sexually transmitted diseases, abortion and contraception.

While the *Gillick* case was primarily concerned with consent to treatment, nevertheless it appears to be the case that this approach would be followed in relation to confidentiality (Montgomery 1987, Grubb & Pearl 1986). In the case of a *Gillick*-competent child, a health professional should not usually disclose information to a third party without that child's consent. This does give rise to some difficult issues as to whether a child has sufficient competence to consent (Ch. 6). Where the child patient is very young, disclosure of information to the parents may be an integral part of the child's care. Nevertheless, the nurse should think carefully before s/he decides to disclose a child's medical information without the child's consent.

THE ADULT LACKING MENTAL CAPACITY

Following the House of Lords decision in *Re F* ([1990] 2 AC 1), it remained uncertain as to whether and to what extent an obligation of confidentiality arose in the context of an adult who lacked capacity. However this matter has now been resolved in the case of *R (on the application of S) v. Plymouth City Council* ([2002] EWCA Civ 388). S was a 26-year-old adult who lacked mental capacity. His mother wanted access to his medical records in her capacity as nearest relative under the Mental Health Act 1983 but was refused access because the Local Authority took the view that disclosure would constitute breach of confidence. Hale L.J. held that:

> Article 8 also confers a right to respect for private life. Adults such as C have that right as much as anyone else. Indeed, many would think them more at risk, and therefore more worthy of respect by the authorities if, because of their mental disabilities, they are unable to protect it for themselves.

Here on the facts of the case she allowed his mother access to the medical records – confirming that what was being asked for was limited access by his mother rather than general disclosure to the world at large.

AFTER THE PATIENT'S DEATH

The obligation of confidentiality continues after the patient's death. When Lord Moran, the physician of Winston Churchill, published a book that discussed the decline of the great war leader (*Churchill – the struggle for survival*) he was roundly condemned by his contemporaries. The Nursing and Midwifery Council (NMC) document *Confidentiality* states that 'The death of a patient/client does not give registrants the right to break confidentiality' (Nursing and Midwifery Council 2006). But while maintenance of confidentiality after death may be part of the professional's ethical obligation, it is less certain whether legal proceedings could be brought in such circumstances. An action for libel and slander cannot be brought after the death of the person who has been defamed. It has been suggested that a court might reject a claim of breach of confidence brought after the patient's death on the basis that the obligation only existed during that patient's lifetime (Kennedy & Grubb 1994). Recent controversy over the protection of health-care confidentiality arose in France with the publication in January 1996, after his death, of a book by a physician to President Mitterand of France that contained information about Mitterand's treatment for cancer that had been withheld from the French public (see further Dorozynski 1996, Mason & Laurie 2006). Initially, further publication was stopped by the French courts but this ban was lifted by the European Court of Human Rights, who held France to be in violation of Article 10 because the injunction was disproportionate to the aim and no longer complied with a 'pressing social need' (*Plon (Societé)* v. *France* Application No 58148/00 18 May 2004).

GROUNDS FOR DISCLOSURE

Patient care would be impossible unless some disclosure of information was made. Certain recognised exceptions do exist. Nevertheless, the nurse should be aware that all disclosures should be carefully justified.

Disclosing with consent

Disclosure is both lawful and complies with professional ethical codes if the patient has given consent to the information being passed on. Such consent must be freely and fully given. However, in practice this may not always be the case. As Mason & Laurie (2006) comment: 'What patient at a teaching hospital out-patients department is likely to refuse when the consultant asks "You don't mind these young doctors being present, do you?" – the pressures are virtually irresistible and truly autonomous consent is impossible.'

It can be argued that when a patient enters hospital s/he impliedly consents to such information as is necessary for his/her treatment being passed to other health-care practitioners. But consent to disclosure should not always be presumed. The nurse must ensure that from the onset of care the patient is aware that some information may be disclosed to third parties who are involved in his/her care. Department of Health guidance states that:

" Where patients have been informed of (a) the use and sharing of their information associated with their health care; and (b) the choices that they have and the implications of choosing to limit how information may be used or shared then explicit consent is not usually needed for information disclosures needed to provide that health care. Even so, opportunities to check that patients understand what may happen and are content should be taken.

Department of Health 2003, para 15

If the patient objects, the need to respect the patient's wishes may mean that it is not possible to offer certain treatment choices (Department of Health 2003, para 15). Where disclosure is necessary then information should be disclosed on a 'need to know' basis.

Public interest exception

The courts have held that in some situations disclosure of confidential information is justifiable in the public interest. The NMC code also recognises a public interest exception.

> " 5.3 If you are required to disclose information outside the team that will have personal consequences for patients or clients, you must obtain their consent. If the patient or client withholds consent, or if consent cannot be obtained for whatever reason, disclosures may be made only where:
>
> - they can be justified in the public interest (usually where disclosure is essential to protect the patient or client or someone else from the risk of significant harm)
> - they are required by law or by order of a court.

Nursing and Midwifery Council 2004

What amounts to disclosure in the public interest by a health-care professional was examined by the courts in *W* v. *Egdell* ([1990] ChD 359). A breach of confidence action was brought against a psychiatrist. He had been commissioned by W's solicitors to make a medical report on W's fitness for discharge from the secure hospital where he had been detained after he was convicted of manslaughter 8 years previously. The report was highly unfavourable to W and W's solicitors withdrew their application to a Mental Health Review Tribunal. Dr Egdell told the solicitors that he believed that a copy of the report should be put on W's hospital file. The solicitors disagreed. Dr Egdell himself sent a copy to the hospital. This fact emerged at a subsequent Mental Health Review Tribunal hearing and an action for breach of confidence was brought against Dr Egdell by W.

The case was first heard in the High Court. Scott J. rejected the claim that Dr Edgell was wrong to have disclosed the information. He noted that W was not an ordinary member of the public. In his opinion the doctor owed a duty not only to W but also to the public. This required him to place before the proper authorities the result of his examination of W. He placed weight upon the fact that while in detention W had been seen by a number of psychiatrists. Each of these owed him a duty of confidence such that they could not, for example, sell the information to a newspaper but, at the same time, the reports compiled about W were on file and were available to the

Home Office. In the view of Scott J. the fact that these reports were on file had not inhibited W in his dealings with these psychiatrists. He did not believe that the report of Dr Egdell should be treated any differently.

W appealed to the Court of Appeal, where his appeal was rejected. Sir Stephen Brown was broadly in agreement with the first instance decision. Disclosure of the information was in the public interest in ensuring the safety of the public as a whole. The effect of suppressing the material contained in the report would have been to deprive both the hospital and the Secretary of State of vital information. The other judge to deliver a full judgment in this case, Bingham J., was more cautious. He stressed that a patient, such as W, who was held under a restriction order had a very great need for recourse to a professional advisor who was independent and discreet. The confidentiality of such patients should only be broken if needed on the basis of the doctor's duty to society. On the facts of this particular case, Bingham J. held that disclosure had been justified. The decisive facts were that:

> " Where a man has committed multiple killings under the disability of serious mental illness, decisions which may lead directly or indirectly to his release from hospital should not be made unless a responsible authority is able to make an informed judgment that the risk of repetition is so small as to be acceptable.

W v. *Egdell* clearly illustrates that confidentiality in law is far from an absolute obligation. In each case the court will balance the public interest in ensuring confidentiality against the public interest in disclosure. In determining public interest the courts will make reference to the guidelines set out by the health-care professionals.

It is fairly certain that disclosure of the fact that your patient has a mental illness that makes him a potential danger to the community to the appropriate authorities will be held to be in the public interest. Similarly, if a nurse was told of child abuse and s/he disclosed this information to an agency such as the National Society for the Prevention of Cruelty to Children it is likely that a court would hold that the disclosure was in the public interest. Nevertheless, there are other situations in which it is not clear whether the public interest justifies disclosure. A nurse who discovers that a patient has committed shoplifting offences should hesitate long before disclosing that fact. Again, the nurse may face a dilemma if a patient tells her/him that he knows the identity of the person who stabbed him but does not want the nurse to give this information to the police because he is frightened of retaliation from a gang of thugs. In such a situation the nurse should attempt to persuade the patient to approach the police himself.

What if a patient who is diagnosed as HIV-positive refuses to tell his wife? Should the nurse or any other health-care professional inform the man's wife? The man may be frightened that his marriage would break up if his wife was told. The General Medical Council has advised doctors that disclosure may be justifiable if there is a serious and identifiable risk to a specific individual (General Medical Council, 1997). The legal position here is unclear but it is suggested that if disclosure did take place a court would be prepared to hold that the breach of confidence was in the public interest.

Disclosure – public interest and press freedom

Safeguarding confidentiality may also conflict with another public interest – that of freedom of the press. We noted above in *X v. Y* that here the court protected patient confidentiality over freedom of expression in the context of health professionals who were HIV-positive. This case was decided before the Human Rights Act was passed. This issue again came before the courts after the Human Rights Act 1998 came into force in the case of *H (a health worker) v. Associated Newspapers Ltd* ([2002] EWCA Civ 195). This case concerned A, a National Health Service (NHS) professional. He was diagnosed as HIV-positive. Department of Health guidelines provided that, where patients had undergone procedures in relation to which there was a risk of infection, they should be notified that they had been treated by a worker who was HIV-positive and they should be offered counselling. The Health Authority wanted to undertake a 'look-back' study and as part of this H was asked to give the Health Authority details of both his NHS and his private patients. He alleged that the first look-back study was unlawful on the basis of clinical confidentiality. In addition he also asked if the Health Authority could be stopped from using information that he had previously supplied. The *Mail on Sunday* newspaper was informed of the case and wanted to publish details that would have identified both H and the Health Authority in question. In reaching their conclusion the Court of Appeal considered Article 8 – the right to privacy and Article 10 – the right to freedom of expression. They held that there was a strong public interest in maintaining confidentiality of the personal medical information of the health professional. They also held that the name of the Health Authority should not be disclosed as this could lead to the identification of the health professional. However they allowed disclosure of his speciality – information that in their view should be made available for public debate. In *Campbell v. MGN*, discussed above, while the Court recognised that there was an interest here in publishing the information about Naomi Campbell in the light of the fact that in the past she had previously lied about her drug addiction, nonetheless the information published about the therapy that she was undergoing and the photographs published were not in the public interest.

Disclosure in the context of disciplinary proceedings

The public interest can also justify the disclosure of information in the context of disciplinary proceedings. This issue arose in the case of *A Health Authority v. X* ([2001] 2 FCR 634), which concerned a Health Authority investigation of a GP's practice because it was claimed that the practice had broken its terms of service. Application was made by the Health Authority for the disclosure of patient records. The Court of Appeal held that disclosure would be justifiable but also agreed with the judge at first instance by imposing restrictions on the scope of disclosure of the records such that if disclosed they should be treated as confidential and in addition any further disclosure of the information must be subject to safeguards requiring confidentiality and prohibiting unauthorised disclosure.

A further example of disclosure of information relating to disciplinary proceedings arose in the context of a nurse in the case of *Woolgar v. Chief*

Constable of the Sussex Police ([1999] 3 All ER 604). Following the death of a patient at a nursing home, W, who was a registered nurse and Y, the nursing home matron, were interviewed by the police. Criminal proceedings were not brought; however, the case was referred to the UKCC, who asked the police for access to information from the investigation. The police stated that authority was needed from the person who had given a statement before it could be disclosed. W objected to disclosure. The police indicated that they would review the contents of the tape to see whether disclosure should be made. W brought legal proceedings to restrain the police from disclosing the information but these were unsuccessful both at first instance and in the Court of Appeal. In the Court of Appeal Kennedy L.J. held that, despite the assurance that information would not be used other than in relation to criminal proceedings, there was here a countervailing public interest that legitimised disclosure being made.

Police enquiries

> A police constable comes into hospital reception. He wants to ask questions of the ward sister and to search through a particular patient's medical records. Can he do this?

First, if the ward sister is asked questions she is under no obligation to answer them. In English law there is no general obligation placed upon any citizen to answer questions put to them by the police (*Rice* v. *Connolly* [1966] 2 QB 416), although if a defendant keeps silent there is a possibility that an adverse inference may be drawn regarding the decision to keep silent (Criminal Justice Act 1994). There are also some exceptional situations in which disclosure is required by statute. For example, under the Terrorism Act 2000, a person can be prosecuted if s/he withholds information relating to acts of terrorism (S19, 20).

Second, the police have no automatic right to demand access to a patient's records. Access to medical records by police conducting enquiries is regulated by statute. Usually, before the police may examine a patient's medical records they must obtain a warrant under the Police and Criminal Evidence Act 1984 (PACE) (s9–s11 and schedule 1). Before a police constable can gain access to premises such as a doctor's surgery or a hospital in order to search for information such as medical records/samples of human tissue, or tissue fluid taken for the purpose of diagnosis/medical treatment or held in confidence, s/he must apply to a circuit judge for a warrant. The police must show that there is a reasonable belief that the information needed is contained on the premises and that prior to the 1984 Act a statute existed under which the police could have obtained the information. There is, however, no duty upon the police when applying for a warrant to inform the person whose confidential information is sought about the application. Only the person who is holding the information – in the case of hospital medical records an administrator – must be told. It is submitted that this is undesirable and that the patient should, wherever possible, have a voice at the hearing. It appears that the courts have been prepared to scrutinise carefully applications for medical records. For example, in R v. *Cardiff Crown Court ex parte Kellam* ((1993) 16 BMLR 76), the court refused to allow police who were investigating a murder of a mental patient to obtain access to records of admission, discharge and leave of patients at the hospital.

The NMC have recently advised that 'In some circumstances, such as accident and emergency admissions where the police are involved, registrants are advised to involve senior staff if they feel unable to deal with the situation' (Nursing and Midwifery Council 2006).

Civil law proceedings

If a patient is injured as a result of what s/he claims is negligent treatment, s/he will need to obtain evidence in the form of, for example, medical reports to establish a case. The patient's lawyers will ask for access to the records. If this is refused, then an application must be made to the court under the Administration of Justice Act 1970 for disclosure of documents. Section 32 makes particular reference to records that are sought in a personal injury action. Here, the court can order that reports are made available to the applicant, to his/her legal advisor or, if the applicant does not have a legal advisor, to his/her medical advisors (s33 and s34 Supreme Court Act 1981). As has been commented (Mason & Laurie 2006, p. 284):

> the court can deal with problems of confidentiality relating to irrelevant conditions – such as a past history of a sexually transmitted disease – by limiting disclosure to the other side's medical advisors who must respect confidentiality save where litigation is affected.

In addition, disclosure of expert reports should be made at the prehearing stage (*Naylor* v. *Preston AHA* [1987] 2 All ER 353). (See Ch. 1 in relation to the encouragement given to broader disclosure and agreement between experts prior to trial following the Woolf report.) There are, however, exceptions to the general requirements of disclosure. For example, communications between a plaintiff and his/her lawyer are usually not required to be disclosed. Such communications are covered by what is known as 'legal professional privilege' (for discussion of the operation of the trial process see Ch. 10). In very limited situations, information may be withheld because it is not in the public interest to disclose that information (*Re HIV Haemophiliac Litigation* [1990] NLJR 1349).

Evidence in court

If a nurse is summoned as a witness in a court case s/he must give evidence. There is no special rule of evidence – no evidential 'privilege' that would entitle the nurse to refuse to testify (McHale 1993, *Duchess of Kingston's case* (1776) 20 State Trials 355). The nurse is protected in disclosing in the courtroom from an action being brought by a patient on the basis of breach of confidence (*Watson* v. *McEwan* [1905] AC 480). If the nurse refuses to disclose any information in response to any question put to her/him, then a judge may find the nurse in contempt of court and may ultimately send him/her to prison.

Public health disclosure requirements

In some situations, disclosure of medical information is required by statute as a public health measure in order to limit the spread of certain diseases. Notifiable diseases include cholera, plague, smallpox, typhus and rabies (s11 Public Health (Control of Disease) Act 1984). Where a registered medical practitioner becomes aware or suspects that a patient s/he is attending is suffering from such an illness, the practitioner must notify the local authority of the patient's name, age, sex, the disease from which the patient is suffering and the date of onset of the disease.

Disclosure required by statute – s60 Health and Social Care Act 2001

A major exception to health-care confidentiality is provided in section 60 of the Health and Social Care Act 2001. This gives the Secretary of State powers to make regulations sanctioning the disclosure of confidential health-care information in the interests of improving patient care or in the public interest (s60(1)). This very broad power is subject to the limitation that before the Secretary of State makes regulations s/he must consult the Patient Information Advisory Committee, which was created under section 61 of the Health and Social Care Act 2001. In addition the regulations are to be compatible with the Data Protection Act and they are to be reviewed on an annual basis to determine whether they continue to be appropriate. Section 60 has proved very controversial (Case 2003). The current regulations which concern the Health Protection Agency and Cancer Registries enable confidential information to be processed without consent where this concerns:

- diagnosis of communicable diseases and other public health risks
- recognition of other diseases and risks and for the control of their spread
- monitoring and management of communicable diseases and incidence of exposure to such disease
- delivery and safety of immunisation programmes and adverse reactions to immunisations and medication (Health Service (Control of Patient Information Regulations SI 2002/1438, reg 4).

Confidentiality and research information

Nurses must always bear in mind that patient information is to be treated as confidential. Research projects may involve highly sensitive clinical information, for example a study examining counselling provision for persons who are HIV-positive. The nurse, as we saw earlier, is obliged by his/her contract of employment and by the NMC professional ethical code to maintain patient confidentiality.

Research may be undertaken using existing medical records. In principle, the patient's consent to disclosure should be obtained. However, if the sample is very large, tracing all patients may be totally impracticable. It is important that information generated during a clinical trial is kept just as confidential as any other clinical information. The researcher must respect the confidentiality of information given to her/him by staff and patients.

Unauthorised disclosure is not only ethically unjustifiable but may also prejudice further research. If a study is undertaken into working practices on the wards, it is important to ensure that nurses can speak frankly. They may not be willing to be so frank without a guarantee of anonymity being provided and adhered to. No individual should be identifiable from the published results without consent.

Use of anonymised information is unlikely to require subsequent consent from the subject. In *R v. Department of Health ex parte Source Informatics* ([2000] 1 All ER 786), the case involved disclosure of data concerning GPs' prescribing habits, which had been anonymised, to a firm that was intended to sell this information to pharmaceutical companies. The Court of Appeal held that here the concern of the law was to safeguard individual privacy and because of the anonymisation of the information there was no invasion of privacy. Some might dispute this, however. While anonymisation removes identity, another aspect of privacy is autonomy – that of control of personal information. An individual may object to the use of their information, for example in a research project, not because of the fact that their identity has been disclosed but rather because they are unable to control the use of that information.

Unauthorised disclosures

Unauthorised disclosures should be minimised. It is unethical to discuss a patient's case outside the clinical setting with friends, or discuss a case with colleagues in public where one may be overheard. In hospital, records should never be left lying around where unauthorised persons may read them. It is important to ensure that safeguards exist against disclosure, particularly where a patient is, for example, suffering from acquired immunodeficiency syndrome (AIDS). A minimal number of clinical staff necessary to facilitate that patient's care should be informed that the patient is HIV-positive.

Occupational health context

Nurses employed by organisations other than the NHS may face some very difficult disclosure dilemmas. Take, for example, the occupational health nurse employed by a large industrial firm. The nurse owes a duty to the employer but at the same time, as a caring professional, s/he is bound by professional ethical code. If the nurse intends that the information given by the patient s/he is treating should be disclosed to the employer, then s/he must make this clear to the patient before undertaking the consultation.

Genetic information and maintaining confidentiality

One category of personal information that has led to particular concern regarding disclosure is that of genetic information. The sequencing of the human genome has been hailed as one of the great scientific achievements in recent years. Nonetheless there has been concern that the enhanced availability of genetic information may lead to individuals being subject to discriminatory treatment by, for example, insurers and employers on the basis that they have some propensity to develop disease in the future. There has been discussion around the prospect of the introduction of specific legislation governing control of disclosure of genetic information (Human Genetics Commission 2002, Nuffield Council on Bioethics 1993). At present insurers do not require individuals to obtain a genetic test before obtaining insurance and there is a voluntary moratorium by insurers on the use of genetic test results to set insurance premiums (Human Genetics Commission 2002). The discriminatory use of genetic information in a situation in which the condition has not yet manifested itself is presently not protected by the Disability Discrimination Act 1995. This may be subject to challenge under the Human Rights Act 1998 in relation to Article 8 of the European Convention on Human Rights – the right to privacy of home and family life.

In the context of the family genetics provides again potential for considerable dilemmas. Take a situation in which a woman is screened during pregnancy and this reveals that she is the carrier of a genetic disorder. This information may be of assistance to her sister, who is contemplating pregnancy. The woman may, of course, be perfectly happy for the information to be disclosed to her sister. But what if she objects? In such a situation, could the midwife legitimately take the decision to breach her patient's confidentiality? One approach is to say that this is not simply an issue of individual confidentiality but that, as the Nuffield Council on Bioethics noted, in certain clearly defined contexts it might be appropriate to treat the family as a unit (Nuffield Council on Bioethics 1993). The Nuffield Council suggested that, where disease would cause grave danger to family members, an attempt should be made to ensure that the information was disclosed voluntarily but that in exceptional situations information could be disclosed by health professionals to other family members despite an expressed wish for confidentiality if, for example, it was to avoid giving rise to grave damage to family members. It remains to be seen how a court would regard such a disclosure. In the past cases have focused on matters such as whether harm will be caused. But can harm here be easily detected? As has been pointed out by Boddington, this differs substantially from a situation in which the disclosure relates to an infectious disease.

> " ...steps to prevent the incidence of genetic disorder in the population consist not exclusively but in the main, not in ensuring that individuals do not acquire the disorder but ensuring that individuals who would have that disorder are not born in the first place. Thus the population is not being protected from an outside danger; it could be said that it is being protected from the costs of bearing certain individuals amongst its number and also that, for certain types of individuals with certain genetic conditions it is itself a bad thing to be born. It is also of course quite fallacious to think of genetic disease as 'spreading' in the population in the way that an infectious disease might spread.

> *Boddington 1994*

The woman may be objecting to disclosure for a number of different reasons. It may be the case that the reason for refusal of disclosure is malicious. But at the same time it could be the case that disclosure would reveal compromising information about paternity. Disclosure could harm the woman not only because of the breach of confidentiality but also because of the impact on the relationship with the man involved. It is also the case that informing the woman's sister may amount to providing her with information that she herself does not want. She may be herself making a conscious choice not to discover certain genetic information. There has been much discussion of the 'right not to know' our genetic information (Chadwick et al 1997). It is worth noting that The Council of Europe, in the Convention for the Protection of Human Rights and Dignity of the Human Being with regard to the Application of Biology and Medicine, provide that 'Everyone is entitled to know any information collected about his or her health. However the wishes of individuals not to be so informed shall be observed.'

Ultimately, of course, these are specific decisions to be made in relation to an individual case. There is no single rule that can be laid down and were the matter to arise in the courtroom the court would obviously take into account all the circumstances in determining whether the public interest here militated in favour of disclosure. Genetics is in its infancy and our approach to such dilemmas may well change as there is greater knowledge of the development of certain diseases and disabilities and if there is the greater prospect for obtaining a cure for such conditions.

Legal obligation to break confidence?

Can the nurse ever be required to disclose information and be held liable in negligence if s/he does not do so? What if a patient tells a nurse of his/her wish to harm another person; should that nurse warn the person who might be in danger? This issue arose in the USA in the case of *Tarasoff* v. *Regents of the University of California* ([1976] 551 P 2d 334). Poddar, a university student, sought out patient care in a psychiatric hospital. He was suffering from deep depression as a result of being rejected by one Miss Tarasoff, with whom he had fallen in love. He told a psychologist at the hospital of his intention to kill Miss Tarasoff. After discussions with psychiatrists, the psychologist decided that Poddar should be detained in a mental hospital. He told the campus police, who detained Poddar but later released him when he appeared to be rational. Two months after the consultation with the psychologist, Poddar killed Miss Tarasoff. The majority in the Californian Supreme Court held that the therapist was under a duty to warn both the victim and the victim's family and was liable for his failure to do so.

The *Tarasoff* case led to an outcry from psychiatric associations in the USA. The court reconsidered its decision some 18 months later. It modified the duty from one to warn the victim to one of exercising reasonable care for the victim's protection and to take steps reasonably necessary in the circumstances. In a memorable phrase it was said that the 'protective privilege ends when the public peril begins'.

There are echoes of *Tarasoff* in the judgment of Scott J. in the English case of *W* v. *Egdell*, a judgment that received the approval of Sir Stephen Brown in the Court of Appeal. Scott J. held that:

> " In my view as a doctor called upon as Dr Egdell was to examine a patient owes a duty not only to his patient, but also to the public. His duty to the

public would require him, in my opinion, to place before the proper authorities the results of his examination if, in his opinion, the public interest so requires.

What did Scott J. mean here by the duty to disclose? Will a court in future be prepared to find that a health-care professional owes a duty of care to the person his patient claims that he is going to kill or seriously injure? At present it seems unlikely that an English court would impose such an obligation. The courts have been unwilling in the past to extend the scope of liability imposed upon third parties (*Smith* v. *Littlewood* [1987] 1 All ER 710). Any obligation to disclose may limit an individual's privacy if practitioners feel that they must go ahead and disclose to avoid being sued in negligence.

Negotiated confidentiality

Confidentiality is an important obligation but determining the boundaries may prove problematic, as has been seen. One suggestion that has been advanced is that the practice of negotiated confidentiality could be adopted (Sieghart 1982, Thompson 1979). Practitioner and patient discuss the extent to which patient information should remain confidential. They negotiate as to what information may be disclosed and what information may not. One major advantage is that negotiation removes much uncertainty. Both parties know the ground rules for disclosure. However, such an approach is not without difficulties. It involves effort and understanding. There is also the danger that when the negotiations were undertaken some criteria relating to disclosure had not been envisaged. Negotiation is also time-consuming and it may not be a practical prospect in many situations.

CONFIDENTIALITY – SPECIFIC OBLIGATIONS

In addition to the general obligations spelt out above, certain specific obligations of confidentiality have been imposed by statute.

Human Fertilisation and Embryology Act 1990

Few statutes expressly require patient confidentiality to be maintained. One exception is the Human Fertilisation and Embryology Act 1990. This Act regulates the provision of new reproductive technology services. Information relating to infertility treatment is particularly sensitive. Section 33 of the 1990 Act places a statutory ban upon the disclosure of information concerning gamete donors and patients receiving treatment under the Act. Unauthorised disclosure of such information by health-care professionals and others has been made a criminal offence (1990 Act s40(1)(5)).

There are certain exceptions to the general obligation. The clinician at the in vitro fertility (IVF) unit may disclose information where the patient has consented to that disclosure to a specific person (1990 Act s33 (6B)) or where it is necessary to disclose the information to a person who 'needs to know' for the purposes of treating the patient or where a medical emergency has arisen or in connection with clinical or accounts audit (1990 Act s33(6c)).

This statutory exception is itself the source of some controversy, particularly in view of the fact that it is now routine practice in IVF clinics to require patients to take HIV tests. It is questionable whether a patient's GP is entitled to know the fact that their patient has tested HIV-positive. This is another instance in which the 'need to know' should be tightly interpreted. The confidentiality provisions of the Human Fertilisation and Embryology Act 1990 are currently under review by the government as part of a broader review of the Act.

Venereal disease

Legislation restricting disclosure of patient information also exists in the area of venereal diseases. The National Health Service Venereal Disease Regulations (SI 1974 No. 29) provide that health authorities should take all necessary steps to ensure that identifiable information relating to persons being treated for sexually transmitted diseases should not be disclosed. Such information may be disclosed where this is for the purpose of communicating the information to a doctor caring for the patient or to a person working under the direction of that doctor to treat that condition or to prevent its spread.

CONFLICTS BETWEEN CONFIDENTIALITY AND THE NEED TO UPHOLD STANDARDS OF CARE – WHISTLEBLOWING IN THE NHS

> A nurse is concerned by the poor staffing levels in her ward and is concerned at the standard of care being provided. She raises some concerns with her colleagues but feels that what she has said has fallen largely on deaf ears. What should she do?

The whole issue of health-care professionals wanting to go public and 'blow the whistle' on what they regard as being unacceptable standards of care has caused a furore over recent years. From, as we shall see below, the well known case of Graham Pink, a nurse in Stockport, to Stephen Boisin, in relation to the deaths of children during cardiac surgery at Bristol Royal Infirmary (Department of Health 2001), incidents of whistleblowing have rarely been far from the headlines.

The NMC code requires the nurse to report circumstances in which the standard of care given has fallen below levels which are acceptable: Clause 8 provides that:

“ As a registered nurse, midwife or specialist community public health nurse you must act to identify and minimise the risk to patients and clients:…

“ 8.2.1 You must act quickly to protect patients and clients from risk if you have good reason to believe that you or a colleague from your own or another profession may not be fit to practise for reasons of conduct, health or competence. You should be aware of the terms of legislation that offer protection for people who raise concerns about health and safety issues.

8.2.2 Where you cannot remedy circumstances in the environment of care that could jeopardise standards of practice, you must report them to a senior person with sufficient authority to manage them and also, in the case of midwifery, to the supervisor of midwives. This must be supported by a written record.

This record may be of importance if subsequent action is taken against the nurse and s/he claims that the actions that s/he took were affected by the fact that there were inadequate resources.

There may be instances in which the obligation of confidentiality owed by nurse to patient may conflict with the nurse's belief that standards of patient care have fallen. This problem arose in the case of Graham Pink. Pink was a charge nurse who believed that standards of hospital services provided to his elderly patients were unsatisfactory. Although he complained within the management structure, he did not believe that his complaints had been addressed. He was concerned about: 'avoidable injuries to patients (including a death); important observations for people on blood transfusions not carried out; patients offered a wash once a day....' (Letter to the chairman of Stockport Health Authority, *The Guardian*, 9 July 1991). Thus, as a result of obtaining no response to his complaints, Pink made the decision to go public about his concerns; he wrote letters to *The Guardian* newspaper and he gave an interview to a local paper. The health authority brought disciplinary proceedings against him on the basis of breach of patient confidentiality. Although the article did not name patients, relatives claimed that a patient could be identified from details of his case given in the press report. Pink was also charged with not reporting an incident in which a patient fell out of bed. At the disciplinary hearing the allegations were upheld against Pink and when he refused to transfer to a post of community nurse he was dismissed (*The Guardian*, 18 September 1991).

As the Pink case shows, the threat of dismissal for breach of confidentiality is a very real one. Pink challenged his dismissal at an industrial tribunal. A claim can be brought before a tribunal for unlawful dismissal on the grounds that the dismissal was unfair (s98 Employment Rights Act 1996). The tribunal decides whether the action taken by the employer was reasonable and assesses the employee's dismissal on the balance of competing equities. Pink's case was ultimately settled before any final decision was made by the tribunal.

If a nurse does not take action about what s/he regards as undesirably low standards then s/he runs the risk of being disciplined by the NMC. The professional practice code of the previous nursing regulatory body, the United Kingdom Central Council (UKCC), was claimed in his defence by Graham Pink. However, as Pink discovered, simply acting in accordance with the UKCC code is by itself no defence should an employee's action breach the duty of employment.

National Health Service 'whistleblowing guidelines'

The government issued a document providing guidance for staff who are considering making complaints about what they regard as being poor standards of care, the latest edition of which was published in 1999 (Department of Health 1999). First, the guidelines stress that procedures should be set up to deal with staff grievances. Informal procedures should be available but where these do not lead to a satisfactory resolution there should be formal procedures in existence to enable concerns to be ventilated. The formal complaints should be made either up the line management chain or to a designated officer, who may be the person designated to receive patient complaints. This has been criticised in that staff may be frightened to make such a reference because of the consequences for their own careers if they are regarded as troublemakers. As *Public Concern at Work* commented in relation to the draft guidelines:

" To require a concerned member of staff to confront his or her line manager on their judgment or priorities in this way is unlikely to be productive or conducive for a good working environment. Only the most exceptional manager would not, in such a situation, want to pull rank over the staff member concerned.

McHale 1994

The guidelines distinguish between those health-care professionals who are in a direct line management relationship and others not in such a relationship, such as consultants. In relation to the latter it is suggested that they discuss their concerns with relevant colleagues and then take the matter up directly with the general manager or chief executive. This difference in approach may be seen as undesirable and indeed as divisive.

The guidelines suggest that if complaints are made to a designated officer and the matter is not resolved then the issue should be referred to the chairman of the authority or trust for action to be taken. There is no external right of appeal, the highest level of appeal being within the existing management framework. The guidelines state that, in some situations, health-care professionals may wish to consult outside agencies. For example, where a nurse is concerned about the welfare of a patient detained under the Mental Health Act 1983 s/he may decide to take the complaint to the Mental Health Act Commission (see page 135 above).

The guidelines make reference to the fact that health professionals may raise concerns with the Health Service Commissioner (the Ombudsman). While at present the Commissioner may not receive general complaints from hospital staff concerning standards, nevertheless he has indicated that he is willing to receive complaints from staff if they are made on behalf of an individual patient, the patient himself is unable to complain, and there is no other person who could claim on the patient's behalf. In his 1991–92 report, the Commissioner commented that he had undertaken an investigation of a complaint brought by a member of staff indicating that the level of care which a patient was receiving was inadequate (Health Service Commissioner 1992). Access to the Commissioner may indeed be a helpful way of ventilating staff concerns. However, the Commissioner's office has only limited resources and it may take a certain amount of time to process a claim.

One welcome provision of the guidelines is the right to consult a professional agency such as a trade union or other representative agency (Department of Health 1999, clause 23). Health-care professionals may also of course raise their concerns with their Member of Parliament. It is only at the very end of the guidelines that the question of disclosure to the media itself is considered. Such disclosure is regarded as a matter of last resort and should the nurse make the decision to 'go public', as did Graham Pink, then the guidelines remind the nurse that s/he is at risk of disciplinary proceedings. The guidelines refer to the duty of confidentiality to preserve patient information and the duty of confidentiality and loyalty to the employer (Department of Health 1999, clauses 8 and 9). Should a nurse find the internal mechanisms inadequate for dealing with concerns then s/he is left with the choice of going public, with the risk of legal and disciplinary proceedings should s/he do so.

The guidelines met considerable opposition when they were originally published. Reg Pyne, former Assistant Registrar at the UKCC, called them 'seriously flawed' and 'oppressive' (Turner 1994). While their publication can in one respect be regarded as an important step recognising that an important issue should be addressed, nevertheless, as was suggested above, in many ways they may be regarded as unsatisfactory.

Safeguarding whistleblowers in employment law – the Public Interest Disclosure Act 1998

In response to the campaigns following celebrated cases such as those of Graham Pink and the establishment of the organisation Public Concern at Work, funded by the Rowntree Trust to support whistleblowers both inside and outside the NHS, specific statutory protection was introduced in the form of the Public Interest Disclosure Act 1998. This safeguards a worker who makes what is known as a 'protected disclosure' under the Act (s43(B) Employment Rights Act 1996). Workers, for the purposes of the Public Interest Disclosure Act 1998, are employees and also independent contractors who provide services outside a professional client relationship (s43K Employment Rights Act 1996). Those who provide general medical, dental, ophthalmic and pharmaceutical services under NHS provision are specifically covered (s43K Employment Rights Act 1996).

Protected disclosures include concerns regarding actual/apprehended breaches of law and dangers to health, safety and environment. Protection was already available in relation to disclosures concerning health and safety matters (Employment Rights Act 1996 ss46 and 100). The worker must have a 'reasonable belief' that this is a protected disclosure (s43(B)(1) Employment Rights Act 1996). Disclosures made are protected if made in good faith to the employer or to a person other than the employer if it relates to that person's conduct or something for which that person has legal responsibility. In addition, disclosure may be made to one of the bodies listed on a list produced by regulations under the Act by the Secretary of State (s43(F) Employment Rights Act 1996).

There is also a second broad category of disclosures; disclosures made to the media are likely to fall into this category. Protection is given to disclosures in this category where the disclosure has been made in good faith, the worker reasonably believes that the information disclosed and any allegations contained in it are substantially true, the disclosure is not made for any personal gain and in all the circumstances of the case it is reasonable for her/him to make the disclosure. In addition, the criteria in subsection (2) must be complied with. These are that the worker reasonably believes that the employer will subject him/her to a detriment if s/he makes the disclosure in accordance with section 43F, s/he reasonably believes that the evidence will be lost or destroyed if s/he makes a disclosure to the employer and there is no person who is prescribed under s43F to whom the worker could disclose in relation to this particular failure.

In this section guidance is given as to what amounts to reasonableness in disclosure. Relevant factors are the person's identity and the seriousness of the failure, whether the failure is continuing or is likely to occur in the future and whether the disclosure has been made in breach of a duty of confidentiality owed to the employer or to any other person.

Special provisions apply under section 43H. The section applies to disclosures that concern failures of an exceptionally serious nature, where the disclosure is made in good faith, the worker reasonably believes that the information that has been disclosed and any allegations contained in it are substantially true, that the disclosure is not made for personal gain and that it is reasonable for her/him to make this disclosure in all the circumstances of the case. In determining the reasonableness of the disclosure for the purposes of this section regard shall be made to the identity of the person to whom the disclosure is made (s42H (2)).

Where a worker has been dismissed for making a protected disclosure then this is automatically an unfair dismissal (s103 Employment Rights Act 1996). Protection is also given against victimisation where this is 'on the ground that a protected disclosure was made' (s47B Employment Rights Act 1996). This applies where the employer subjects the employee to actions that are to his detriment, including failing to act – as, for example, in refusing promotion. The employer has the task of establishing the ground on which s/he subjected the employee to a detriment (s48(2) Employment Rights Act 1996). There is no limit on the award of compensation under the 1998 Act.

Following the 1998 Act, the Department of Health amended their guidance on whistleblowing in the NHS (Department of Health 1999). This requires Trusts to have local policies and procedures in place to ensure that they comply with the Public Interest Disclosure Act. These include, first, a senior manager or non-executive director who is to have the task of dealing in confidence with concerns raised outside the normal management chain. There should also be guidance to enable staff who have concerns regarding malpractice to raise these concerns. In addition the guidance states that there should be a clear commitment to ensure that concerns are taken seriously and investigated and that those staff who raise concerns should be protected against the prospect of victimisation. Furthermore, it states that gagging clauses are to be prohibited. Staff are to be made aware of policies and procedures and their 'responsibilities for raising genuine concerns in a reasonable and responsible way'.

Gagging clauses

One of the concerns in the debate in the 1990s regarding whistleblowing in the NHS was the proliferation in the number of so called 'gagging clauses'. These were contractual clauses imposed on NHS employees with the aim of stopping them from 'going public'. Such clauses are now prohibited by the Public Interest Disclosure Act 1998, to the extent to which they stop a worker making a protected disclosure (section 43 J Employment Rights Act 1996).

HEALTH-CARE RECORDS – ALLOWING PATIENT ACCESS

In this section, the extent to which patients may access their own records is considered, and the particular obligations placed upon the nurse to maintain the security of these records against unauthorised disclosure to third parties. The 1980s saw a dramatic shift in the policy of allowing patients access to their medical records. In the past, there was considerable opposition to patient access. There were several reasons for this. First, it was argued that the patient would have difficulty in understanding the records because they might have been compiled using technical terms or medical shorthand. Second, if health-care professionals knew that a patient could gain access, they would not be so candid in their comments when compiling the records. Third, it was argued that to allow access might be against the patient's interests because records might contain information that had been deliberately kept from the patient, for example, showing a terminal prognosis. But these arguments met with criticism. It was claimed that access to records is a fundamental part of patient autonomy and that denial of access in the patient's best interests is a paternalistic approach. It was said that a blanket ban was wrong because, while some patients might be unable to cope with the information, this did not mean that all patients were unable to cope. If health-care records were incomprehensible to patients this was not a basis for denying access; rather, it should be ensured that the records are comprehensible.

Statutory rights of access to health-care records

Access to Medical Reports Act 1988

The Access to Medical Reports Act 1988 grants a statutory right of access to reports compiled for the purposes of employment or insurance (s2). This right covers only those reports made by a person who has had clinical care of the patient, and would exclude a one-off examination specifically under-taken for the purposes of insurance by a clinician previously unknown to the patient. The patient who has requested that such a report be drawn up has the right to see the report. If the patient does not request the report it cannot be sent for 3 weeks (s4). If s/he believes it to be inaccurate, the patient may ask the doctor to amend it (s5). If the doctor refuses, then the patient can either refuse to allow the report to be sent to the employer or insurer or can have his/her own comments added to the report. Information may be withheld if the information would cause serious harm to a patient's physical or mental state or that of another person (Access to Medical Reports Act 1988 s17).

Data Protection Act 1998

Prior to 2000, access to health-care records was regulated predominately under the Access to Health Records Act 1990 and the Data Protection Act 1984.

The Access to Health Records Act applied to manually stored records created after 1991, while the Data Protection Act 1984 related to those records which were stored electronically. The position has now changed (Data Protection Act 1998(Commencement) Order 2000 SI 2000/183). The Data Protection Act 1998 gave effect to the European Directive on Personal Data and repealed the Data Protection Act 1984 and most of the Access to Health Records Act 1990 (HSC 2000/009). It applies to access to both electronic and manual health records. Manual records are those that are part of a relevant filing system. This refers to information that is structured by reference to individuals (s1(1)). It may be criteria relating to individuals such that specific information that relates to individuals is accessible. Information is also covered where this is part of an 'accessible record' that includes health records, defined in section 68(2) as:

" any record which –

(a) consists of information relating to the physical or mental health of the individual, and
(b) has been made by or on behalf of a health professional in connection with care of that individual.

'Health professionals' include doctors, nurses, dentists, opticians and pharmacists (s69).

The legislation covers processing of 'personal' data regarding 'data subjects' by 'data controllers'. 'Personal data' must relate to a living individual and must identify that individual.

Data controllers are required to comply with what are known as 'data protection principles', for example in relation to the purposes for which data is processed, its accuracy and the fact that personal data shall be processed in accordance with the rights of data subjects under the legislation.

Enforcement

The legislation is subject to enforcement by the Information Commissioner. Data subjects who believe that there is some error in the legislation may ask for the register to be rectified (s14), may claim compensation for damage and distress (s10) and can prevent processing of data that is likely to occasion distress or damage. In the case of a disputed decision between a person on whom a notice has been served and the Information Commissioner there is the provision for an appeal to the Data Protection Tribunal within 28 days of the notice relating to the disputed decision being served on the applicant (Data Protection Tribunal (Enforcement Appeals) Rules 2000 SI 2000 No 189). At such an appeal hearing, the burden is on the Commissioner to satisfy the Tribunal that the decision should be upheld.

Access rights

The data subject may apply for access to information under section 7 of the Act. The data controller must supply the information requested 'promptly' and there is a time limit imposed of 40 days (s7(8) and (10)). In a situation in which this information is not supplied then s/he may be required to do so by the court (s7(2)(a). A fee may be requested, subject to a statutory maximum. Transitional provisions were applicable in situations where records were not exclusively automated or so intended up to 24 October 2001. The maximum fee where a permanent copy of the information is supplied is £50. However where the request applies simply to data that forms part of a health record, and it was created in the 40 days that preceded the request and no permanent copy is going to be made, then no fee should be charged (Data Protection (Subject Access) (Fees and Miscellaneous Provisions) Regulations 2000, SI 2000 No 191). The subject may request a copy of the information, which may include an explanation of any terms that have been used.

Limitations on access rights

As with the Data Protection Act 1984 and the Access to Health Records Act 1990, access rights are not absolute. Access to health-care records may be withheld in a situation in which the information may cause serious harm to the patient's physical or mental health or condition or that of another person. Where the data controller is not a health professional s/he must either consult the health professional who has responsibility for the patient's care or, if that person is not available, another health professional with sufficient experience and qualifications to advise on these matters. Access to information regarding the provision of treatment services and those born as a result of such treatment services and the keeping and use of gametes and embryos under the Human Fertilisation and Embryology Act 1990 is also restricted (Data Protection (Subject Access Modification) (Health) Order 2000 SI 2000 No. 413).

This clinical privilege needs to be exercised with considerable sensitivity if the rights of the patient are to be adequately protected. As Brazier (2003) notes: 'What should not be forgotten is that a patient who genuinely would rather not know what was wrong with him will never ask for access to his records'.

Information concerning identifiable third parties

Information relating to an identifiable third party may be withheld (s7(4)). There are exceptions where that person has given their consent or that it is reasonable in the particular circumstances to disclose without consent. (s7(5)).

General exemptions

Data processed for research, statistical or historical purposes are exempt from the access rights where these data are not being processed for the purpose of supporting measures or decisions in relation to specific persons. In addition, the processing itself must not be undertaken in such a way that it causes the patient 'substantial damage or distress'. Finally, in the case of research, any results of that research should not be made available in a form in which the patient is identifiable (s33). Professional regulatory bodies, such as the NMC, are given some protection from access provisions where this is likely to prejudice the proper discharge of their functions (s31(2)(a)(iii), s31(4)(b), s31(4)(a)(iii)).

Patients lacking mental capacity

In contrast to the Access to Health Records Act 1990, in which specific provisions related to the child patient, under the 1998 Act the situation regarding adults lacking mental capacity and child patients is problematic because neither group is dealt with specifically in the legislation. It is unclear whether persons other than the data subject may make an application for access under the legislation.

Residual access rights under the Access to Health Records Act 1990

While the majority of the provisions in the Access to Health Records Act 1990 have been superseded by the 1998 Act, access to the health records of a deceased person are not covered by the 1998 Act. Personal representatives (s3(1)(f)) or persons claiming in relation to the deceased's estate (s5(4) will have to make an application under the Access to Health Records Act 1990.

Ensuring the security of records

The nurse must ensure that patient records are kept secure from unauthorised access. This is particularly important in view of the fact that so much information today is held on computer.

Unauthorised access to information held on computer may constitute a criminal offence under the Computer Misuse Act 1990, although there are certain exceptions in relation to a situation in which a person accidentally exceeds his/her permission. The need to maintain controls over disclosure of computerised records has now further been developed with the Caldicott review and subsequent developments.

The electronic patient record and the Caldicott review

At present there are major developments within the NHS in relation to the use and transfer of patient information. The electronic patient record is being formulated along with the 'NHS net' which is an 'intranet' for exchanging business and clinical data. An initial pilot study defined the electronic patient record as 'a dynamic collection of messages, held electronically, created by healthcare professionals principally to inform themselves and others about the provision of health care to an individual patient'. It is envisaged that eventually patients will possess an electronic health record that will operate during the whole of their life. While such developments have considerable potential, they may also raise dilemmas concerning access to and security of health information. The Caldicott Committee was established to undertake a review of the uses of patient-identifiable information flowing from NHS organisations to NHS and other bodies for purposes other than direct care, medical research or where there is a statutory requirement for information (Department of Health 1997). It recommended that data flows within the health service should be tested against basic principles of good practice. Individuals should be designated 'guardians' of health-care information. Protocols were to be developed governing the sharing of information between NHS and non-NHS bodies. In addition, the identity of persons who were responsible for monitoring the sharing and transfer of information should be clearly communicated. Guardians should document all routine uses of person-identified information. Access to records would be on a strictly need-to-know basis with confidentiality 'heath checks' to be undertaken each year.

The Committee's recommendations were accepted by the government and Caldicott guardians were established nationwide. The document *Protecting and using patient information: a manual for Caldicott guardians* (National Health Service Executive 1999) provides that the guardian should be either a member of the existing management board, a senior health professional or an individual responsible for promoting clinical governance. A series of principles are set out in the document. The proposed use and transfer of patient information must be justified. The second principle states that patient information should not be used save where this is absolutely necessary. Third, the minimum amount of identifiable patient information should be used. Principle 4 provides that patient information should be available on a strictly need to know basis. Principle 5 states that all persons who handle patient information should know their responsibilities. Finally, they should understand and comply with the law. All HA/Special Health Authorities NHS trusts and Primary Care groups were required to appoint a Caldicott Guardian no later than 30 March 1999 (HSC 1999/012).

The intention was that during the first year there should be an audit by the management of procedures for protection and use of patient information. Issues to be considered included reviewing existing flows of patient-identifiable information. The guidance emphasised that all NHS bodies must have active policy for informing patients regarding the purposes for which information about them is collected and persons to whom such information may be passed. Protocols should be drawn up governing the disclosure of patient/client-identifiable information to other organisations. Where an individual wants information to be withheld the guidance states that this wish should be respected. Protocols should govern both the disclosure of the information and its security. The guidance also notes the need to maintain security within the individual organisation. These guidelines are to be commended as a step in the right direction, alongside the safeguards of the Data Protection principles contained in the 1998 Act. Nonetheless, the boundaries of disclosure are something that does need to be carefully monitored. The NMC has recently stated that:

" The principle of the confidentiality of information held about patients/ clients is just as important in computer-held records as in all other records, including those sent by fax. All registrants are professionally accountable for making sure that whatever system is used is fully secure. Clear protocols should be implemented at local level to specify which staff members have access to computer-held records. National and local information technology support agencies should be consulted to install a cascade system giving appropriate access to specific members of staff. Managers should be able to inform staff as to the level of access they, or other members of the health care team and other ancillary or administration staff have. Such a system ensures that access is only available to authorised users.

Liability for unauthorised disclosure of health information

There have been suggestions that, if a health-care professional goes ahead and discloses confidential information without the consent of that patient, the health-care professional may be held liable in negligence for that disclosure. Carson & Montgomery (1990) give an example of a case in which a doctor was held to be liable in negligence for revealing to the husband of his patient the fact that he considered that she was paranoid. He had not told the patient directly because he thought that this would cause harm to the patient's mental state and to the doctor–patient relationship. It was held that the harm that took place was reasonably foreseeable in nature, even though the circumstances in which the husband revealed the information were not.

Should patients be allowed to retain their own records?

Health-care records are usually held in hospitals, health centres or surgeries, although certain trials have been conducted to ascertain the feasibility of patients being given their own records on 'smart cards' – small cards on which data are electronically stored and which may be accessed by a special machine. However, the fact that a patient is simply given a smart card by itself will not facilitate access to records, because access is dependent upon the patient having the means to access the information on that card.

But if the general principle of patient access is accepted then why not allow patients to keep hold of their own records? There is, of course, the risk that patients would lose them, but studies undertaken seem to suggest that this is not the case (Gilhooley & McGhee 1991) There are considerable advantages in patient-held records. For example, nurses would have immediate access to records if visiting patients at home; there would be no delay in transferring records when the patient moved GP; time would be saved in GPs' surgeries storing records; it would assist patients in correcting inaccuracies in records. It might also increase trust between patients and health-care professionals.

CONCLUSIONS

Reforming the law

The present law concerning patient confidentiality can only be gleaned by reference to a number of disparate sources. The boundaries of disclosure for the nurse are unclear. There have been a number of proposals for reform in the area. In 1981 the Law Commission suggested that the law concerning breach of confidence should be placed upon a statutory footing (Law Commission 1981). In 1995 the British Medical Association produced a draft Bill on confidentiality. The Bill was the result of deliberations by a working party, which included nursing input from the UKCC. A version of this Bill was introduced into the House of Lords by Lord Walton in 1996 and was given a second reading. This Bill applied to information relating to an individual's physical or mental health that is in the control of a health service body or qualified health professional. It set out the basis on which information could be lawfully disclosed, and made unauthorised disclosure a criminal offence.

The Bill ultimately fell and, at present, comprehensive legislation in the area appears unlikely.

While the Human Rights Act 1998 has rooted confidentiality in privacy, the boundaries of confidentiality still remain to be ascertained on a case-by-case basis. Ultimately the best safeguard of patient confidentiality is good professional norms.

REFERENCES

Boddington P 1994 Confidentiality in genetic counselling. In: Clarke A (ed.) Genetics counselling practice and principles. Routledge, London

Brazier M 2003 Medicine, patients and the law. Penguin, London

Carson D, Montgomery J 1990 Nursing law. Macmillan, Basingstoke

Chadwick R, Levitt M, Schickle D (eds) 1997 The right to know and the right not to know. Avebury, Aldershot

Case P 2003 Confidence matters: the rise and fall of informational autonomy in medical law. Medical Law Review 11: 208–236

Department of Health 1999 Whistleblowing in the NHS. HSC 1999/198. Department of Health, London

Department of Health 2001 Learning from Bristol: the report of the Public Inquiry into children's heart surgery at the Bristol Royal Infirmary 1984–1995. Stationery Office, London

Department of Health 2003 Confidentiality: NHS code of practice. Department of Health, London

Department of Health 2004 Best Practice Guidance for doctors and other health professionals on the provision of advice and treatment to young people under sixteen on contraception, sexual and reproductive health. Department of Health, London

Dorozynski A 1996 Mitterand book provokes storm in France. British Medical Journal 312: 201

General Medical Council 1997 Serious communicable diseases. GMC, London

Gilhooley M, McGhee SM 1991 Medical records; practicalities and principles of patient possession. Journal of Medical Ethics 17: 138–143

Grubb A, Pearl D 1986 Medicine, health, family and the law. Family Law 101: 25

Health Service Commissioner 1992 Annual Report for 1991–92. HC 82. HMSO, London

Human Genetics Commission 2002 Inside information. HGC, London

Kennedy I, Grubb A 1994 Medical law, text with materials. Butterworths, London

Law Commission 1981 Breach of confidence. Law Commission, London

Mason JK, Laurie G 2006 Mason and McCall Smith's Law and Medical ethics, 7th edn. Oxford University Press, Oxford

McHale JV 1993 Medical confidentiality and legal privilege. Routledge, London

McHale J 1994 Whistleblowing in the USA. In: Hunt G (ed.) Whistleblowing in the health services. Edward Arnold, London

McHale J, Gallagher A 2004 Nursing and human rights. Butterworth Heinemann, London

Montgomery J 1987 Confidentiality and the immature minor. Family Law 101: 26

National Health Service Executive 1999 Protecting and using patient information: a manual for Caldicott Guardians. NHSE London

Nightingale F 1859 Notes on nursing. Reprint, 1974. Blackie, Glasgow

Nursing and Midwifery Council 2004 NMC Code of Professional Conduct: standards for conduct, performance and ethics. NMC, London

Nursing and Midwifery Council 2006 A–Z advice sheet: confidentiality. NMC: London

Nuffield Council on Bioethics 1993 Genetic screening: ethical issues. Nuffield Council: London

Department of Health 1997 Report on the review of patient-identifiable information: the Caldicott Committee. Department of Health, London

Sieghart P 1982 Professional ethics: for whose benefit? Journal of Medical Ethics 8: 25–32

Siegler M 1982 Confidentiality in medicine – a decrepit concept. New England Journal of Medicine 307: 1518–1521

Thompson IE 1979 The nature of confidentiality. Journal of Medical Ethics 5: 57–64

Turner T 1994 Paradox in practice. Nursing Times 90(21): 18

Clinical research and the nurse

Jean McHale

Nurses increasingly participate in clinical trials (Parabor 1997). The nurse may run his/her own trial or may undertake research as part of a diploma qualification or for a higher degree. The nurse may be involved in a trial being run by a medical practitioner or by another nurse. A nurse may be a member of a research ethics committee, which has the task of scrutinising proposals for clinical research in a particular area. Research is integral to good clinical practice. As the Nursing and Midwifery Council (NMC) Code of Professional Conduct provides: '6.5 You have a responsibility to deliver care based on current evidence, best practice and, where applicable, validated research when it is available' (Nursing and Midwifery Council 2002).

Awareness of legal and ethical issues in research is therefore important for reflective practice (Royal College of Nursing 2004). While research is necessary for scientific development and clinical practice it can also prove controversial, as illustrated by the recent press reports concerning six volunteers involved in an anti-inflammatory drugs trial at Northwick Park Hospital in London, who suffered a severe reaction and multiple organ failure within hours of taking the drug (BBC Newsonline 2006). This chapter provides an account of the legal regulation of research and the obligation of the researcher to the research subject.

The first section of this chapter considers the manner in which clinical research is regulated. In the second section, the role of research ethics committees in scrutinising clinical trials and legal principles regulating clinical trials are discussed. In the final section the question of negligence actions brought against nurses and others where research subjects are injured in a clinical trial are considered, along with the role of the nurse in policing unethical researchers.

FRAMEWORK OF REGULATION

The human rights abuses of clinical research in Nazi Germany and in Japan during the middle years of the 20th century resulted in pressure for the regulation of clinical research. Concern to safeguard the human rights of the individual has played an important part in structuring responses to research regulation (McHale & Gallagher 2004). International guidelines were developed, most notably the Nuremberg Code in 1949 and the Declaration of Helsinki, originally produced in 1964 (Plomer 2004). In this country there is no one piece of legislation governing the conduct of all research activity, although certain legislation does govern specific areas such as animal research (Animals (Scientific Procedure) Act 1986) and research undertaken on embryos (Human Fertilisation and Embryology Act 1990). Most recently the European Union Clinical Trials Directive has led to major changes in the legal regulation of drug trials in this country through the Medicines for Human Use (Clinical Trials) Regulations 2004.

A number of guidelines have been published, for example by the Department of Health in the form of the Research Governance Framework (Department of Health 2005a) and the Guidelines for NHS Research Ethics Committees (GAfREC, Department of Health 2001), the Royal College of Physicians (1996) and the Royal College of Nursing (1993). While these guidelines are not legally binding, they suggest conduct that amounts to good research practice and may be referred to in subsequent legal proceedings. The law governing research derives from general principles of civil law and criminal law, along with certain specific statutory provisions such as the Medicines Act 1968 and the Medicine for Human Use (Clinical Trials) Regulations 2004 (SI 2004/1031). Clinical research is undertaken across a vast area of scientific activity.

Below is a brief overview of some of the areas of current regulatory activity. Certain research gives rise to particularly difficult ethical issues, requiring careful consideration, for example embryo research, the use of fetal tissue and the research into gene therapy. Embryo research was considered by the Warnock Committee Embryo research is regulated by the Human Fertilisation and Embryology Authority under the Human Fertilisation and Embryology Act 1990. Embryo research was eventually sanctioned after a heated ethical debate regarding the status of the embryo. As with abortion, ethical objections were raised to the use and consequent destruction of embryos for research purposes. The Act represents in many respects a compromise of views allowing controlled research for a limited period of time in the early stages of development of the embryo. The Authority issues licences to researchers to undertake such research as falls within the criteria set out in the legislation. Researchers may undertake embryo experimentation if this comes within the criteria set out in the Human Fertilisation and Embryology Act 1990, which includes promoting advances in the treatment of infertility, increasing the knowledge of congenital disease, increasing knowledge about the cause of miscarriages, developing more effective means of contraception or developing methods for detecting the presence of gene or chromosome abnormalities in embryos before implantation. The Act bans certain forms of experimentation such as keeping or using an embryo after the appearance of the primitive streak (after 14 days of development), placing an embryo in an animal or replacing the nucleus of a cell of an embryo with a nucleus taken from a cell of any person, embryo or subsequent development of an embryo (cloning through nuclei substitution) (s3(3) Human Fertilisation and Embryology Act 1990). As we shall see in Chapter 9, this area is currently under review by the government (Department of Health 2005b). (For general discussion on one particular issue consequent upon such research – cloning, see Chapter 9.)

Xenotransplantation is regulated by the Xenotransplantation Interim Regulatory Advisory Authority (see Ch. 10). Gene therapy is overseen by a specially created government body, the Gene Therapy Advisory Committee, which imposes stringent requirements on researchers. This chapter focuses upon those clinical trials in which nurses are at present most likely to be directly involved, and discusses general principles of research activity on human subjects. As we shall see below, the conduct of most clinical trials is subject to the consideration of non-statutory bodies – local research ethics committees.

Drug trials and innovative therapies

Before medicines are made used in a clinical trial the use must be 'authorised' by the Medical and Healthcare Products Regulatory Agency (Medicines for Human Use (Clinical Trials) Regulations 2004, regs 17–21). Although safeguards in the form of licensing exist in relation to experimental drug therapy, there are at present no equivalent safeguards as regards innovative therapy, such as keyhole surgery. It has been suggested that, in view of the fine line between innovative therapy and research, innovative therapy should be classed as medical research in situations in which the main purpose of therapy is to acquire knowledge, as opposed to care for the patient. In the light of much public concern regarding the use of certain new therapeutic techniques, notably keyhole surgery, the government indicated that it was considering the introduction of legislation in this area (*The Times*, 21 February 1995). The safety of medical interventions is now the subject of consideration by the National Institute for Health and Clinical Excellence (http://www.nice.org.uk/page.aspx?o=whatwedo). NICE undertakes technology appraisals which include the assessment of new surgical procedures. This includes taking into account clinical evidence as to how well the new procedure will work in addition to looking at economic evidence as to the extent to which this can be seen as constituting value for money.

Animal research

The Animals Scientific Procedures Act 1986 states that, before research can be undertaken on animals, researchers must obtain a licence from the Home Secretary. A Home Office committee examines whether the benefits to be gained from research being undertaken upon these animals justify the suffering that may be occasioned. The practice and ethics of these procedures go beyond the scope of the book and the reader is referred to further sources (see, for example, Fox 1995).

REGULATION OF RESEARCH: GENERAL PRINCIPLES

This section considers the basis of regulation of clinical research involving human subjects and legal principles governing the operation of clinical trials, as well as the criteria that the nurse should satisfy before embarking on a clinical trial. The principles of consent to treatment applicable in the context of research are considered, and the particular issues that arise in the context of certain groups of research subjects such as children and adults lacking mental capacity. This section concludes by examining the role and obligations of the nurse researcher on the wards. Issues of confidentiality and research are considered in Chapter 7.

Local research ethics committees

Before a trial is undertaken, the researcher should obtain approval for the conduct of the trial from a research ethics committee. Where the trial concerns medicinal products the Medicines for Human Use (Clinical Trials) Regulations provide that it is an offence to begin such a trial without ethics committee approval (reg 49). The main guidelines governing the operation of such committees are GAfREC (Department of Health 2001). These recommend that there should be a maximum of 18 members (para 6.1). The Committee should have a mixture of 'expert' and 'lay' members (para 6.3). The expert members should be drawn from persons with:

- relevant methodological and ethical expertise in:
  - clinical research
  - non-clinical research
  - qualitative or other research methods applicable to health services, social science and social care research
- clinical practice including:
  - hospital and community staff (medical, nursing and other) general practice
  - statistics relevant to research
  - pharmacy (Department of Health 2001, para 6.4).

At least one-third should be 'lay members' (Department of Health 2001, para 6.5). Of these GAfREC provides that at least half must be 'persons who are not, and never have been, either health or social care professionals, and who have never been involved in carrying out research involving human participants, their tissue or data' (Department of Health 2001, para 6.7). The members of a research ethics committee must act as individuals and not as a representative of the group from which they have been drawn (Department of Health 2001, para 6.8).

Multicentred research ethics committees

Although such committees operate predominantly on a 'local' basis, in recent years there have been increasing attempts to facilitate consistency in approach. Where it is proposed to undertake a trial over a number of research centres in different parts of the country the proposal should be referred to one of a number of multicentred research ethics committees governing the approval of multicentred trials (Department of Health 2001, part 8.)

Regulation of research ethics committees

Until recently, research ethics committees were not subject to central co-ordination save through the production of guidelines by the Department of Health. This has, however, changed somewhat. The operation of research ethics committees in England is today governed by the Central Office for Research Ethics Committees (COREC) (http:www.corec.org.uk). From 1 April 2005 the operation of COREC became part of the National Patient Safety Agency (http://www.npsa.nhs.uk).

As a result of the Medicines for Human Use (Clinical Trials) Regulations 2004 the government was also required to establish the UK Ethics Committee Authority (2004 Regulations, part II). This organisation is required to establish, recognise and monitor ethics committees in order that they comply with the Clinical Trials Regulations.

Assessing the risk

A researcher must satisfy the committee that the project is ethical and that any risk posed to research subjects is of an acceptable level. Factors that the committee must consider include any discomfort or distress the project may cause the research subject, any hazards that may arise during the project and precautions that should be introduced to deal with them, and the extent to which the research subject's health will be affected by involvement in a trial. The Royal College of Physicians 1996 guidelines state helpfully the following:

> " Benefit may be weighed against risk in two different ways. First and most obviously the patient may benefit. This is typified in a therapeutic trial where at least one of the treatments offered may be beneficial to the patient. Benefits may be considerable, for example, in cancer treatment and may counter balance even high risk to the individual. Second, society rather than the individual may benefit. In such situations however large the benefit to expose a participant to anything more than a minimal risk needs very careful consideration and would rarely be ethical.

> *Royal College of Physicians 1996, para 7.3*

What if a volunteer is prepared to accept a risk that is more than minimal of participation in a clinical trial? Some people will take risks of a very high order for altruistic reasons. A person may volunteer to be involved in a trial to help researchers develop a cure for a condition suffered by a close relative. It is unclear whether it is lawful for a research subject to consent to involvement in a very high risk trial. As was noted earlier in relation to consent to treatment, English law does not allow a person to consent to any harm. If a research subject included in a high-risk trial dies, then there is the possibility that a researcher would be prosecuted for manslaughter.

Inducements to participate

Many trials are undertaken using volunteers. While some may be willing to give up their time out of altruism, many trials would simply not go ahead unless some inducements were given. A small financial inducement may be given to compensate for time spent and potential inconvenience caused. But while payment of small sums may be acceptable, there is a danger that an unethical researcher may offer large sums to encourage participation in a trial imposing an undue risk. Similarly, some payments to researchers may be unethical.

If the researcher receives payment on the basis that the more patients are recruited the larger the fee, there is a danger that researchers may place undue pressures on patients and others to be included in the research. Nonetheless, the level of any inducement given to the NHS body, health professionals, researchers or subjects to participate in clinical research is a factor that will be considered by a local research ethics committee when considering whether to approve a clinical trial (Department of Health 2001, para 9.15, k). Inducements to research subjects may of course be other than financial. For example, pressure may be put on nurses by nurse researchers to participate in clinical trials because it is something that is expected of them. Such pressure is unjustifiable. It is important to ensure that subjects give full and free consent to entry into any trial.

Consent

As with any clinical procedure, it is vital to obtain consent from a research subject before a trial commences. The nurse may have the task of obtaining a patient's consent to participation in a trial or, even if not involved in initially obtaining consent, the nurse may be drawn into the process if a patient later approaches her/him and asks questions about the trial. Ensuring that research subjects are given adequate information is an important part of the role of a research ethics committee. What information must be given to the research subject in a clinical trial? A distinction should be drawn between therapeutic and non-therapeutic trials. Therapeutic research is research intended to benefit an individual patient. Non-therapeutic research is research that is unlikely to or will not benefit the research subject (whether a patient or healthy volunteer) personally. The consent guidelines were revised following controversy concerning one particular clinical trial.

In May 2000 the UK government announced that they would be conducting a review into the consent process for clinical research in the NHS. This was in response to the study that was undertaken at the North Staffordshire hospital NHS Trust by Professor David Southall. A trial was conducted upon neonates who suffered respiratory failure, considering the effect of treatment using continuous negative extrathoracic pressure rather than standard ventilation. Parents whose two children received the procedure complained. The first died while on a ventilator and 10 months later a second child was discovered to have brain damage. In neither case, it was claimed, had it been explained to the patients that this was an experimental procedure. The review of the trial conducted by Professor Rod Griffiths, a director of public health in the West Midlands regional office of the National Health Service Executive, was highly critical (Griffiths 2000). It stated that 'the apparent lack of adequate explanation, of choice and consequent properly elicited and recorded consent and involvement in later decision making' was unacceptable. The professor heading the trial had not 'ensured that each member of staff who might be involved in the project was trained or supervised to ensure that they were doing what the research project said they should'. The ethics committee that approved the trial was also the subject of criticism. It was claimed that the committee had not examined the proposal sufficiently. In fact, it was the case that failures of management and supervision were, in the view of the report 'virtually built into the design'. The report commented that: 'In effect the combination of a slightly complacent local research ethics committee, an enthusiastic and assertive researcher, and a vacuum in research governance in the trust led this trial to run in a less than adequate way'. Both consultants were subject to disciplinary action, and it appears that nurses who were involved in the trial were also subject to investigation by the UKCC. The report has recommended that formal guidance on research governance within the NHS should be developed. Until this is developed at NHS level the report recommended that the Trust should develop its own guidance. They also recommended that there should be cooperation between the Department of Health and professional and regulatory bodies to consult and produce agreed guidelines that clarify issues of consent for participation in clinical trials.

GAfREC requires research ethics committees to consider the informed consent process (Department of Health 2001, para 9.17). It requires that there must be:

" a. full description of the process for obtaining informed consent, including the identification of those responsible for obtaining consent, the time-frame in which it will occur, and the process for ensuring consent has not been withdrawn
b. the adequacy, completeness and understandability of written and oral information to be given to the research participants, and, when appropriate, their legally acceptable representatives
c. clear justification for the intention to include in the research individuals who cannot consent, and a full account of the arrangements for obtaining consent or authorisation for the participation of such individuals
d. assurances that research participants will receive information that becomes available during the course of the research relevant to their participation (including their rights, safety and well-being)
e. the provisions made for receiving and responding to queries and complaints from research participants or their representatives during the course of a research project.

Department of Health 2001, para 9.17

Information provision and the randomised controlled trial

Providing full information recognises the autonomy of the research subject. Without informed consent, research subjects may not realise that they are being subjected to procedures aimed at benefiting future patients rather than themselves. However, there are certain situations in which researchers may wish to withhold information from patients. Take randomised controlled trials: some patients included in a trial recover not because of the effect of new medication but simply because they think that they have been given a new drug. This is known as the 'placebo effect'. In an attempt to overcome this problem, researchers undertake randomised controlled trials. Research subjects are divided into two groups: one group is given the treatment, the other is given a placebo or dummy treatment. The patient does not know whether s/he is receiving the real or the dummy treatment. A variant on this is the 'double-blind' trial: in this type of trial, neither the clinician nor the research subject knows whether the patient has been given the treatment or an inert substance. It is particularly important for patients to appreciate that they are being entered into a randomised clinical trial and that there is a risk of missing out on a standard course of treatment. When providing information about the trial, researchers must ensure that all subjects are told that they are free to withdraw at any stage.

The law and information provision in clinical research

There are no statutes or decided cases in English law stating how much information should be given to subjects in clinical research. A research subject may claim that provision of inadequate information constitutes the tort of battery. As stated earlier in relation to consent to medical treatment, the courts have stated that as long as a patient gives general consent to an operation being undertaken then health-care professionals will not be liable in battery (*Chatterson* v. *Gerson* [1981] QB 432 at 443). But would the same test be applied to clinical research? In the Canadian case of *Halushka* v. *University of Saskatchewan* it was held that the failure of researchers to provide the subject with full information constituted a battery, Hall J.A. said: 'The subjects of medical experimentation are entitled to a full and frank disclosure of all the facts, probabilities and opinions which a reasonable man might be expected to consider before giving consent' ([1965] 53 DLR (2d) 436 at 438).

It is suggested that the adoption of such an approach, requiring a broad duty of disclosure to those entering a non-therapeutic trial, is desirable. What of patients included in therapeutic trials? The difficulty here is that if patients included in trials had to be given a full explanation this would give such patients the right to receive more information than a patient receiving any other therapy. At present it seems likely that the courts would hold that a patient is entitled to the same level of disclosure whether therapy is given as part of treatment or as therapeutic research.

It may be necessary to undertake research using patients brought unconscious into Casualty who are in a critical condition. Research projects involving such patients should be examined with particular care. If it is possible to anticipate that a patient may be subject to an unexpected event, such as complications during childbirth, then the researchers should obtain the patient's consent before labour begins.

Duty to inform – negligence

While a research subject may have been given some information as to the trial such that an action in battery may be difficult to establish, a research subject may claim that a researcher acted negligently because inadequate information was provided as to the risks posed by involvement in the trial. In the context of medical treatment, we noted that, while for many years the courts were prepared to hold that a health-care professional was not negligent as long as s/he gave the patient such information as would have been provided by a responsible body of professional nursing opinion (*Sidaway* v. *Bethlem Royal Hospital Governors* [1985] AC 871), in recent years the courts have indicated that they may be moving towards a 'prudent patient' test (*Pearce* v. *United Bristol NHS Trust* (1999) PIQR P53). Does the duty differ in relation to clinical research?

Two alternative approaches could be taken. Given the uncertain nature of clinical research and the risks involved, a different standard of disclosure could be adopted for treatment and therapeutic research. The research subject could be entitled to receive more information than the patient. But the dividing line between therapeutic treatment and therapeutic research is a very fine one and this may be regarded as an unjustifiably narrow distinction to draw. Alternatively, a complete reassessment could be made of the legal obligation to disclose information to patients. It appears unlikely that the courts or Parliament will attempt such a reform in the near future. Such judicial or legislative reform may not prove necessary given the move in clinical practice towards providing patients routinely with more information regarding the risks of treatment (Ch. 5).

A strong argument can be made in favour of full disclosure of all risks in the case of non-therapeutic trials. If a research subject is subjected to scientific tests for the benefit of the community as a whole and not for his/her own personal benefit then s/he should be told of the risks run by involvement in the project. What must be emphasised is that to simply provide a large amount of information about potential risks of entry into a clinical trial may be of little value. A nurse will not comply with his/her legal obligation by simply providing a patient with an information sheet.

The nurse can independently observe what information the patient has been given. S/he may be of the view that the information that has been given is inadequate. In such a situation, the nurse should raise the concerns with the researcher. It is certainly arguable that in a research situation the nurse may be justified in personally providing the research subject with more information. However, the nurse should only contemplate providing the patient with more information directly after having ascertained the position regarding disclosure. The question of unethical researchers is explored further in the section on policing trials below. See also discussion of conflicts between nurses and other health-care professionals over information disclosure on page 115.

Where a research subject asks questions about the research project, again whether the researcher has to fully answer such queries is unclear. It is submitted that, as with medical treatment, any refusal to provide information would require careful justification in the case of a therapeutic trial, and that such a refusal would be unjustifiable in the case of a non-therapeutic trial.

Can patients be compelled to participate?

Consider a patient asked to participate in a clinical trial. The trial offers the prospect of a cure for what is otherwise an incurable condition. The patient refuses to be involved. Could the patient be compelled to participate? The law states that a competent adult patient has the right to refuse treatment, even if as a consequence the patient dies (e.g. *Re B (adult: refusal of medical treatment)* ([2002] 2 All ER 449), see also Chs 5 (p. 108) and 10 (p. 224)). Nonetheless, it is doubtful whether any court would authorise the inclusion of a competent but protesting adult in a research trial even if the trial was clearly therapeutic. Indeed, to sanction such involvement would, it is submitted, represent an unjustifiable limitation on individual autonomy.

If a nurse or doctor in charge of a project appears to be putting pressure on a patient to participate, the nurse acting as patient advocate should make the patient aware of his/her right to refuse to be included in the trial. The nurse should also protest to the researcher about what s/he regards as bad practice. If a researcher continues to act in flagrant disregard of legal obligations, then the nurse should bring the matter to the attention of the appropriate bodies, including the research ethics committee.

Children and clinical trials

Wherever possible, clinical trials should be conducted using competent adults. But in some situations it is necessary to include children in a clinical trial, for instance if the trial involves a study into childhood diseases or the suitability for administration to children of a drug that is currently used to treat adult patients. A research ethics committee assesses the risk level of trials. The risk to a child of participation in a trial is something that the research ethics committee will be particularly concerned to assess.

Particular difficulties surround non-therapeutic trials. The GAfREC guidelines emphasise that to expose a child in a non-therapeutic trial to a risk that is other than merely negligible may be to act unlawfully. But is this right? We noted earlier that some are of the view that it is legitimate to include children in non-therapeutic procedures as long as this is 'not against' their best interests. It has been argued that, just as parents are lawfully entitled to expose their children to certain quite risky activities they should be entitled to expose them to the risks surrounding entry into a clinical trial (Nicholson, 1985). One approach is to limit the entry of child patients to those trials where there is minimal risk, an approach favoured by, for example, the Royal College of Paediatrics and Child Health (2000). But there is scope for disagreement as to what constitutes 'minimal risk'. A scientist may rate a procedure as having a lower risk than would a patient assessing the same procedure (Nicholson 1991). Research ethics committees need to be extremely sensitive to the different weightings that may be placed on risk levels by scientists and research subjects in scrutinising research protocols.

If it is proposed to include a child in a clinical trial, from whom should patient consent be obtained – parent or child? As already discussed, in law, a child over 16 years can give consent to medical treatment and a child under that age may be competent to give consent (s8 Family Law Reform Act 1969). In *Gillick* v. *West Norfolk and Wisbech AHA* ([1985] 3 All ER 402), the House of Lords held that whether a child under 16 years was capable of consenting to medical treatment was dependent upon an assessment of the child's maturity. It seems likely that the *Gillick* approach would be adopted by a court if it was asked to consider whether a child could consent to involvement in a therapeutic research project. Application of this test is not straightforward. Researchers must carefully assess each child individually to determine his/her capacity to consent to be involved in a particular trial. It would be good practice for researchers to ensure that they have the written consent of those with parental responsibility, even if the child is competent to consent to involvement in the trial.

It is uncertain whether a child can consent to being included in a non-therapeutic trial. The courts may be prepared to adopt the *Gillick* test of competency and hold that a competent child may give a valid consent to involvement in a non-therapeutic research project. But would a child be competent to make that choice? It is important not to underestimate a child's powers of comprehension.

Compelling a child to be involved

What can a nurse do if a child tearfully refuses to be involved in the project? Can the child be compelled on the grounds that it is in his/her best interests to be involved? The courts have indicated that, if a competent child refuses treatment, the parents may authorise treatment on the child's behalf. Compelling a child's involvement in any clinical procedure is a very serious step. Were such conflicts to arise and the issue go to court, then it is submitted that a court is unlikely to authorise a child to be forcibly involved in a therapeutic trial, save perhaps in an exceptional situation where the child is suffering from a condition with a terminal prognosis and the treatment represents the child's only chance of life. Even here, it would be exceedingly controversial to compel involvement. Can a very young child be forced to take part in a clinical trial? The Department of Health guidelines do not deal with this question. The legal position is uncertain. Certainly, as far as possible, the wishes of even a very young child should be given serious consideration in making this decision.

Adults lacking mental capacity

The nurse may be involved in a research project including mentally incapacitated adults. Wherever possible, adult participants with mental capacity should be used. But, as with the child participant, there may be situations in which research is inevitable, including those lacking mental capacity because it relates to a condition specific to this subject group, such as, for example, research into a particular mental illness or the effects of a particular treatment. For example, a study into the side effects of antipsychotic drugs must be undertaken using clients who are receiving such medication. However, researchers must not forget that, while persons may have some mental impairment, this does not mean that they are totally unable to give consent. The majority of psychiatric patients are as capable of giving consent as other patients (Royal College of Psychiatrists 1990). Admittedly, some patients will never reach that level of capacity. Nevertheless, including such patients in a research project may be of very real benefit to them or to groups of other patients in the future.

As stated in Chapter 6, at common law relatives and other persons have no power to give consent in law on behalf of an adult lacking mental capacity. The House of Lords in *Re F* ([1990] 2 AC 1) stated that treatment may be given where the health professionals believe that it is in the best interests of an incompetent patient. While the question of therapeutic research was not discussed in *Re F*, it appears likely that such research may be justified if it can be shown that it is treatment for 'life, health, well-being'. The difficulty lies in determining what amounts to treatment in the 'best interests' of the patient. In *Re F*, Lord Brandon said:

> " The operation or other treatment will be in the best interests of such patients if, but only if, it is carried out either in order to save their lives or in order to ensure improvement/prevent deterioration in their physical/mental health.

The court have sanctioned the conduct of experimental therapy upon an adult without capacity in *Sims* v. *Sims and an NHS Trust* ([2002] EWHC 2743). Here the case concerned teenagers in the advanced stages of Creutzfeldt–Jakob disease. The court confirmed that an experimental form of treatment that had been subject to some animal testing but had not yet been tested on humans could be authorised. In determining that this was in the individual's best interests the court did emphasise that this was an exceptional case in the context of an otherwise fatal condition.

As far as non-therapeutic research is concerned, at present it appears that at common law it is unlawful to undertake non-therapeutic research on a mentally incompetent patient. It can be argued that such research is not in the best interests of an adult lacking mental capacity within the definition of the House of Lords in *Re F*.

Concern as to the vulnerability of the adult lacking mental capacity, and the need to ensure that procedures were undertaken only when necessary, was reflected in the report of the Law Commission on mental incapacity (Law Commission 1995). It accepted that in certain limited situations non-therapeutic research could be undertaken, but subject to safeguards, which included the creation of a specifically created new committee – a mental incapacity research committee. The committee was to approve trial proposals in principle. Involvement of a particular individual in a trial was a matter to be assessed separately. If the individual was unable to give consent themselves, consent could be given by court approval, consent of an attorney or manager, or a certificate from a doctor not involved in the research that the person's participation was appropriate or that the research was designated as not involving direct contact (draft Bill clause 11(1)(c) and (4)).

This final consideration refers to covert observation, photography or the inspection of written records. Allowing automatic approval for such observational studies is exceedingly controversial. Much may depend upon the condition of the individual patient. Any decision to include a person in such a project should be made on the basis of what constitutes that person's best interests.

In its document *Who decides*, issued in 1997 (Lord Chancellor's Department 1997), while the government announced its intention to enact some of the provisions of the Law Commission, it was not convinced of the fact that there was the need for an additional committee, although it did consult on this issue (para 5.41).

The Council of Europe Convention on Human Rights and Biomedicine (1997) now provides that non-therapeutic research on incompetent patients may be undertaken if:

" i) the research has the aim of contributing, through significant improvement to the understanding of the individual's condition, disease or disorder, to the ultimate attainment of results capable of conferring benefit to the person concerned or to other person in the same age category or afflicted with the same disease or disorder or having the same condition

ii) the research entails only minimal risk and minimal burden for the individuals involved

" and that in addition research of comparable effectiveness cannot be undertaken on a competent adult and that the appropriate consent has been obtained.

At present the UK has not become a party to this convention but it is likely to have some influence, at the very least in the context of directing ethical guidelines in this area in the future.

The Mental Capacity Act 2005 will have a considerable impact in the future upon the conduct of research involving adults lacking mental capacity. Interestingly, the draft Mental Incapacity Bill introduced in 2003 did not make specific reference to research, very much in line with the consultation documents that followed the Law Commission report. However the Joint Select Committee that reported on the Bill took the view that the inclusion of statutory provisions governing this research would enable ethical require-ments that would underpin research involving persons with incapacity to be clearly enshrined in statute. The Committee recommended that the Bill should set out key provisions as in the Declaration of Helsinki. In addition, it recommended that codes of practice should set out specific issues that ethics committees should be obliged to consider when any research involved persons who might lack capacity. Following their recommendations the final redrafted Mental Capacity Bill that was introduced in summer 2004 did include provisions relating to research including adults lacking mental capacity.

Section 30 of the Mental Capacity Act 2005 now provides that 'intrusive research' undertaken on a person lacking mental capacity is unlawful unless it is undertaken as part of a research project approved by an 'appropriate body' (s30(1)(a)) and is in accordance with sections 32 and 33. Section 30(3) expressly excludes those clinical trials that are regulated under the provisions of the Clinical Trials Regulations (see below). 'Intrusive research' is defined as follows:

" S30(2) Research is intrusive if it is of a kind that would be unlawful if it was carried out

(a) on or in relation to a person who had capacity to consent to it, but
(b) without his consent.

In contrast to the Clinical Trials Regulations there is no requirement for con-sent to be given by a personal or professional legal representative. Research must comply with the requirements set out in section 31. This provides that the 'appropriate body' must be satisfied that various criteria will be complied with. Research must be approved by an 'appropriate body'. The Explanatory Notes to the Act state that this is likely to be a research ethics committee, although it remains unclear whether this will be a standard local research ethics committee or a specialist ethics committee. If the former, then there will remain problematic issues of consistency in determining issues involving approval of such trials across the country. Section 31 goes on to provide that:

> (2) The research must be connected with –
>> (a) an impairing condition affecting P, or
>> (b) its treatment.
>
> (3) 'Impairing condition' means a condition which is (or may be) attributable to, or which causes or contributes to (or may cause or contribute to), the impairment of, or disturbance in the functioning of, the mind or brain.
>
> (4) There must be reasonable grounds for believing that research of comparable effectiveness cannot be carried out if the project has to be confined to, or relate only to, persons who have capacity to consent to taking part in it.
>
> (5) The research must –
>> (a) have the potential to benefit P without imposing on P a burden that is disproportionate to the potential benefit to P, or
>> (b) be intended to provide knowledge of the causes or treatment of, or of the care of persons affected by, the same or a similar condition.

In relation to non-therapeutic research this may only go ahead where there is only 'negligible risk' and must not interfere with the individual's freedom of action or privacy in a significant way nor be 'unduly invasive or restrictive' (s31(5). The Mental Capacity Act 2005 now makes reference, in section 32, to the need to consult carers. This is a right to consultation but not a right to consent. It should be noted, however, that the requirement to consult carers is not absolute and therefore may not apply, for example, in an emergency situation. These provisions of the Mental Capacity Act 2005 are to be particularly welcomed as providing clarification for researchers in an area that was otherwise notable for its uncertainty.

Clinical trials involving medicinal products

The conduct of one particular type of clinical trial – that concerning medicinal products – has been considerably affected by the EU Clinical Trials Directive (Directive 2001/20/EC) and the subsequent passage of the Medicines for Human Use (Clinical Trials) Regulations 2004, which places the conduct of such trials on a statutory basis in English law.

As a consequence of the Directive and Regulation 14(6) of the Medicines for Human Use (Clinical Trials) Regulations, clinical trials involving medicinal products must be approved by a research ethics committee and should a researcher proceed without such approval s/he would commit a criminal offence (regs 12 and 49). Research ethics committees that scrutinised such trials must in turn be approved by the new UK Ethics Committee Authority that has been established. Trials must be approved subject to specific time limits and the regulations also set out the factors research ethics committees must consider when approving such a trial, including the trial design, anticipated risks and benefits, the reason why persons who lack decision-making capacity should be included and provisions in relation to recruitment and for compensation should harm occur (reg 15(5)).

In relation to children and adults lacking mental capacity the regulations provide that the trial 'must be designed to minimise pain, discomfort, fear and any other foreseeable risk' (sch 1 part 4, para 14 (children) and sch 1 Part 5, para 13, adults lacking mental capacity). In the case of the adult lacking mental capacity there is a requirement that consent for their inclusion in the clinical trial must be obtained from a 'legal representative'. This introduces for the first time a proxy decision maker in relation to the involvement of the adult without capacity in the clinical research process.

Research involving human tissue samples

Much valuable clinical research would be impossible without the use of data from human tissue samples. The retention and use of tissue and organs has attracted much controversy, as it has been discovered over the last few years that hospitals up and down the country maintained large stores of bodily parts, allegedly without patient consent. The question of retention of such materials after a coroner's post mortem has been ordered and undertaken was been considered by the Bristol Interim Inquiry and by Michael Redfern QC's inquiry into the retention of children's organs at Alder Hey hospital in Liverpool (Kennedy 2000, Redfern 2001). This led to the government issuing a consultation document *Human Bodies: Human Choice* in 2002 and finally to a new Human Tissue Act 2004, which received Royal Assent in November 2004. This legislation is due to come wholly into force by autumn 2006. The Act is discussed further in the context of organ transplantation in Chapter 10. Space precludes a detailed examination here of what is complex legislation and we provide an overview. For further discussion see the growing literature in this area, including Price 2005; Liddell & Hall 2005 and McHale 2005.

The Act sanctions the use of human material for a wide range of purposes, including research. Human material is given a very broad definition in section 53 of any material consisting of, or including, human cells. There are, however, exclusions; for example, material regulated under the Human Fertilisation and Embryology Act 1990 and also hair and nail from a living person fall outside the scope of the legislation.

Relevant material must only be used where 'appropriate consent' has been given (s1). Specific provision is made for children (s2) and adults lacking mental capacity (s6). A person may entrust the decision regarding the use of their material after their death to a 'nominated representative' (s4). One feature of the legislation is that use of material without 'appropriate consent' or for a purpose other than sanctioned by the legislation is subject to explicit criminal penalties (see ss5 and 8). In addition, there is a specific offence in relation to the unauthorised use of DNA (s45). This area is to be regulated by a new body, the Human Tissue Authority, which is to have powers to license the use of human material, for example in the context of tissue banks. The Human Tissue Authority is also empowered to issue codes of practice – including a code on consent (s.26).

Some issues regarding consent remain unclear. For example, should consent be general – generic – or is specific consent required for each use? Generic or 'blanket' consent allows for future unspecified use of the registered materials. An alternative approach is that of obtaining separate 'specific' consent for each study for which it is proposed to use materials. The advantage of the former is that it gives control and consequently greatest flexibility to the researchers. In contrast, specific consent might be seen as supporting individual decision making autonomy and recognising that, while some individuals may be happy for their human material to be used for one particular research purpose(s) they would not necessarily sanction all forms of research using their excised material because, for example, of some religious/cultural objection. There is the prospect that generic consent may be subject to subsequent human rights challenges under the Human Rights Act 1998, in particular Article 8 – the right to privacy – which also concerns autonomy, and also Article 9, which concerns respect for freedom of religious beliefs.

The Human Tissue Act 2004 does not resolve these uncertainties. While section 1 of the 2004 Act makes use of the term 'appropriate consent', whether consent should be specific or generic is not addressed in the legislation, despite suggestions during the Parliamentary debates that generic consent would be sufficient. The current version of the Human Tissue Authority code of practice (HTA 2006) provides that:

> 79. If identifiable tissue is to be used for research, patients should be told about any implications this may have. For example, they may be contacted by researchers, given feedback, or be asked for access to their medical records. Patients should be told whether the consent is generic (i.e. for use in any future research project approved by a REC) or specific. If it is the latter, detailed information about the research project should be provided, in line with good practice.

> 80. Patients should be told if their samples will or could be used for research involving the commercial sector. They should be given appropriate information on the range of activities and researchers which may be involved and whether these include commercial pharmaceutical companies.

Further uncertainties will remain following the Human Tissue Act. One notable issue is the extent to which the human material removed from a person can be regarded as 'property'. The legal issues surrounding this whole area are complex. There is no property in a dead body (*R* v. *Kelly* [1998] 3 All ER 741) and yet it is the case that property interests have been recognised in bodily parts and products (*R* v. *Welsh* [1974] RTR 478; *R* v. *Rothery* {1976] RT 478). Particular difficulties are likely to arise in the future in the form of the retention and use of materials extracted from body tissues in DNA banks (Martin & Kaye 1999, McHale 2004). There is the risk that the English courts may be faced, as in the USA, with patients challenging the use of their bodily materials without their consent, particularly in situations in which there has been commercial exploitation of such bodily materials (*Moore* v. *University of California* (1990) 793 P 2d 479).

Intervention with care of the patient on the ward

While observing practice on the ward, the nurse researcher may come across situations in which patient care falls below what is regarded as being an acceptable standard (Dines 1995):

" A nurse researcher is interested in the feeding problems of stroke patients. She is using non-participant observation as her research method. She is seated inconspicuously wearing a white coat in the ward; it is a meal time. A stroke patient nearby is propped up against his pillows and reaches for his milky tea. He takes the spouted beaker to his lips but spills the drink down his pyjama jacket. No nurse is in sight, what should the nurse researcher do?

" Some time later the sister appears; she is updating the fluid balance charts. Observing the empty beaker she congratulates the patient on drinking his tea and charts the fluid intake. What should the nurse researcher do?

Should the nurse intervene? As Dines notes, the nurse faces a dilemma. By intervening she would be unable to observe what action the ward sister would take in that situation, a matter that is part of her research. But if the nurse failed to act and the patient became dehydrated, would she be negligent? In this situation a court would have to consider whether she owed a duty to the patient on that ward. The nurse is not responsible directly for the clinical care of that patient. There is no general duty to act as a 'good Samaritan'. If the nurse researcher was held to be under a duty in such a situation, the court would assess whether the conduct was negligent by reference to a responsible body of professional practice. Some guidance to the approach of one body of professional opinion in such a situation can be gleaned from a publication of the Royal College of Nursing (RCN). The College (Royal College of Nursing 1993) suggests that:

" The nurse who is undertaking a research project in an exclusively research role has no responsibility for the service, care, treatment or advice given to patients or clients unless stipulated within the design of the research. Otherwise, any intervention in a professional capacity should be confined to situations in which a patient or client requires to be protected or rescued from danger.

But it is uncertain what is meant here by 'protection from danger'. Does this mean immediate danger or something which becomes dangerous because it is repeated – the patient regularly spilling his/her drink and losing fluid?

The RCN (Royal College of Nursing 1993) has said: 'A nurse in a research situation still holds expert knowledge and may at times feel impelled to action for a patient's benefit'.

Whether the nurse is held to be negligent may depend on factors such as the risk to the patient of her non-intervention. Take the example given at the start of this section. If the nurse continued to observe the patient losing fluids and that no check was made by the sister, and the patient was placed at grave risk of dehydration, then it is arguable that by not acting to warn the nurse on the ward the nurse researcher would be negligent.

COMPENSATING RESEARCH SUBJECTS AND POLICING TRIALS

This section considers liability of nurses, whether as researchers or as ethics committee members, when trials go wrong (Guest 1997). Also discussed is the role of the nurse in policing unethical behaviour in a trial. As noted above, the general principles of law apply to clinical trials. If a research subject is not told of a particular risk of involvement in a trial and that risk materialises and the subject is injured s/he may bring an action in negligence or battery against the researcher. If a research subject is injured during a trial because of the researcher's lack of care, then again an action for negligence may be brought.

No national scheme of compensation exists for those injured in clinical trials. Researchers must be adequately insured. However, some special compensation provision exists for certain trials. The Association of British Pharmaceutical Industries (ABPI) guidelines provide that researchers should make contractually binding undertakings with research subjects in non-therapeutic trials to pay compensation in the event of injury. The Association does not require contractually binding undertakings to be made with research subjects, although it suggests that assurances should be given that compensation would be paid in the event of harm resulting. While there are no contractual sanctions for breaking an undertaking, to break it would lead to criticism and would make it very difficult for the researcher to arrange insurance cover from the Association in the future. This scheme has not, however, met with universal approval.

There has been some criticism of the operation of indemnity schemes by the ABPI in that it has installed threshold limits before claims can be brought (Barton et al 1995). If the research is commissioned by the Medical Research Council there is no automatic entitlement to compensation, although the Council has indicated that compensation payments may be made on an ex gratia basis.

Liability of ethics committee members

If a research subject is injured in a clinical trial then it is possible that an action could be brought against individual members of the research ethics committee on the grounds that they were negligent in approving the conduct of the trial. It has been suggested that, at least in theory, each individual ethics committee member owes a duty of care to each research subject (Brazier 1990). Any costs of legal proceedings brought against a nurse employed by the NHS who sits on a research ethics committee will be covered by NHS indemnity insurance. The Department of Health has stated that it will cover the costs of a research ethics committee member as long as s/he has not been guilty of misconduct or gross lack of care. It should be noted that, although an action in negligence is a theoretical possibility, in practice bringing such a claim may be difficult. A research subject would have to show that it was the negligence of a particular committee member in approving the trial that caused the injury that s/he suffered.

What can be done if it is thought that the trial is being conducted unethically?

If the nurse believes that a trial in which s/he is involved is being conducted unethically, the nurse may raise this with the person in charge of the trial. But what if no notice is taken of what the nurse has said? S/he can draw the matter to the attention of the research ethics committee who approved the trial. The committee may decide to take action, but in practice it has few powers. It may ask the researchers to report to them and then withdraw authorisation from the trial. If the unethical researcher is a nurse, it may be thought appropriate to refer the researcher's conduct to the NMC, which may decide to take disciplinary proceedings. In the case of a doctor, misconduct may be referred to the General Medical Council. As in the report over the research undertaken by Professor David Southall, conduct of a particular trial may also be the subject of an inquiry.

Following up the conduct of a trial

If a nurse conducting a trial departs from an agreed trial protocol and has acted unethically it may limit the nurse's chances of obtaining approval for another clinical trial. GAfREC provides that researchers should not deviate from the clinical trial protocol without informing the research ethics committee and will require prior written approval unless the reason for the change is to eliminate an immediate risk of harm to research participants (Department of Health 2001, paras 7.23–7.24). In addition, it is for the research sponsor to have arrangements to 'review significant developments' in relation to the conduct of the research and also to approve modification (Department of Health 2001, para 7.25). Researchers are required to provide annual reports and a final report to the research ethics committee (Department of Health 2001, paras 7.26–7.27.) There is also specific provision for reports if the research ends early or if there are 'unusual or unexpected results raising questions about the research (Department of Health 2001, paras 7.28 and 7.30). However, other than through these reports research ethics committees have no monitoring responsibilities. That is the role of the NHS institution itself (Department of Health 2001, para 7.33). While some committees have follow-up procedures and write to the researcher to find out how the project has progressed, others do not. It is arguable that the rights of the subject in the trial are being neglected. Neuberger (1992) has suggested that new powers be given to committees to carry out spot checks. In addition, perhaps questionnaires could be given to research subjects to discover how a trial has been conducted. But to expect the research ethics committee to undertake detailed policing of the many trials that they scrutinise is unrealistic. Committee members are unpaid. Systematic scrutiny with spot checks, etc. would really require full time officers to be appointed. The administrative workload would

Clinical research and the nurse

increase, as would the cost. In an NHS subject to considerable budgetary restraints, such innovations are unlikely, at least in the immediate future.

REFORMING THE RESEARCH ETHICS REVIEW PROCESS

In the last few years the structures for research review have proliferated, but some now think that we have gone too far. Researchers are complaining that the proliferation of research governance guidelines is severely inhibiting research. So is there now a case for reform? Expressed concerns led to proposals for reform of the system in the report of the Ad Hoc Advisory Group on the reform of research ethics committees (Department of Health 2005c). The Committee did not share the view of some of the submissions 'that research is a good in itself and that research ethics appraisal is in some way a distraction from or unjustifiable interference in medical research' (para 2.6). The Group made a number of recommendations. They suggested that there should be reconsideration of the remit of NHS research ethics committees and that such things as surveys should be excluded where they do not raise 'material ethical issues'. In addition, the group took the view that the decisions of research ethics committees should not cover scientific matters. This has already proved the source of some controversy. It has been suggested that to totally separate scientific and ethical review is in practice impossible (Dawson 2005). A further controversial recommendation was that there should be fewer research ethics committees with greater reliance on electronic communication and the suggestion that members of research ethics committees time commitment being recognised through payment either directly or through the compensation to their employers. In effect this would result in breaking the 'local link' of research ethics committees. The prospect of paid research ethics committee's has also come under criticism. It has been suggested that the proposal is insufficiently discussed and there are concerns both that it may not be feasible to combine this extended role with a full time job and there are also concerns that payment may be seen to impact on the perceived impartiality of research ethics committees (Dawson 2005). The Ad Hoc Group was also concerned to ensure that membership of research ethics committees represented a wider mix of society. One concern is the alleged inconsistency in decision making of research ethics committees. The Ad Hoc Group suggested that this needed to be addressed and proposed the use of better training and quality assurance. A further concern was the inconsistency of approach across jurisdictions and the Group recommended that there should be consideration of better harmonisation of governance arrangements. At the time of writing COREC is consulting as to how to take these recommendations forward (Central Office for Research Ethics Committees 2006).

BBC Newsonline 2006 Six taken ill after drug trial. 15 March. Available online at: http://news.bbc.co.uk/1/hi/england/london/4807042.stm

Brazier M 1990 The liability of ethics committee members. Professional Negligence 6: 186

Barton JM, Macmillan MS, Sawyer L 1995 The compensation of patients injured in clinical trials. Journal of Medical Ethics 21: 166–169

Central Office for Research Ethics Committees 2006 Implementing the recommendations of the Ad Hoc Advisory Group Consultation. National Patient Safety Agency, London

Dawson AJ 2005 The Ad Hoc Advisory Group's proposals for research ethics committees: a mixture of the timid, the revolutionary and the bizarre. Journal of Medical Ethics 31: 435

Department of Health 2001 Governance arrangements for NHS research ethics committees (GAfREC). Department of Health, London

Department of Health 2005a Research governance framework for health and social care. Department of Health, London

Department of Health 2005b Review of the Human Fertilisation and Embryology Act: a public consultation. Department of Health, London

Department of Health 2005c Report of the Ad Hoc Advisory Group on the Operation of NHS Research Ethics Committees. Department of Health, London

Dines A 1995 An ethical perspective – nursing research. In: Tingle J, Cribb A (eds) Nursing law and ethics. Blackwell Scientific, Oxford

Fox M 1995 Animal rights and wrongs: medical ethics and the killing of non-human animals. In: Lee R, Morgan D (eds) Death rites: law and ethics at the end of life. Routledge, London

Griffiths R 2000 Report of the Review into the Research Framework in North Staffordshire. Available online at: http://www.doh.gov.uk/wmro/northstaffs.htm

Guest S 1997 Compensation for subjects of medical research; the moral rights of patients and the power of research ethics committees. Journal of Medical Ethics 23: 181–182

Human Tissue Authority 2006. Code of Practice: consent. HTA, London

Kennedy I 2000 Bristol Inquiry interim report: removal and retention of human material. Available online at: http://www.bristol-inquiry.org.uk

Law Commission 1995 Mental incapacity. Report No. 231. HMSO, London

Liddell K, Hall A 2005 Beyond Bristol and Alder Hey – the future regulation of human tissue. Medical Law Review 13: 170–223

Lord Chancellor's Department 1997 Who decides. LCD, London

McHale JV 2004 Regulating genetic databases: some legal and ethical issues. Medical Law Review 12: 70–96

McHale JV 2005 The Human Tissue Act 2004 – innovative legislation, fundamentally flawed or missed opportunity? Liverpool Law Review 26: 169–188

McHale J, Gallagher A 2004 Research and rights. In: Nursing and human rights. Butterworth Heinemann, London, Ch 7

Martin P, Kaye J 1999 The use of biological sample collection and personal medical information in human genetics research. Wellcome Trust, London

Neuberger J 1992 Ethics and health care: the role of the research ethics committee. Kings Fund Institute, London

Nicholson R 1985 Medical research and children. Medical Research Council, London

Nicholson R 1991 The ethics of research with children. In: Brazier M, Lobjoit M (eds) Protecting the vulnerable. Routledge, London

Nursing and Midwifery Council 2002 Code of professional conduct. NMC, London

Parabor K 1997 Nursing research: principles, process and issues. Macmillan, Oxford

Plomer A 2004 The law and ethics of medical research: international bioethics and human rights. Cavendish, London

Price D 2005 The Human Tissue Act 2004. Modern Law Review 68: 798–821

Redfern M 2001 Report of the Inquiry into the Royal Liverpool Children's Hospital (Alder Hey) (2001). (Alder Hey Report.) Available online at: http://www.rclinquiry.org.uk

Royal College of Nursing 1993 Ethics relating to research in nursing. Scutari Press, London

Royal College of Nursing 2004 Research
ethics: RCN guidance for nurses. RCN,
London

Royal College of Paediatrics and Child
Health 2000 Ethics Advisory Committee
guidelines for the ethical conduct of
medical research involving children.
Archives of Disease in Childhood
82: 177–182

Royal College of Physicians 1996
Guidelines on the practice of ethics
committees in medical research involving
human subjects, 3rd edn. Royal College
of Physicians of London, London

Royal College of Psychiatrists 1990
Guidelines for psychiatric research
involving human subjects. Psychiatric
Bulletin 14: 48

Reproductive choice

Jean McHale

Today, patients have an increasing range of reproductive choices and increasingly these 'choices' are phrased in terms of reproductive rights, particularly in the light of the Human Rights Act 1998 (McHale & Gallagher 2004). The nurse may play a direct part in guiding some of these choices, for instance the case of the teenager who approaches the nurse for advice regarding contraception, or the mother wondering whether her daughter who has learning disabilities should be sterilised. In others, the nurse may not be a direct participant in the process unless a patient specifically approaches her/him for advice. Nevertheless, it is important for the nurse to be aware of the legal framework within which these choices are made and clinical procedures are undertaken. This chapter begins with an examination of the legality of the provision of contraceptive services and the question of sterilisation of adults with learning disabilities. Second, we consider the regulation of the new reproductive technologies such as in vitro fertilisation (IVF) and the prospects for cloning. Third, the role of the law in regulating conduct during pregnancy is explored. Finally, the legality of abortion and the involvement of the nurse in the abortion process are discussed.

PROVISION OF CONTRACEPTIVE SERVICES

The nurse may be involved in providing contraceptive advice and treatment, whether as in a family planning clinic or in the hospital setting. Statute states that the Secretary of State for Health has a duty to meet reasonable requirements relating to the provision of contraceptive advice/treatment of persons in England and Wales (s5(1)b National Health Service Act 1977).

While in the past the legality of undertaking sterilisation operations for contraceptive purposes was questioned, today such operations are generally accepted to be lawful (*Bravery* v. *Bravery* [1954] 3 All ER 59 at pp. 67–68). As with any surgical procedure, before sterilisation is undertaken the patient's consent must be obtained. Consent must be obtained from the patient him/herself. His/her spouse/partner has no rights to participate in the consent process and may not veto the operation. The implications of the operation and the fact that there is a possibility of failure are indicated on the NHS consent form, but these should also be drawn explicitly to the patient's attention, otherwise there is the possibility that a negligence action will result (*Thake* v. *Maurice* [1986] 1 All ER 497).

One major point of controversy concerns the provision of contraceptive advice and treatment to teenagers. As seen in the section on children and confidentiality in Chapter 7, this issue came before the courts in the case of *Gillick v. West Norfolk and Wisbech AHA* ([1986] AC 150) and was confirmed in the recent *Axon* case (see Ch. 7). If a young girl approaches a nurse seeking contraceptive advice/treatment, the nurse must assess whether the girl has sufficient maturity to appreciate the nature of the advice/treatment sought and whether she is capable of making an informed choice.

Sterilisation and adults lacking mental capacity

A mother is worried that her daughter, who is in her early teens and has learning disabilities, is vulnerable to seduction. She believes that her daughter should be sterilised for her protection. She discusses her concerns with the district nurse who is helping her to care for her daughter. What should the nurse do?

The mother genuinely believes that sterilisation is in her daughter's best interests. However, while the girl may have the mental age of a young child she may develop maternal feelings and in the future be capable of being a loving mother. There is also a danger in assuming that sterilisation will be a panacea when in fact by removing the risk of pregnancy the girl may be placed at risk of undetectable abuse. If parents and health-care professionals disagree as to whether sterilisation should be undertaken, this issue should be referred to the court. The court will determine whether the proposed sterilisation operation is lawful, by assessing whether the procedure is in the girl's best interests.

Use of a 'best interests' test leaves much discretion in the hands of the courts. In *Re D*, D, an 11-year-old child from a poor background, suffered from Sotos' syndrome ([1976] 1 All ER 326). This condition results in accelerated growth during infancy, epilepsy, generalised clumsy appearance, behaviour problems and certain aggressive tendencies. She had reached puberty and, while she had not shown any marked interest in the opposite sex, her protective mother was concerned about the consequences if she became pregnant. She wanted her daughter sterilised and her opinion was supported by her doctor.

Heilbron J. refused to authorise the sterilisation. She said that the evidence showed that there had been improvement in D's mental and physical condition. Her future prospects were unpredictable. Nevertheless, it was likely that in the future she would be able to make her own choice. Should she then realise the impact of what had happened to her, she might feel frustration and resentment. The judge emphasised that a decision to undertake sterilisation for non-therapeutic purposes on a minor was not a matter for clinical judgment alone.

In cases following *Re D* the courts have, however, shown far less hesitation before authorising sterilisation. In *Re B* ([1987] 2 WLR 1212), B was a 17-year-old woman who had a mental age of 5–6 years and was epileptic. Evidence was given to the effect that she did not understand and was unable to learn the causal connection between intercourse, pregnancy and the birth of children. However, she had the sexual inclinations of a normal 17-year-old. It was claimed that there was only a 40% chance of establishing an acceptable regime with oral contraceptives and there would be side effects. Because she suffered swings of mood and had considerable physical strength, administration of a daily dose of medication might be impossible. B was also obese and this, coupled with the irregularity of her periods, might make early detection of pregnancy difficult. B's mother and the local authority sought an order from the court authorising sterilisation. The court granted the order. Lord Hailsham said that the case was clearly distinguishable from *Re D*. He said:

> " To talk of a basic right to reproduce of an individual who is not capable of knowing the causal connection between intercourse and childbirth, the nature of pregnancy and what is involved in delivery, unable to form maternal instincts or to care for a child is to wholly part company with reality. (p. 216)

Lord Templeman stated that in his opinion sterilisation of a woman under 18 years should only be undertaken with the leave of the High Court. In this case it would, he said, be cruel to expose her to an unacceptable risk of pregnancy. Lord Oliver also distinguished *Re D*. He said:

> " the right to reproduce is only valuable if accompanied by the ability to make a choice and in the instant case there is no question of the minor being able to make a choice or indeed to appreciate the desire to make one. All the evidence indicates that she will never desire a child and that reproduction will be positively harmful to her.

The decision of the House of Lords in *Re B* has been the subject of much critical comment. For example, Lee & Morgan (1989) have asked why B was able to manage the hygienic mechanics of menstruation but not contraception, and why she was able to understand the link between pregnancy and babies but not that between sex and pregnancy. Emphasis was placed in the case upon B's mental age. But it has been suggested that this hides the complexity of the issue. For instance, a woman may have a mental age of 5 years in relation to some functions while at the same time having far higher comprehension levels in relation to other tasks. Reference was made in *Re B* to a Canadian case, *Re Eve* ([1986] DLR (4t) 1), in which the court had held that non-therapeutic sterilisation of a mentally incompetent adult was never justifiable. The House of Lords, however, disagreed and said that it was wrong to draw a distinction between therapeutic and non-therapeutic sterilisation. It is perhaps ironic in view of this that, as we shall see below, later courts appear to have drawn just such a distinction when considering whether all sterilisation operations should require judicial approval.

There are perceptible advantages in the postponement of the sterilisation decision until a teenager with learning disabilities is older. Assessment of her physical and mental development may then be made on the basis of conclusive evidence, as opposed to guesswork. In B's case there was some urgency in performing the operation before she reached her 18th birthday because at that time the legality of treatment of adults who lacked mental capacity was unclear. This issue was finally resolved 1989 by the House of Lords in *Re F* ([1990] AC 1) The House of Lords held that an adult woman lacking mental capacity could be sterilised if it was in her best interests, but it stated that it would be desirable for the medical team to obtain a declaration from the court before such an operation was undertaken.

The majority of the cases concern females however in *Re A (Medical treatment: male sterilisation)* ([2000] FCR 193), the Court of Appeal was asked to rule upon the sterilisation of a 28-year-old man with Down's syndrome. He was assessed as borderline between significant and severe intelligence impairment. While incapable of making a decision regarding sterilisation himself, he was sexually aware and active. His mother supported his sterilisation. The Court of Appeal held that the sterilisation should not at present go ahead. Dame Elizabeth Butler-Sloss P. indicated that, at a time when there was soon to be direct application of the European Convention of Human Rights in English law, the court should be slow to take a step that may infringe the rights of those who are unable to act for themselves. The Court of Appeal emphasised that the patient's best interests was something that was different from the interests of carers or others but left open the extent to which the interests of third parties should be weighed in the balance when determining what was in the patient's best interests. It was noted that such a decision should not be authorised on eugenic grounds. Moreover a decision to sterilise a female patient involved different considerations and that in the context of a man there were no direct consequences other than the fact that he might contract a sexually transmitted disease.

The courts have indicated that sterilisation of an adult woman lacking mental capacity, undertaken for therapeutic purposes, such as the performance of a hysterectomy upon a woman suffering from extensive menstruation, does not require judicial approval (*Re E (a minor)* [1992] 2 FLR 585). Cases involving non-therapeutic sterilisation will, however, continue to be referred to the courts. It is important to ensure that such decisions are made on the basis of the woman's best interests rather than what is convenient for the carers.

In a number of cases the courts, when authorising sterilisation, emphasised the possibility of surgical reversal of the sterilisation operation (*Re P (a minor) (wardship: sterilisation)* [1989] 1 FLR 182, [1989] Fam Law 102 and *Re M (a minor) (wardship: sterilisation)* [1988] 2 FLR 497). But as Brazier (1990) has argued, while leading experts may achieve a high level of reversals this does not mean that all clinicians can achieve this. Also, it is highly questionable whether an operation to reverse the sterilisation of an adult with severe learning disabilities will be a priority in a financially constrained NHS.

The nurse acting as patient advocate may play an important role, particularly in ensuring that, in those situations in which sterilisation has not been referred to the courts, it is being undertaken for therapeutic purposes and is in that patient's best interests. In the future such decisions will be subject to the provisions of the Mental Capacity Act 2005, discussed in Chapter 5. The decision to go ahead with a sterilisation must be in the patient's best interests. The Draft Mental Capacity Act Code of Practice 2006 provides that it is envisaged that 'the proposed non-therapeutic sterilisation of a person lacking to capacity to consent (e.g. for contraceptive purposes)' will be among the serious health-care decisions which will require judicial approval after the Act comes into force (Department for Constitutional Affairs 2006, para 7.17).

Developments in medical technology have, in the last half century, given much hope to the infertile. For example, a woman who is unable to conceive may receive IVF. This involves the egg being fertilised outside the womb and then implanted into it. But use of such techniques has not been free of controversy. In response to debate generated, the government established a committee, the Warnock Committee, to examine the use of new reproductive technologies. This Committee reported in 1984 (HMSO 1984). It recommended that use of these technologies be subject to regulation. Today, modern reproductive technologies are regulated by statute in the form of the Human Fertilisation and Embryology Act 1990. This Act established the Human Fertilisation and Embryology Authority (HEFA), whose functions include the licensing of clinics providing fertility treatment (s5 and schedule 1 Human Fertilisation and Embryology Act 1990; Lee & Morgan, 2001). It also grants licences for the conduct of embryo research. Not all forms of assisted conception must be licensed by the Authority, for example artificial insemination of a woman with her partner's sperm. There are a series of limitations on what may be licensed. For example, human embryos may not be placed in an animal, nor can 'cloning' by cell nuclear replacement (where this amounts to replacing the nucleus of an embryo with the nucleus of another cell or embryo) be undertaken (s3(3)). Attempts to create 'designer babies' are subject to regulation.

A right to access to assisted reproduction services?

The Human Rights Act 1998 provides recognition for reproductive rights in Article 8, the right to privacy of home and family life, with its scope for safeguarding autonomy-based interests, and also in Article 12, the right to marry and to found a family. These rights, however, are not absolute in nature and are qualified by public interest considerations. The courts have confirmed that there is no automatic right of access to reproductive technology services (*R (Mellor)* v. *Secretary of State for the Home Department* [2002] QB 13.) A woman seeking access to IVF would have to satisfy the clinic that she was a suitable case for receiving such treatment. Her eligibility is determined by reference to criteria set out in the code of practice produced by the HEFA (Human Fertilisation and Embryology Authority 2004) and this is in turn structured by the Human Fertilisation and Embryology Act 1990. Section 13(5) provides that:

" s. 13 (5) A woman shall not be provided with treatment services unless account has been taken of the welfare of any child who may be born as a result of the treatment (including the need of that child for a father), and of any child who may be affected by the birth.

In addition to the child's need for a father, the Code of Practice directs them to consider the applicants' medical histories and their commitment to bringing up children (Human Fertilisation and Embryology Authority 2004). That does not mean that single women would be precluded from access to infertility treatment, but the clinic would scrutinise the application and determine whether there would be any male influences in the child's upbringing. Criteria imposed by individual clinics include restrictions by reference to the age of the woman seeking treatment. Many clinics do not allow women over 35 years of age access to infertility treatment on the grounds that the success rates of treatment on older women are limited. Debates have also centred around access to IVF services for gay and lesbian couples. The HFEA Code of Practice does give a considerable degree of discretion to clinics in determining who they accept for treatment. Recently the current chair of the Human Fertilisation and Embryology Authority, Dame Suzie Leather, has suggested that section 13(5) as currently drafted can be seen as outdated in today's society, with different conceptions of what constitutes a family relationship. The House of Commons Science and Technology Committee recommended its abolition, commenting that 'it discriminates against the infertile and some sections of society, is impossible to implement and is of questionable practical value in protecting the interests of children born as a result of assisted reproduction' (House of Commons Select Committee on Science and Technology 2005, para 107).

Although they recognised that there should be some checks and balances there should be a 'minimal threshold principle' which should be 'the risk of unpreventable and serious harm' (House of Commons Select Committee on Science and Technology 2005, para 101). As we shall see below, this provision is currently under consideration as part of the Department of Health's consultation exercise on the HFEA (Department of Health 2005).

While there is the potential for persons denied access to IVF services to challenge this refusal in the courtroom, in practice such challenges are unlikely to be successful. For example, in R v. *Ethical Committee of St Mary's Hospital, Manchester* ([1988] 1 FLR 512), R was unable to conceive. Her appliation to adopt a child had been rejected because of her criminal record relating to prostitution and brothel keeping. She sought IVF treatment. A consultant at the IVF clinic rejected her application. This decision was supported by the hospital's infertility ethical committee. (Bodies undertaking infertility treatment must establish ethical committees to which problematic decisions relating to access to such treatments may be referred.) Schiemann J. said that the committee was in essence an informal body. If the committee in a particular case refused to give advice to a consultant or did not come to a majority view on a decision, he didn't see that the court could compel it, either to give advice or to enter into a particular investigation. Schiemann J. did not rule out the possibility of judicial review:

" If the committee had advised, for instance, that the IVF unit should in principal refuse treatment to anyone who was a ... Jew or coloured, then I think that the court might well grant a declaration that that was illegal.

But he stressed that the committee was a talking shop for professionals and a court should be cautious before intervening. It appears that such challenges are unlikely to be successful in the future unless they are manifestly unreasonable/indefensible. This was illustrated in the later case of *ex parte Seale* (1994 unreported). S, a 36-year-old woman, was denied IVF treatment. It was said that there was a need to ration resources and treatment was generally less effective in those women who were over 35 years of age. The court was not prepared to overrule the clinic's decision to refuse her treatment on the basis that it was irrational.

The 'consent' principle and reproductive rights

The Human Fertilisation and Embryology Act 1990 is rooted in the principle of consent to use stored sperm, eggs and embryos. In the case of stored embryos, consent is required from both parties who provided the gametes – consent from one is not sufficient. But what if one party claims that by refusing consent the other is stopping them from ever reproducing in the future? Is there a right to reproduce even in the face of the opposition of a woman's ex-partner?

This issue arose in the case of *Evans* v. *Amicus Health Care* ([2004] 2 FLR 767). It concerned a dispute over a stored embryo between women and their former partners. The embryos had been created from the women's eggs and their former partners' sperm. Both women wanted to use the embryos while their former partners were opposed. In the case of one of the litigants, Natalie Evans, she was unable to have any more genetically related children following her treatment for ovarian tumours. The other woman, Mrs Hadley, had difficulties conceiving but the chances, while remote, did not render it impossible. Their claim was rejected in the English courts. At first instance Wall J. held that the Human Fertilisation and Embryology Act 1990 was quite clear that consent was required from both parties in relation to stored gametes. Furthermore he also rejected her challenge on the basis of the provisions of the European Convention of Human Rights. It was claimed that the embryos were protected under Article 2 of the ECHR – which safeguards the right to life. This claim was rejected. It was held that, given that a right to life was not afforded to the fetus, it was difficult to see how an embryo could be granted such a right. Although he recognised that Article 8 rights were engaged here, so too were those of the ex-partner. Interference with a person's private life must be necessary and proportionate and this was a case in which the courts were prepared to award a generous margin of appreciation. Regarding Article 12 of the ECHR which provides that there is a right to marry and found a family it was held that this either wasn't engaged here or if it was the interference was justifiable. It was also argued that the refusal of the claim to use the embryos contravened Article 14 – the prohibition on discrimination – because the argument was made that they were being discriminated against because of their inability to conceive. However it was held that the 1990 Act did not distinguish between women on the basis of disability; rather it distinguished on the basis of those who had changed their minds regarding the decision to go ahead with IVF treatment. Wall J. rejected the argument that a woman whose egg was used to create an embryo that was frozen and then stored was in the same position as someone who was pregnant without the use of modern reproductive technologies and who wanted to continue with the pregnancy despite the opposition of her partner.

The approach of Wall J. was confirmed by the Court of Appeal. Mrs Hadley decided not to take her claim further; however, Ms Evans took her case to the European Court of Human Rights (ECHR) in Strasbourg but again was unsuccessful (*Evans* v. *UK* 2006). The ECHR upheld the approach taken in the English courts. The case illustrates the difficulties in attempting to use what are essentially very broad brush human rights principles to determine complex issues of policy and conflicting rights.

The question of posthumous conception arose in the case of Diane Blood, who wanted to be artificially inseminated with her deceased husband's sperm (*R* v. *Human Fertilisation and Embryology Authority ex parte Blood* [1997] 2 All ER 687). The HFEA refused to allow the treatment to go ahead because they stated that the treatment was not sanctioned under the 1990 Act because the Act required that prior consent be obtained from her deceased husband for use of the sperm after death. However this refusal was subject to challenge using European law principles. The Court of Appeal held that the HFEA had failed to take into consideration the application of European Community law and in particular the free movement principles, and referred the decision back to the HFEA to reconsider their decision. The HFEA ultimately exercised their discretion and allowed the sperm to be exported to Belgium, where Diane Blood was treated and ultimately gave birth to a son.

The *Blood* case is instructive as it illustrates the difficulty of effectively regulating reproductive services on a single jurisdictional basis. Individuals denied treatment in the UK because, for example, they are considered unsuitable for treatment whether through age or because a particular controversial procedure such as sex-selection is not available, may ultimately simply bypass national restrictions and go overseas for treatment. A recent illustration of this was in May 2006 when it was announced that a 63-year-old English psychiatrist was pregnant, having travelled abroad to receive treatment in Romania and becoming potentially the oldest mother to give birth in the UK.

The code of practice issued by the HFEA provides that couples contemplating use of reproductive technologies should be given counselling as to the implications of undertaking such therapy (Human Fertilisation and Embryology Authority 2004, Ch. 6). The nurse may be involved in such counselling.

Conscientious objection

A nurse may object on religious or cultural grounds to participation in the use of certain techniques, such as IVF, that involve gamete or embryo manipulation. Section 38 of the 1990 Act gives nurses and other health professionals the right to refuse to participate in such treatments by expressing a conscientious objection to participation.

Cloning

One of the most heated recent debates in relation to the use of new human reproductive technologies has arisen in the context of cloning. In 1997 Ian Wilmut cloned Dolly the sheep at the Roslin Institute in Edinburgh. Cloning involves various techniques. One such technique is 'embryo splitting'. This is the replication of the process that occurs naturally and leads to the production of twins. Embryonic cells are separated at a very early stage before they have had a chance to differentiate. Another method is that of nuclear replacement.

Cloning may be undertaken for therapeutic purposes, such as tissue and organ replacement (Ch. 10), and for reproductive purposes – the creation of a new human being. Although the Human Fertilisation and Embryology Act 1990 prohibits cloning where this is the replacement of the nucleus of an embryo, uncertainty remained as to the extent to which other cloning technologies were sanctioned under English law.

Following Dolly, a House of Commons Select Committee on Science and Technology was established. Its report was published in March 1997. It proposed that Parliament should confirm a ban on reproductive cloning. It also proposed that the 'creation of experimental human beings' should not be sanctioned. This was supported by the Minister of State for Health in June 1997.

There are a number of reasons why there has been opposition to cloning; first, the fact that it is a costly technology and one that is likely to lead to considerable wastage of eggs and a high degree of risk. Dolly was the only normal lamb that was born from 276 similar attempts. In only 29 cases did they lead to implantable embryos and all of these except Dolly resulted in defective pregnancies and grossly deformed births. Other concerns relate to the life expectancy of the clone, which may be reduced as a result of the fact that a clone could be born prematurely aged because its genetic material would already be as old as the person from whom it had been removed. Some concerns have also been expressed that that cloning might produce resultant health defects. In 1999 a 2-month-old cloned calf died after it developed blood and heart problems (British Medical Journal 1999). Moreover, the clone may be born with a reduced life expectancy. Numerous ethical and social issues have also been identified. It has been suggested that cloning may amount to using individuals as means to end and as such is wrong. Could cloned children in effect be regarded as commodities? Human rights/ dignity might be infringed by the prospect of there being two or more persons in existence with an identical genetic composition. However, it has been argued that nature provides for monozygotic twins, which have identical composition. Clones would also not be identical. It has also been suggested that a clone would not be identical to the individual from which it was cloned because this does not take into account social, cultural and environmental issues, which play a very important part in an individual's development (Harris 1998)

There has been considerable opposition to reproductive cloning. Warnock was of the view that it should not be permitted. In introducing the report of the Human Genetic Advisory Commission and the Human Fertilisation and Embryology Authority, Sir Colin Campbell stated that 'We want to stop the wild and irresponsible notion of cloning whole human beings but allow procedures that in 5 to 10 years time may lead to the curing of diseases'. Ruth Deech, the chair of the HEFA, suggested that:

" The Human Fertilisation and Embryology Act 1990 empowers the HEFA to forbid human reproductive cloning in the UK and we have no intention of changing our minds on that decision. Nevertheless the government may wish to consider the possibility of legislation explicitly banning reproductive cloning.

At the same time as the UK debate was being undertaken the international response to cloning has been hostile. In January 1998, 19 members of the Council of Europe signed an agreement in Paris to the effect that it prohibited 'any intervention seeking to create a human being genetically identical to any other human being, whether living or dead, by whatever means'. In 1998 the European Union called upon member states to ban cloning.

Cloning has been seen by some as constituting a serious violation of human rights, as contrary to principle of equality, permitting eugenic and racist selection and offending against human dignity. In July 1999 the UK government confirmed that in their view human reproductive cloning was ethically unacceptable. However, an advisory group chaired by the Chief Medical Officer supported the development of stem cell cloning technology (Chief Medical Officer 2000). Stem cells are the master cells of the body, which have the ability to develop into any cell type. Cloning through stem cell technology gives rise to the prospect of cures for a wide-range of conditions. It also raises the prospect of growing tissue and organs using the genetic material from the person it is intended to transplant the organ into, which reduces the prospect of rejection. Following this report the government enacted regulations that extended the purposes for which the HFEA could approve embryo research projects to include stem cell cloning (Human Fertilisation and Embryology Research Purposes Regulations 2001 SI No 188). The decision by the HFEA to license cloning for therapeutic purposes was subject to challenge by a pro-life group, CORE – Comment on Reproductive Ethics (*R (ex parte Quintavelle)* v. *Secretary of State for Health* HL [2003] 2 All ER 113). The issue was whether cloning through cell nucleus transfer – the technique used in relation to Dolly the sheep – was regulated by the legislation. It was argued that it was not and that this technique fell outside the Act. CORE won at first instance. Panic ensued – the consequence of the decision was that some types of cloning were not banned by the 1990 Act nor were they capable of being regulated by the HFEA. There was thus the prospect that someone might try and clone a human being. This issue was resolved by the government rapidly passing the Human Reproductive Cloning Act 2001, which now clearly places a legislative ban on undertaking reproductive cloning. On appeal, the courts overturned the decision at first instance and construed the legislation to enable regulating of stem cell cloning. Nonetheless, this decision was controversial and in many ways can be seen as the court stretching the law to 'fit' a difficult issue through the use of purposive interpretation. This in itself is controversial, and indeed it can be argued that, if the law is not really capable of dealing with new ethical dilemmas, this should be a matter for Parliament rather than individual judges to determine.

Reforming the Human Fertilisation and Embryology Act 1990

The *Quintavelle* decision was illustrative of the problems of the 1990 Act not being able to deal really effectively with the fast moving area of reproductive technology and embryo research. In 2005 the Department of Health published a consultation document setting out the proposals for the reform of the law in the area (Department of Health 2005). This is a wide-ranging document that looks in detail at the whole Act. Some of the changes in this area have been prompted by the EU Tissue Directive, which has required the establishment of a regulatory body for cells and tissues. The HFEA is to be merged by 2008 with the new Human Tissue Authority as part of the response to this change, to form a new body, the Regulatory Authority for Tissues and Embryos (Department of Health 2005; see also Ch. 10).

Other reasons for reviewing the law concern the debates as to what extent, if at all, it is legitimate to regulate such issues in the future. To what extent should, for example, s13(5) – the requirement of clinics to consider the welfare of the child – be retained? Should reference also be made to the need of the child for a mother, in addition to a father – recognising the situation in which a child may be born to a gay male couple through use of a surrogate? To what extent should the law sanction the creation of 'designer babies'? Pre-implantation genetic diagnosis is currently sanctioned where there is a significant risk of a serious genetic disorder in the embryo (Human Fertilisation and Embryology Authority 2004, para 14.21). The HFEA has already sanctioned the performance of tissue typing to enable the creation of a sibling in order that stem cells can be extracted from the umbilical cord to cure a sick sibling – but exactly how far should this extend? (See further *R (ex parte Quintavelle)* v. *Secretary of State for Health* [2003] 3 All ER 257 and in the House of Lords [2005] 2 All ER 257.) The government is presently consulting on this issue (Department of Health 2005, para 2.35).

A further question is as to whether sex selection should be allowed. There is concern that this may lead to gender discrimination and at present sex-selection is not sanctioned for social reasons, only as a means of screening out disease. The government is consulting, however, as to whether it should be allowed for family balancing purposes (Department of Health 2005, para 5.32).

Surrogacy

A surrogate is the term used to describe a woman who carries the child of another. This practice has been undertaken for centuries. Recently, however, surrogacy been linked with modern reproductive technologies. It is argued that surrogacy can be both a necessary and helpful method of alleviating infertility. It may assist women who have suffered repeated miscarriages and might be appropriate in a situation in which a woman was medically unable to cope with the trauma of pregnancy although she was capable of caring for a child once born. In practice, it appears that surrogacy is regarded as appropriate only in exceptional cases. The British Medical Association has recommended that surrogacy 'should only be considered as a last resort where the commissioning couple suffers from infertility due to a medically recognised disorder and where all appropriate means for enabling them to have a child have been tried and failed' (British Medical Association 1990).

There are several reasons why surrogacy is seen as problematic. First, there may be conflicts between the natural mother and the commissioning parents, with the surrogate seeking to keep the child. Second, much discussion around surrogacy has concerned the commercialisation of the practice. It has been argued that making money out of the surrogate process is ethically unacceptable. The Warnock Committee was opposed to the commercialisation of surrogacy. The Surrogacy Arrangements Act 1985 provides that it is an offence to arrange a commercial surrogacy agreement (s2(1)) or to advertise surrogacy services (s3). No prosecutions have yet been brought under the Act. The legislation is targeted at surrogacy agencies. The commissioning mother and the surrogate do not commit an offence under this statute (s2(2)). While the law does not ban surrogacy agreements, they are, however, unenforceable. For instance, if a surrogate decided to keep the child, the commissioning parents could not demand that the child was handed over by her (s36(i) Human Fertilisation and Embryology Act 1990).

A number of non-profit-making surrogacy agencies have been established following the legislation, notably the agency COTS. Some surrogates were being paid considerable sums of money in the form of expenses. The legitimacy of such payments was the subject of consideration in a review commissioned by the Department of Health and chaired by Professor Margaret Brazier (DOH 1997). The review was opposed to the commercialisation of surrogacy and argued that expenses could be recoverable, but proposed that expenses should be reclaimable where these were documented relating to costs consequent to pregnancy and birth. As part of the review of the Human Fertilisation and Embryology Act 2005, the government is presently consulting as to the approach that should be taken to regulation of surrogacy in the future.

REGULATING THE CONDUCT OF THE MOTHER DURING PREGNANCY

Nurses and midwives have long played an important role during pregnancy and in childbirth. Today, midwives are involved not only in the delivery itself but through antenatal classes in the process of health education regarding birth. While over time the guidance and advice given to pregnant women has increased, few active constraints are imposed during pregnancy. While there is an active debate in the USA as to the extent to which women should be constrained by law during pregnancy, attempts in the UK to use the law to regulate behaviour in the period prior to birth have been unsuccessful (Robertson 1995). This is illustrated by the case of *Re F (in utero)* ([1988] 2 All ER 193). The court was faced with the issue of whether a fetus could be made a ward of court. F's mother had led a nomadic existence around Europe. She had disappeared and those caring for her were concerned that the fetus in her womb would suffer harm if the woman did not seek medical attention. The court, however, refused to make the child a ward of court, stating that the court's jurisdiction under wardship did not extend to an unborn child.

It is unlikely that at present English law will be used to compel behaviour during pregnancy (although contrast the attitude of the law regarding childbirth itself, below). Were such compulsion to be sanctioned, this would require radical revaluation of the role of the nurse and midwife in caring for the mother.

Freedom to choose where to give birth

During the last century the birth process has become increasingly medically dominated. Much use is made of technological interventions in pregnancy.

Today only around 1% of women give birth in their own homes. There are a number of reasons why this is the case. It may be regarded as 'safer' for the mother. Hospital births may be more convenient for the hospital team. Some suggest that the increase in surgical interventions during pregnancy is motivated by fear of a 'malpractice crisis', with doctors increasingly prepared to advise patients to undergo caesarean section to avoid the risk of litigation should the pregnancy prove problematic. Indeed, the need for the number of caesarean sections presently undertaken has been questioned. In some instances a caesarean section may be the only alternative, otherwise mother, child or both may be at risk of death. A child may be in the breech position and, if the child's head becomes stuck, brain damage may result. At the same time, there are risks attached to the performance of a caesarean section. Evidence has been given to the effect that, for example, the operation may put a woman at a six to 11 times increased chance of death during childbirth or haemorrhage. In addition, if the woman becomes pregnant again, the risk of rupture of the scar on the uterus may mean that another caesarean operation will be required (Anderson & Strong 1988).

There is some evidence of a shift in policy regarding the conduct of childbirth. A report issued by a House of Commons Committee stated that 'the policy of encouraging all women to give birth in hospital cannot be justified on grounds of safety' (House of Commons Health Committee Session 1991–92 Maternity Services). A government committee chaired by Lady Cumberlege published a report in 1993 called *Changing Childbirth: Report of the Expert Maternity Group* (Cumberlege 1993). The report identified three key principles. The woman should be the focus of maternity care provision. Maternity services should be readily and easily accessible to all, and services must be effective and efficient.

Birth plans and compelling a caesarean section

Today it is common for women to agree with their midwife a plan for the conduct of their birth. This states such matters as whether a woman would receive pain relief, etc. But what if in a particular situation a midwife believes that it is necessary for the health of the woman to depart from the birth plan? Treating in the face of a previously stated refusal may, as we saw earlier, render the midwife or doctor liable in the tort of battery (Ch. 5). However, in some situations this may not prove practical. A woman states her wishes as regards a natural 'low tech' birth, but then complications develop; should the birth plan be followed? It could be argued that it should not if all the possible eventualities have not been foreseen. Any birth plan that is drawn up should be undertaken only after the implications of refusal of certain types of treatment and the problems if an emergency arises have been pointed out to the woman. Where it is proposed to go ahead in the absence of express consent, then, wherever possible, a court order should be sought.

Take a situation in which it is discovered late in pregnancy that a caesarean section is required. The woman says that she is a Jehovah's Witness, she is opposed to being given a blood transfusion and she does not want a caesarean section. What if the consequence of the patient's refusal of a medical procedure such as a caesarean is that both woman and fetus will die? Such a problem came before the English courts in the 1992 case of *Re S* ([1992] 4 All ER 671). S was 6 days overdue giving birth. The health-care team wanted to undertake a caesarean section because, as the fetus was in transverse lie, any attempt at a normal birth carried a very grave risk of rupture of the uterus. S, who was a born-again Christian, refused the operation. This was because it would have involved a blood transfusion, which was against her religious beliefs. The hospital sought a declaration from the court, which was granted by Sir Stephen Brown. The decision – notable for its brevity – has been criticised (Grubb 1993), not least for the fact that Sir Stephen Brown made reference to a US case, *Re AC* ([1990] 573 A.2d 1235 at 1240), in which a court had been prepared to authorise a caesarean section on a pregnant woman. While some courts in the USA have been prepared to order enforced treatment upon pregnant women, *Re AC* is very far from a clear authority supporting the use of an enforced caesarean. On appeal in that case, after the death of the woman on whom the caesarean had been ordered, the court stated that the operation should not have been authorised. The Royal College of Obstetricians and Gynaecologists (1994) published a consultation paper stating that:

> " It is inappropriate and unlikely to be helpful or necessary to invoke judicial intervention to overrule an informed and competent woman's refusal of a proposed medical treatment even though her refusal may place her life and that of her fetus at risk.

Despite this, in a number of subsequent cases judicial intervention was sought and the courts authorised the performance of caesarean sections upon women who had refused such procedures. (*Tameside* v. *Glossop* [1996] 1 FCR 753; *Rochdale NHS Trust* v. *C* [1997] 1 FCR 274; *Norfolk & Norwich NHS Trust* v. *W* [1996] 2 FLR 613). These cases attracted a storm of controversy and thus it was hardly surprising when attempts were made to challenge these decisions in the courts. The Court of Appeal was given an opportunity to rule upon this issue in *Re MB* ([1997] 2 FLR 426). MB attended an antenatal clinic when she was 33 weeks pregnant. She refused to have blood taken from her because she had a fear of needles. She subsequently agreed to a caesarean section when she found that her fetus was in the breech position and was at risk of harm due to oxygen starvation. However she then refused consent, then she subsequently agreed to the anaesthetic and then later refused it again. The hospital then sought a court order, which was given by Hollis J. He found that MB was incompetent because of the effects of the needle phobia on her decision-making powers. An appeal that night to the Court of Appeal was rejected. The caesarean operation was carried out the following day.

Subsequently MB challenged the legality of the procedure. In the Court of Appeal (Butler-Sloss, Saville and Ward L.J.J.) the right of the competent patient to refuse treatment was confirmed. The Court of Appeal upheld earlier cases such as *Re F* (in utero), *Paton* v. *British Pregnancy Advisory Authority* ([1978] 2 All ER 987) in confirming that the fetus has no independent status in English law. They were of the view that Sir Stephen Brown in *Re S* had reached an incorrect conclusion. The Court of Appeal stated that:

> " Although it may seem illogical that a child capable of being born alive is protected by the criminal law from intentional destruction, and by the

Abortion Act from termination otherwise than as permitted by the Act, but is not protected from the (irrational) decision of a competent mother not to allow medical intervention to avert the risk of death, this appears to be the present state of the law. (p. 441)

Thus even at the point of birth itself the court could not intervene in the face of refusal of medical intervention by a competent woman with the aim of safeguarding the position of the fetus.

Nonetheless it was also recognised that, in an emergency, treatment could be given where a patient lacks capacity, as long as this was on the basis of necessity, the procedure not extending beyond what was reasonably required by the patient. It was noted that difficult issues arose regarding the determination of capacity. Butler Sloss L.J. quoted from Lord Donaldson in *Re T* that the doctor must assess carefully whether in that case the patient had the capacity relative to this particular decision.

In *Re MB* the Court of Appeal upheld the decision of the judge at first instance to the effect that *MB* lacked capacity. While MB was competent to consent to the caesarean section itself she was not competent to make the actual refusal as she was 'at that moment suffering an impairment of her mental functioning that disabled her. She was temporarily incompetent'. In this case it was her phobia of needles that impaired her ability to decide.

Having found MB to be temporarily incompetent, the Court of Appeal then considered whether the procedure itself could be authorised, by reference to the test of best interests set out by the House of Lords in *Re F* [1990]. Here best interests equates to what a responsible body of medical practice would regard as being in the 'best interests' of the patient in accord with the *Bolam* test (*Bolam v. Friern Hospital Management Company* [1957] 2 All ER 118). In *Re MB*, Butler-Sloss L.J. stated that:

" In considering the scope of best interests, it seems to us that they have to be treated on similar principles to the welfare of a child since the court and the doctors are concerned with a person unable to make the necessary decision for himself. (p. 439)

The Court of Appeal held that the treatment was in MB's best interests in this emergency situation. It took into consideration the fact that agreement had initially been given by MB for the caesarean section. Furthermore, evidence from the consultant psychiatrist was to the effect that, if the child had been born handicapped or had died, MB herself would have suffered long-term harm. In contrast, little harm would be caused by the administration of the anaesthetic against her wishes.

While the decision of the Court of Appeal in *Re MB* does confirm the pregnant woman's autonomy in principle, it does leave open a number of important issues. How will temporary issues of capacity be addressed? What is the scope of the best interests test today and what are the differences in practice between children and incompetent adults? Nonetheless one of the most important aspects of the decision in *Re MB* is that it provides guidance for future cases in this area, in that it sets out the procedure that should be undertaken. This includes the requirement that the woman should be represented in all cases save where, in exceptional circumstances, she does not wish to be (p. 445). This recommendation goes some way to meet concerns as to the manner in which such proceedings have been brought.

Caesarean sections and the Mental Health Act

In parallel to the cases discussed above regarding caesarean sections there have been a number of cases involving the use of the Mental Health Act 1983. Section 63 of the Act provides that 'The consent of a patient shall not be required for any medical treatment given to him for the mental disorder from which he is suffering'. But how far does this provision extend? Would it sanction the Act being used to authorise the performance of a caesarean section? This issue came before the courts in *Tameside and Glossop Acute Hospital Trust* v. *CH* ([1996] 1 FLR 762) (see also Grubb 1996). CH was detained under section 3 of the Mental Health Act 1983. She was suffering from paranoid schizophrenia. She was then discovered to be pregnant. It was held that she lacked capacity to consent or refuse treatment. The caesarean section could be authorised as the performance of a caesarean section was treatment for 'mental disorder' and thus fell within the scope of section 63 of the Mental Health Act 1983. If a stillbirth had occurred her health would have deteriorated. In addition, she needed strong antipsychotic medication. This could not be given to her when she was pregnant. The court followed the approach in *B* v. *Croyden HA* ([1995] 1 All ER 683), namely that section 63 of the 1983 Act encompassed matters that related to the 'core treatment'. In *B* v. *Croyden* the court authorised the force-feeding, through a nasogastric tube, of a patient with a personality disorder and intended self-harm.

However a more restrictive approach was taken by the Court of Appeal in the case of *St Georges NHS Trust* v. *S* ([1998] 3 WLR 936). S was diagnosed as suffering from severe pre-eclampsia when she registered as a patient at a new NHS practice when 8 months pregnant. She was advised that she should have an early delivery. S, who had intended a home delivery, refused treatment. She asserted that nature should take its course, although she was informed as to the risk of death and disability to herself and the fetus. Her GP then called a psychiatrist and approved social worker. S was detained in hospital under section 2 of the Mental Health Act 1983 and was subsequently transferred to another hospital. She repeated her refusal both orally and in writing. She sought legal advice. Without the knowledge of S, or of her legal advisors, the hospital authority made an *ex parte* application to the High Court for a declaration to the effect that it would be lawful to undertake treatment, including a caesarean section. Meanwhile, S had been in touch with solicitors with the intention of bringing an appeal before a Mental Health Tribunal.

The declaration was granted. It appears that the judge was under what was an incorrect impression that S had been in labour for 24 hours. S gave birth to a daughter. The detention under the Mental Health Act was terminated. S discharged herself. While detained in hospital S was not offered treatment for her mental disorder. An action was subsequently brought for judicial review to challenge the legality of the action taken.

As in *Re MB*, the Court of Appeal (Butler-Sloss, Judge and Robert Walker LL.J.) again emphasised the fact that the competent adult is entitled to refuse treatment. They addressed the question of the status of the fetus. Judge L.J. stated that:

9

> " In our judgment while pregnancy increases the personal responsibilities of a woman it does not diminish her entitlement to decide whether or not to undergo medical treatment. Although human and protected by the law in a number of different ways as set out in the judgment in *Re MB* ... an unborn child is not a separate person from its mother. Its need for medical assistance does not prevail over her rights. (p. 957)

The Court held that a battery had been committed on S. Judge L.J. asked: '...how can an enforced invasion of a competent adult's body against her will even for the most laudable of motives (the preservation of life) be ordered without irredeemably damaging the principle of self-determination?' (cf. 953).

The Court examined the provisions of s2(2) of the Mental Health Act 1983, which had been used to authorise the admission of S. The Court of Appeal emphasised that the criteria for detention under the section were cumulative. In this case, the doctors had been justified in their assessment that the woman was suffering from depression, which constituted 'mental disorder'. However, S was not being detained in order that treatment be given for her mental disorder. It was stated that 'For the purposes of section 2(2)A such detention must be related to or linked with the mental disorder. Treatment for the effects of pregnancy does not provide the necessary warrant'.

Thus the courts have affirmed that treatment to be lawful under section 63 it must be crucial to the mental disorder. In this case, the treatment was not treatment for mental disorder within the provisions of the statute. However, as Bailey Harris has commented (1998), it is the case that questions regarding the connection between the disorder and the treatment proposed are likely to arise in the future. One further point here was that there had also been an irregularity in the documentation used by the hospital. Forms had not been completed when the woman was transferred between hospitals as was required under section 19 of the Mental Health Act. This would, in any event, have entitled S to discharge herself from hospital. S was thus competent, she had been unlawfully detained and the procedure was a battery. The fact that her refusal might be regarded by some as unjustifiable or even irrational did not mean that it was of no legal validity. The Mental Health Act cannot be used as a means of circumventing the pregnant woman's right to refuse a caesarean section. Finally, the Court of Appeal criticised the procedure adopted in the case of the *ex parte* application, the application was made without the knowledge of S and her legal advisors and, as in *Re MB*, they set out guidelines regarding the conduct of proceedings for a declaration.

Both *Re MB* and *St Georges NHS Trust* v. *S* provide what may be regarded as a welcome clarification of the legal position in the area. The autonomy of the patient is confirmed. The operation of the Mental Health Act 1983 in such cases is made clear. The refusal of treatment by the competent pregnant woman is upheld. Guidance is provided as to the correct procedures that should be adopted when making an application for a declaration. These decisions highlight the need for information to be given to the pregnant woman and her advisors. In too many cases the woman has been without

Reproductive choice

legal advice or, as in *St Georges NHS Trust* v. *S*, is simply not informed of the steps that are being taken. Admittedly there is a danger that the involvement of the legal process may be regarded as detracting from patient care, leading to the polarisation of views of the parties, women, midwives and doctors. However it could be argued that reference of what appear to be insurmountable differences for judicial determination constitutes a recognition that there are certain decisions that, because of their inherently difficult nature, cannot be left for resolution by the parties. The decision-making process may in fact be benefited by the involvement of an independent arbiter.

We should not underestimate also the acute dilemma facing health-care professionals in such a highly emotionally charged situation, in which they realise that medical intervention will almost certainly enable the fetus to be born healthy. It also provides safeguards for the patient in ensuring account-ability. Difficulties are, however, likely to arise in the future regarding the definition of incapacity itself and those situations in which a pregnant woman is declared to be incompetent, enabling treatment to be given without her consent.

Patient refusing care with dependant family

No English court has yet been faced with the question of whether to authorise treatment on the basis that the patient who is refusing care has a dependent family. The issue has arisen in the USA, where the courts have been prepared to uphold the right of the patient to refuse treatment regardless of the impact upon the patient's family (*Norwood Hospital* v. *Munoz* [1991] 564 NE 2d 1017). It is submitted that this is the correct approach to take and that, whatever the consequences, if a competent patient makes a clear refusal of treatment that refusal should be respected.

Postnatal care

The nurse or health visitor may be involved in providing antenatal care to mother and baby. What if the nurse believes that a mother s/he is attending is abusing drugs and that the home is unsuitable? In this situation, the nurse should bring the matter to the attention of the social services. They may decide to take action and, if necessary, use one of the orders available to them under the Children Act 1989 (for fuller discussion, see Ch. 6).

Liability for injuries in relation to conception and childbirth

Negligence of health professionals, whether in providing advice regarding sterilisation or during the conduct of childbirth, may lead to litigation. The process of childbirth is fraught with difficulties and mistakes are easily made. In the debates on the existence of a malpractice crisis in health care, obstetrics and gynaecology are frequently cited as examples. The general principles of negligence are discussed in Chapter 2. Here a few specific points are considered briefly.

Where a child is born handicapped as a result of conduct that it is claimed is negligent, then a claim may be brought against a nurse or doctor.

The Congenital Disabilities (Civil Liability) Act 1976 allows an action to be brought by a child who has suffered a disability (s1(3)). This Act was passed following the debate and legal action that arose from the use of the drug thalidomide. This drug had been given to pregnant women to counteract morning sickness, and it was alleged that as a consequence children had been born handicapped. An action can only be brought under the 1976 Act if the child is born alive and has lived at least 48 hours (s4(2)). It must be shown that the disability that the child has suffered was the result of an occurrence that affected the mother/father's ability to have a child, or affected the mother during pregnancy or affected mother or child during birth. Situations in which an action may be taken include a child being born handicapped as a result of negligence during the birth. To bring a claim under the Act, it must be shown that the nurse or midwife owed the mother a duty of care (s4(2)). Any damages awarded under the Act may be reduced if the parents were contributorily negligent in the harm caused.

In practice, it seems that liability is difficult to establish, with few claims having been brought. Many of these claims will fall on the grounds that the negligence itself did not cause the harm suffered. It is perhaps of interest, in view of the earlier discussion as to the obligation of the pregnant woman towards her fetus, that an action may not be brought by a child against her mother for negligent conduct under the 1976 Act. The one exception to this is in a situation in which the fetus is injured by negligence of the mother when driving a car and the mother knew or ought reasonably to have known that she was pregnant (s2 Congenital Disabilities (Civil Liability) Act 1976).

An action at common law cannot be brought on behalf of the child on the basis that the injuries the child suffered were such that s/he would be better off never having been born. The Court of Appeal rejected such a 'wrongful life' claim in the case of *McKay* v. *Essex Area Health Authority* ([1982] 2 All ER 771), on the basis that the court could not assess the award of damages satisfactorily to assess the difference between never having been born and a life of disability. In addition, it was argued that to allow such damages here could encourage health-care professionals to advise on an abortion rather than risk subsequent litigation where a child was born handicapped. Parents can, however, bring claims for the cost of bringing up an infant born severely disabled as a result of medical negligence during pregnancy or childbirth. The possibility of such litigation illustrates the importance of risk management and following protocols where available (Ch. 10).

ABORTION

Background to the existing law

Abortion is one of the most controversial of all clinical procedures (Keown 1988, Dworkin 1993). It was made a criminal offence in England by the Offences Against the Person Act 1861 ss58 and 59. In addition, the Infant Life Preservation Act 1933 made it an offence to destroy the life of a child capable of being born alive. This remained the position until 1967, subject to a limited exception being recognised for abortions undertaken to preserve the life of the mother or to ensure that she was not rendered a 'physical and mental wreck' (*R v. Bourne* [1939] 1 KB 687). In 1967, after much heated debate, the Abortion Act was passed, largely through the efforts of the Liberal MP David Steel. This legislation was amended in 1990 by clauses inserted into the 1967 Act by the Human Fertilisation and Embryology Act 1990. The introduction of abortion legislation was accompanied by a heated ethical debate. On the one hand the use of abortion was strongly advocated by those who supported a 'pro-choice' approach. Abortion was, however, opposed by those who can be loosely grouped under the heading 'pro-life' and who regarded the abortion process as that of the killing of a human person or potential person (Dworkin, 1993). The legislation, as can be seen below, has provided no absolute rights to any of the parties to the abortion process. There is no right to abortion on demand, the father has no rights and nor has the fetus. In many respects the abortion decision can be viewed as one characterised by medical determination and domination.

The nurse should be broadly aware of the law as it relates to abortion, and particularly the Abortion Act 1967, for a number of reasons. Acting in his/her role as patient advocate, the nurse may be involved in counselling and advising a woman who is contemplating an abortion. Also, the nurse may have fundamental religious objections to abortion. When can s/he legitimately refuse to participate?

When is an abortion lawful?

An abortion is lawful if authorised by two registered medical practitioners who are of the opinion, held in good faith, that one of the four grounds laid down in the Abortion Act 1967 has been met.

Social abortions

First, an abortion is allowed if the woman is less than 24 weeks pregnant and continuation of the pregnancy would involve a risk, greater than if the pregnancy were terminated, of injury to her physical or mental health or that of any child in her family (s1(1)a). This category – the so called 'social ground' – is the provision under which most abortions are authorised. It leaves considerable room for the exercise of medical discretion. For example, there is controversy as to whether the psychological pressure placed upon women in certain cultural groups to have a male child provides sufficient justification for the abortion of a female fetus. 'Social' abortions can only be undertaken in the first 24 weeks of pregnancy, but the Act does not state from when this time runs. There are a number of possibilities (Murphy 1991), such as the date of the woman's last period, date of implantation or date of fertilisation.

Other grounds for abortion

The other grounds for abortion under the 1967 Act are not subject to an express time limit. An abortion may be undertaken if termination of pregnancy is necessary to prevent grave permanent injury to the physical or mental health of the pregnant woman (s1(1)b). An abortion is also lawful if continuation of the pregnancy involves a risk to the life of the pregnant woman greater than if the pregnancy were terminated (s1(1)c). Finally, an abortion may be undertaken if there is a substantial risk that if pregnancy were to continue the child would be born seriously handicapped (s1(1)d). The statute does not define 'seriously handicapped'. It is unclear whether this refers to a handicap that the child would be born with if the pregnancy continues, or if it extends to conditions such as Huntington's chorea, which will not develop until a person is around 40 or 50 years old (Morgan 1990, Sheldon & Wilkinson 2001). A recent challenge concerned a Church of England curate, Joanne Jepson, who challenged the decision of West Mercia police not to investigate an allegation that a fetus had been aborted because otherwise it would have been born with a cleft palate (*Jepson* v. *Chief Constable of West Mercia* [2003] EWCA 3318). In 2005 the police decided not to prosecute this further because they were of the view that the doctors concerned had acted in good faith.

Emergency abortions

The Act states that an abortion must be authorised by two medical practitioners (s1(1)). However, one doctor may authorise an abortion if it is the only way of averting an immediate risk to the woman's life or grave permanent injury to her (s1(4)).

No right to an abortion

It must be stressed that there is no right to abortion on demand. The ultimate decision regarding the performance of an abortion is a matter of clinical judgment after discussion between the doctor and the patient. Just as a woman has no right to demand an abortion, neither does her husband/partner have any legal right to be consulted or to veto the abortion decision (*Paton* v. *Trustees of the British Pregnancy Advisory Service* [1978] 2 All ER 987, *C* v. *S* [1988] QB 135). Also, English law does not recognise the fetus as possessing legal rights (*Paton* v. *British Pregnancy Advisory Service* (1987) 2 All ER 987). The Human Rights Act 1998 provides for a 'right to life' in Article 2 of the European Convention on Human Rights – however the ECHR has confirmed that this does not confer protection on the fetus separate from the mother (*Paton* v. *UK* (1980) 3 EHRR 408; *Vo* v. *France* ECHR [2004] 2 FCR 577).

Selective reduction

The development of IVF treatment led to a difficulty relating to abortion. In the course of IVF treatment, in order to increase the chance of a successful implantation, more than one embryo is usually transferred into the womb. In some situations, this may result in a number of embryos becoming implanted. Such a multiple pregnancy may constitute a serious risk to the mother's health. The amendments made to the Abortion Act 1967 in 1990 included a provision to the effect that it was lawful to remove one or more embryos as long as one of the grounds for abortion under the 1967 Act had been met (s5(2)). These provisions do not only apply to multiple pregnancies arising as a result of infertility treatment. There was controversy regarding a press

Reproductive choice

report that a consultant had performed selective reduction on a woman with twins who sought an abortion under the 'social' grounds of the legislation (*The Guardian* 1996).

Abortion and patients lacking mental capacity

While a competent adult patient can clearly consent to an abortion, difficulties may arise if it is proposed to undertake an abortion upon a teenager or an adult with learning disabilities. A teenager may be competent to consent herself if she is regarded as of sufficient maturity under the test in *Gillick* (Ch. 6). But what if she refuses an abortion? While in theory the parental power of consent may override the refusal of a competent child, if a teenager wanted to keep her baby then any dispute between her and her parents should be immediately referred to the court. It would, it is suggested, be unlikely that the court would force a girl to undergo an abortion.

While it may be seen as good practice to seek court approval before an abortion is performed on a mentally incompetent woman, there is, strictly speaking, no need for such an order to be made before the abortion goes ahead (*Re SG* [1991] 6 BMLR 95 (Fam Div)). The decision to undertake an abortion upon a mentally incompetent adult must be reached on the basis of what are her best interests. The nurse as patient advocate may play an important role in ensuring that the patient's interests are properly taken into account in making this decision.

The Law Commission, in its report on *Mental Incapacity* (1995), expressed concern that abortions were being undertaken on young women with learning disabilities without proper investigation into their ability to consent, and best interests. It suggested that, before an abortion is performed upon a mentally incompetent woman, there should be a requirement for a certificate to be obtained from an independent medical practitioner that the abortion is in the woman's best interests (para 6.10). The government, in its document *Who decides* (Lord Chancellor's Department 1997), was not convinced by this solution and was of the view that the existing legislative safeguards were adequate: the new Mental Capacity Act 2005 does not make specific provision for abortion.

Where should the abortion be carried out?

Section 1(3) of the Act provides that abortions must be undertaken in an NHS hospital or in a place that has been approved by the Secretary of State for the purposes of undertaking abortions. This provision created difficulties in relation to the abortion pill, the drug RU486. It was intended that this would be administered to patients at GPs' surgeries. To cover this, section 1(3)(a) was enacted, which provides that:

> " The power under subsection (3) of this section to approve a place includes a power in relation to treatment consisting primarily in the use of such medicines as may be specified in the approval and carried out in such manner as may be so specified, to approve a class of places.

This power has not yet been exercised; thus at present RU486 may be lawfully administered to patients only in hospital.

Role of the nurse in prostaglandin abortions

While the 1967 Act provides that the pregnancy must be terminated by a registered medical practitioner, the nurse plays a major role in certain abortion procedures. In prostaglandin abortions, the doctor inserts a catheter into the womb via the cervix in order to create a space between the womb and the amniotic sac containing the fetus. This may cause abortion. If not, various other steps are undertaken, such as attaching a catheter to a pump propelling prostaglandin into the womb. These are mostly carried out by a nurse or midwife. However, the legislation made no reference to the nurse, simply referring to the doctor's role in the process. The Royal College of Nursing went to court to obtain an order to clarify the legality of the nurse's involvement in the abortion process (*RCN* v. *DHSS* [1981] AC 800). The House of Lords held that the doctor need not do everything with his own hands. Lord Diplock stated that Parliament had contemplated that, as with other hospital treatment, abortion would take place as a team effort: junior doctors, paramedics, nurses and other members of the health-care team would each undertake those tasks that would be, in accordance with a responsible body of medical practice, entrusted to a member of staff possessed of their respective skills. The involvement of the nurse in the process was lawful.

Conscientious objection

Abortion is an exceedingly sensitive ethical issue on which many people hold very strong beliefs. The 1967 Act itself takes account of this. Section 4 of the 1967 Act provides that:

" no person shall be under any duty whether by contract or by any statutory or other legal requirement, to participate in any treatment authorised by this Act to which he has a conscientious objection: Provided that in any legal proceedings the burden of proof of conscientious objection shall rest on the person claiming to rely on it....

The section does, however, go on to provide that:

" Nothing in subsection (1) of this section shall affect any duty to participate in treatment which is necessary to save the life or to prevent grave permanent injury to the physical or mental health of a pregnant woman.

Thus, a nurse who is a devout Roman Catholic may refuse to participate in an abortion procedure save in an exceptional situation, such as where a woman is brought in bleeding profusely from the uterus and it is clear that without an abortion she will die.

While the Act gives the nurse the right to refuse to be involved in clinical procedures, the statutory right of conscientious objection does not extend to those persons more remotely connected to the abortion process. In *Jannaway* v. *Salford AHA* ([1988] 3 All ER 1079) a secretary who was a Roman Catholic refused to type a letter referring a pregnant woman to a consultant with a view to securing an abortion. Ultimately she was dismissed. She claimed that the dismissal was unfair and that the conscientious objection provision under section 4 protected her. Her claim was rejected in the House of Lords. Lord Keith said that 'participation' for the purposes of section 4 meant actual participation in the treatment administered in a hospital or other approved place.

Liability if the 1967 Act is not complied with

There has been some discussion as to whether the procedure set out in the 1967 Act has to be complied with before, for example, an intrauterine device is inserted after intercourse or before the 'morning after pill' is given. In some situations, failure to comply with the Abortion Act 1967 may result in a criminal prosecution. Section 58 of the Offences Against the Person Act 1861 states that it is an offence to use an instrument with the intention of procuring a miscarriage. What constitutes 'carriage' for these purposes is somewhat unclear (Montgomery 1997, p. 362). The courts have confirmed that administration of the morning-after pill does not have to comply with the Abortion Act 1967 because at that point the embryo is not implanted (*R (on the application of Smeaton)* v. *Secretary of State for Health* (2002) 2 FLR 146). Today, abortion may also be undertaken through administration of the drug RU486. This drug is clearly abortifacient, since it operates after the ovum has become implanted. It is almost certain that it must be given in accordance with the 1967 Act.

Failure to comply with the 1967 Act may also place those performing the abortion at risk of prosecution under the Infant Life Preservation Act 1929 for the offence of child destruction. Section 1(1) of this Act provides that:

> " Any person who with intent to destroy the life of a child capable of being born alive by any wilful act causes the child to die before it has a life independent of its mother shall be guilty of the offence of child destruction and shall be liable on conviction to life imprisonment.

> " But that no person shall be found guilty under this section unless it is proved that the act which caused the death of the child was not done in good faith for the purpose only of preserving the life of the mother.

No offence will be committed under this Act as long as the provisions of the Abortion Act 1967 have been complied with. Were a prosecution to be brought under this section, a court would have to consider whether the fetus was 'capable of being born alive'. Some guidance as to what this term means has been given in the case of *C* v. *S* ([1988] QB 135). Here, the court rejected the claim that a fetus of 18–21 weeks was 'capable of being born alive'. Lord Donaldson said that, while at 18–21 weeks the cardiac muscle is contracting and primitive circulation is developing – and therefore the fetus could be said to be developing real and discernible signs of life, nevertheless it was unable to breathe either naturally or with the aid of a ventilator.

The mature fetus

If a hysterectomy is undertaken in the later stages of pregnancy, the fetus may be born alive. An infant who has taken breath and shown signs of life after being expelled from the womb is entitled to a full birth certificate and to be fed and cared for. If a nurse leaves the infant to die, a prosecution for murder or manslaughter may result. For example, in *R* v. *Hamilton* (*The Times*, 16 September 1983), an infant was discovered after abortion to be 33 weeks rather than 23 weeks old. The infant – clearly alive after delivery – was left in the sluice room for some 15 minutes before being transferred to the intensive care unit. The infant survived. Dr Hamilton was charged with attempted murder although, ultimately, the magistrates decided that there was no case to answer. The nurse as patient advocate should be concerned to safeguard the rights of the infant patient. If the nurse finds that a baby has been born and is at risk of death, s/he must immediately take steps to secure the infant's survival. The nurse should also report the condition in which the infant was found and any perceived deficiencies in care.

There is a greater chance that the fetus will be born alive in a situation in which an abortion is undertaken late in pregnancy. One reason why abortion may be undertaken late in pregnancy is because of delay in the initial referral. Clarke quotes a Royal College of Gynaecologists study, which found that 20.5% of women who had abortions between 20 and 23 weeks had been referred at 12 weeks but had then experienced delay in obtaining a consultation and appointment for treatment (Clarke 1987). As far as possible, any delay from the initial point at which a woman sees her doctor to any abortion should be minimised.

REGISTRATION OF BIRTHS AND STILLBIRTHS

When a woman gives birth, whether to a living infant or to a stillbirth, then the doctor or the midwife who has attended the woman is under a statutory duty to inform the responsible medical officer of that fact (s124 NHS Act 1977; Notification of Births and Deaths Regulations 1982; SI 1982 No 286). A stillbirth is the term used to describe a child born dead after 24 weeks of pregnancy which did not breathe or show any sign of life (s41 Births and Deaths Registration Act 1953, as amended by the Still Birth Definition Act 1992).

The Births and Deaths Registration Act 1953 requires the mother or father to inform the Registrar of a birth within 42 days (s2). If either of them is unable to do so, then there is a duty upon the occupier of the house, any person present at the birth or any person who has charge of that child to give the Registrar that information (s2(1)(2)). A midwife may be such a person. If the birth has not been registered within 42 days then the Registrar can compel any qualified informant to come before him to provide information and to sign the Register, having first given them 7 days' notice in writing. Where a stillbirth is being registered, the informant must provide the Registrar with a certificate stating that the child was not born alive. This certificate should have been signed by a registered medical practitioner or by a certified midwife who was present during the birth or who subsequently examined the dead body. A birth is classified as a stillbirth where the fetus is more than 24 weeks old. (Still Birth (Definition) Act 1992).

REFERENCES

Anderson G, Strong C 1988 The premature breech; caesarean section or trial of labour. Journal of Medical Ethics 18: 18

Bailey Harris R 1998 Pregnancy, autonomy and refusal of medical treatment. Law Quarterly Review 550: 550–555

Brazier M 1990 Sterilisation: down the slippery slope. Professional Negligence 6: 25

British Medical Association 1990 Surrogacy: ethical considerations. Report of a working party on human infertility services. BMA, London

British Medical Journal 1999 Cloning may cause health defects. British Medical Journal 318: 1230B

Chief Medical Officer 2000 Stem cell research: medical progress with responsibility. Chief Medical Officer's Expert Group Report. Office of the CMO, London

Clarke L 1987 Abortion – a rights issue. In: Lee R, Morgan D (eds) Birthrights. Routledge, London

Cumberlege JF 1993 Changing childbirth: report of the Expert Maternity Group. Department of Health, London

Department for Constitutional Affairs 2006 Mental Capacity Act: draft code of practice. Stationery Office, London

Department of Health 1997 Surrogacy: Review for health ministers of current arrangements for payments and regulation – report of the review team. Department of Health, London.

Department of Health 2005 Review of the Human Fertilisation and Embryology Act 1990: a public consultation. Department of Health, London

Dworkin R 1993 Life's dominion: an argument about euthanasia and abortion. Harper Collins, London

Grubb A 1993 Treatment without consent: adult. Medical Law Review 1: 931

Grubb A 1996 Treatment without consent: pregnancy(adult) – Tameside and Glossop Acute Services Trust v. C.H. Medical Law Review 4: 193–198

The Guardian 1996 'No new issue' in abortion of twin. 5 August

Harris J 1998 Clones, genes and immortality. Oxford University Press, Oxford

HMSO 1984 Report of the Committee of Inquiry into Human Fertilisation and Embryology (Warnock Committee Report). Cmnd 9314. HMSO, London

House of Commons Science and Technology Committee 1997 The cloning of animals from adult cells. Science and Technology Committee Fifth Report of Session 1996–7. (HC 373–1). HMSO, London

House of Commons Select Committee on Science and Technology 2005 Human reproductive technologies and the law. Stationery Office, London

Human Fertilisation and Embryology Authority 2004 Code of practice. HFEA, London

Keown J 1988 Abortion, doctors and the law. Cambridge University Press, Cambridge

Law Commission 1995 Mental incapacity. Report no. 231. HMSO, London

Lee R, Morgan D (eds) 1989 A lesser sacrifice: sterilisation and the mentally handicapped woman. In: Birthrights: law and ethics at the beginnings of life. Routledge, London

Lee R, Morgan D 2001 Regulating the reproductive revolution, 2nd edn. Blackstone Press, London

Lord Chancellor's Department 1997 Who decides? LCD, London

McHale J, Gallagher A 2004 Rights and reproduction. In: Nursing and human rights. Butterworth Heinemann, Edinburgh, Ch 2

Montgomery J 1997 Health care law. Oxford University Press, Oxford

Morgan D 1990 Abortion – the unexamined ground. Criminal Law Review Oct: 687–694

Murphy J 1991 Cosmetics, eugenics and ambivalence; the revision of the Abortion Act 1967. Journal of Social Welfare and Family Law 1: 375

Robertson J 1995 Children of choice. Princeton University Press, Princeton, NJ

Royal College of Obstetricians and Gynaecologists 1994 A consideration of the law and ethics in relation to court-authorised obstetric intervention. RCOG, London

Sheldon S, Wilkinson S 2001 Termination of pregnancy for reason of foetal disability: are there grounds for a special exception in law? Medical Law Review 9: 85–109

The end of life

Jean McHale

The nurse frequently plays an important role in caring for patients at the end of life whether, for instance, in the area of palliative care and the hospice movement or in the intensive care unit. Many difficult issues arise at the end of life. A patient who is terminally ill and who is in considerable pain may tell the nurse that he wants to die. What should the nurse do? The midwife presents a mother with a child who is severely handicapped and the mother screams for the child to be taken away from her. How far is the medical team required to keep that child alive? A young man is killed in a road accident, and the man's father approaches the nurse for advice as to whether his son's organs could be used for transplantation. While the nurse may be the primary carer and required to take primary responsibility at the end of life, in many situations s/he will be acting as part of a treatment team. This area also gives rise to a number of difficult issues for the nurse as patient advocate.

This chapter considers a number of important legal questions at the end of life. It begins by examining the approach taken in English law to issues of active and passive termination of life. There is much discussion as to whether there is a 'right to die'. As will be seen, in English law there is only a right in the sense that a patient can choose to end his or her own life – English law does not sanction active euthanasia, though in certain situations withdrawal of treatment is lawful. The second section considers the definition of death. In the final section the legal regulation of organ transplantation is examined and some proposals for law reform are considered.

ENDING LIFE – CRIMINAL LIABILITY

> A seriously ill patient may plead with a nurse that he has suffered enough and that he wants someone to 'put him out of his misery'. What action should the nurse take?

However grave his agony, if the nurse complies s/he may be prosecuted for murder.

English law does not recognise active euthanasia. In *R* v. *Carr* (*Sunday Times*, 30 November 1986) Dr Carr had injected a massive dose of phenobarbital (phenobarbitone) into a patient with inoperable lung cancer. The judge, Mars J., emphasised that every patient was entitled to every hour that God had given him, however seriously ill that patient might be. The jury eventually acquitted Dr Carr.

However, in 1992 Dr Cox was prosecuted and convicted of attempted murder (*The Times*, 22 September 1992). (He was not charged with murder because, at the time of the investigation, the body of the alleged victim had been cremated and thus the exact cause of death could not be established.) Dr Cox had been treating a 70-year-old woman terminally ill with rheumatoid arthritis and also suffering from gastric ulcers, gangrene and pressure sores. She expressed a wish to die. When repeated doses of heroin did not ease her agony, Dr Cox gave her a dose of potassium chloride – a poison. Dr Cox was convicted and sentenced to a year's imprisonment suspended for 12 months. Dr David Moor was charged with the murder of an 85-year-old retired ambulanceman, George Liddell, in July 1997 (British Medical Journal 1999a, 1999b). It was alleged that he had caused the death through the administration of a large dose of morphine. In a TV interview Dr Moor had said that he had been involved in helping patients to die. He had stated that he 'would be very surprised if I had to defend myself in court'. At the trial Mr Liddell's relatives spoke up in support of the doctor. His 66-year-old son said at the trial: 'When I eased him forward he started to cry. It was a long and protracted cry. This was more than I could stand. I have never heard anything like it before.' Dr Moor was acquitted. The judge told the jury that 'You may consider it a great irony that a doctor who goes out of his way to care for George Liddell ends up facing the charge he does'.

In *R* v. *Arthur* (*The Times*, 5 November 1981) the non-treatment of an infant resulted in a criminal prosecution. A baby, John Pearson, was born with Down's syndrome but apparently suffering no other complications. Dr Arthur, a paediatrician caring for the child, wrote in the notes, 'Parents do not wish it to survive, nursing care only,' and he prescribed a strong pain killing drug, DF118 – a drug not normally given to infants. The baby died a few hours later. Dr Arthur was charged with murder but this was later reduced to a charge of attempted murder. While he was eventually acquitted, the case left open many difficult issues as to what care a child must be given and whether the health-care professional could cease treatment if it is believed that further care is hopeless. The judge in *R* v. *Arthur* described the doctor's conduct as being a 'holding operation'. However, it has been suggested that the administration of the drug DF118 – an appetite suppressant – amounted to a positive act. This case must now be considered in the light of the *Bland* decision, where the court indicated that a decision to cease life-sustaining treatment will not necessarily give rise to criminal liability (see below).

Generally, there will only be liability in criminal law where a nurse or doctor has undertaken a positive action. The law does not usually impose liability for omissions. Nonetheless, as will be seen below, there may on occasions be only a narrow line between these two categories.

The nurse as whistleblower where a doctor has deliberately ended a patient's life

A nurse strongly suspects that that a doctor has deliberately ended the life of an elderly patient on her ward. What should the nurse do?

In two cases in which doctors were prosecuted for allegedly ending the life of the patient, the prosecutions followed action taken by the nursing staff. Dr Arthur was prosecuted after a nurse who was a member of a pro-life organisation made a report. Dr Cox's prosecution followed a report made by a nurse, Sister Hart, regarding his conduct. She stated that she was required by the then United Kingdom Central Council for Nursing, Midwifery and Health Visiting (UKCC) code to speak out. The nurse may be subject to disciplinary proceedings if she fails to report such an incident (Fletcher et al 1995, p. 210). Today the nurse is also given some statutory protection under the Public Interest Disclosure Act 1998 (see Ch. 7).

What should a nurse do if, as in the case of Sister Hart, she knows that the patient's life has been ended but that the patient expressed a wish to die? Does the duty that the nurse owes to the patient mean that s/he should take into account the fact that this patient had expressed a wish to die? While the nurse is obliged to act in the patient's interests, it must be the case that the nurse should be prepared to report what is a serious breach of criminal law.

Parental obligations to their children

The law places parents under particular obligations in relation to the care of their children and holds them accountable not only for their actions but also for their omissions. If parents, perhaps motivated by some personal ethical belief, fail to seek medical care for a gravely ill child and as a result the child dies, they may be prosecuted under s1 of the Children and Young Persons Act 1933, which makes it an offence to neglect the care of the child. A prosecution may also be brought for murder or manslaughter. In *R* v. *Senior* ([1899] 1 QB 283), the parents were members of a religious sect that objected to the use of medical assistance and medicines. Their child fell ill but they did not seek medical help. The child died of diarrhoea and pneumonia. Evidence was given to the effect that had the child received medical treatment then she would probably have lived. Although no medical care had been given, the child had been generally well treated. It was held that the parents' actions amounted to neglect under section 1 of the Prevention of Cruelty to Children Act 1896 – the statutory predecessor to the 1933 Act, which provided that: 'If any person… who has the custody, charge or care of a child… wilfully neglects… such child in a manner likely to cause such child injury to its health that person shall be guilty of a misdemeanour'.

In this case the parents were found guilty of manslaughter because their actions had caused or accelerated the child's death. But, more recently, the courts have held that neglect by itself will not necessarily mean that a prosecution for manslaughter will succeed (R v. *Lowe* [1973] QB 70). However, in 1993, parents who believed in homeopathic remedies and who failed to seek conventional medical help for their child, who subsequently died, were convicted of manslaughter (*The Independent*, 29 October 1993).

Administration of pain-killing drugs

The nurse charged with ending the life of a suffering patient cannot plead that this was a 'mercy killing'. No such defence is recognised in English law.

But, in some situations, administration of strong pain-killing drugs is justifiable even though repeated doses will, over time, have the effect of cutting short the patient's life. In *R v. Bodkin Adams*, Dr Bodkin Adams was prosecuted for murder ([1957] Criminal Law Review 365). Dr Adams had cared for many elderly patients and had been a beneficiary in the wills of a number of those patients. One 81-year-old widow who had suffered a stroke was prescribed heroin and morphia by Dr Adams and later died. Dr Adams was named as a beneficiary under her will. At the trial the judge, Devlin J., said that there was no special defence of mercy killing. But a doctor was entitled to do all that was proper and necessary to relieve his patient's suffering, even if the measures used had the effect of incidentally shortening that patient's life. Brazier (2003, p 441) has stated that: 'This analysis introduces into the law the double-effect principle much debated in philosophical circles, whereby if an act has one of two inevitable consequences, one good and one evil, the act may be morally acceptable in certain circumstances.'

The doctrine of double effect has been used in the context of abortion. The approach taken in *R v. Bodkin Adams* has been questioned. In evidence to the House of Lords Select Committee on Euthanasia, the UKCC (House of Lords Select Committee on Medical Ethics 1994) commented that: 'to prohibit euthanasia… yet permit the use of narcotics to alleviate pain even at doses which will dramatically shorten life or even bring it to a close within a very short period, is no longer a sustainable position'.

Reg Pyne, former assistant registrar of the UKCC, suggested that nurses generally saw the doctrine of double effect as hypocritical (House of Lords Select Committee on Medical Ethics 21–4, 1994). The first duty of the nurse and other health care professionals is to care for the patient. A decision to administer strong pain killing drugs is not to be taken lightly. However, if that decision is made and the incidental effect is that a patient's lifespan is reduced then, at present in English law, that will not amount to murder. The status of the double-effect doctrine has now been questioned following the decision of the House of Lords in *R v. Woolin* ([1999] AC 82). There it was stated that 'intention' should be assessed in considering whether death was a 'reasonably foreseeable consequence' of the action. An action was regarded as intentional if the actor was 'virtually certain it would occur', which would suggest that the double-effect doctrine would not be applicable in the context of pain relief because it can be argued that when the pain relief is increased it is virtually certain that death will result. The legal position remains uncertain, although it was considered in *Re A (children) (conjoined twins: surgical separation)* ([2001] Fam 147) where Ward L.J. noted the difficulty with *Woolin* while suggesting that the doctrine might be applicable in the case of the administration of pain-killers to deal with extreme pain (see further discussion of this case in Ch. 6).

Suicide

While euthanasia is unlawful, a patient may take his/her own life. Suicide has not been a crime in this country since the Suicide Act 1961 came into force. As noted in Chapter 5, a patient may refuse life-saving treatment, and indeed to treat a patient who has refused such treatment without his/her consent may lead to an action in the tort of battery and possibly to a criminal prosecution. But if the patient asks a nurse to bring some lethal drug and to sit with her/him while s/he dies, the nurse must not do so. Section 2(1) of the Suicide Act 1961 provides that assisting suicide is an offence. To establish a prosecution it must be shown that the defendant knew that the person was intending to commit suicide, assented to this and encouraged them in their attempt (*AG* v. *Able* [1984] 1 All ER 277).

One interesting issue is the extent to which section 2 of the Suicide Act could be seen as contravening fundamental respect for human rights and contravening the Human Rights Act 1998 (McHale & Gallagher 2004). A human rights challenge was brought in relation to section 2 in the House of Lords and ultimately in the European Court of Human Rights in the case of *R (on the application of Pretty)* v. *DPP* ([2002] 1 All ER 1). Mrs Dianne Pretty was 42 years old and was suffering from a degenerative condition, motor neurone disease. She was confined to a wheelchair and was paralysed from the waist down. Unable to take her own life she asked the Director of Public Prosecutions (DPP) for an assurance that if her husband assisted her to die he would not be prosecuted. The DPP refused to provide this assurance. She challenged the DPP's decision and also argued that section 2(1) of the Suicide Act 1961 infringed the European Convention on Human Rights as incorporated in the Human Rights Act 1998. The action was rejected at first instance in the Divisional Court. On appeal to the House of Lords, three issues were raised: first, did the DPP have the power to undertake not to prosecute in advance of a proposed assistance in suicide? Second, if he did have that power, taking into account Articles 2, 3, 8, 9 and 14 of the European Convention on Human Rights was he required not to prosecute? Third, if not, was section 2(1) of the Suicide Act 1961 incompatible with Articles 2, 3, 8, 9 and 14 of the European Convention on Human Rights?

Mrs Pretty's action failed in the House of Lords. Her counsel argued that Article 2, the right to life, also included her right to determine when her life should come to an end. This was, however, rejected in the House of Lords. Their Lordships held that the right to life did not extend to a right to self-determination in relation to a person's own life and death. Second, it was argued that to deny Mrs Pretty assistance in dying would be to contravene Article 3 – the prohibition on torture and inhuman and degrading treatment. However, the House of Lords held that Article 3 did not impose obligations on the UK such that they were require to ensure assistance in dying for a competent, terminally ill person who is unable to end his/her own life. Article 8, the right to privacy, was also argued in the context that there was a right to autonomy and that this included a guarantee as to when to choose to die. This was rejected by the House of Lords. First it was held that, while Article 8 prohibited interference with the manner in which a person conducts their life, it did not relate to the manner in which they wanted to die. Moreover, even had Article 8 been applicable, arguments of public policy including protection for the elderly and vulnerable would preclude its application. An argument that Article 9, freedom of conscience and religious belief, would apply was also rejected by the House of Lords. It was held that Article 9 did not allow Mrs Pretty to manifest her belief in assisted suicide by being given assistance in ending her own life. Finally, it was argued that Article

14, the prohibition on discrimination, was applicable. It was argued that Mrs Pretty was discriminated against because she was unable to end her own life and, while an able-bodied person could end his/her own life by committing suicide, Mrs Pretty was unable to do so. However this claim too was rejected because it was held that Article 14 could not operate on its own and only in conjunction with other rights and that, as none of the other Articles had been violated, thus an Article 14 claim would not be applicable.

Mrs Pretty continued her legal fight before the European Court of Human Rights (*Pretty* v. *UK* [2002] 2 FCR 97). There she also failed. In contrast to the House of Lords, the ECHR was prepared to hold that Article 8 was engaged. They found that decisions concerning the nature and time of death were indeed matters that fell within Article 8 of the European Convention on Human Rights. However, they nonetheless went on to find that any infringement of Article 8 was justifiable. Article 8 rights were qualified in a situation in which the limitation was 'necessary in a democratic society' in a situation where this was for legitimate reasons for the objectives of the legislature and the state was given a 'margin of appreciation'. Here the law prohibiting assistance in suicide was justifiable because it safeguarded the position of the vulnerable in society. Mrs Pretty died of natural causes in a hospice on 11 May 2002 after the ECHR had delivered its ruling. However, the debate as to whether the law should allow assistance in dying still continues, as we shall see below.

Refusing treatment

In the same period in which Dianne Pretty's case was being heard before the House of Lords and ECHR the English courts were faced by another case of a woman who wanted to end her own life – the case that came to be known as that of 'Ms B'. (*Re B (adult: refusal of medical treatment)* [2002] 2 All ER 449.). Ms B was quadriplegic. She was supported on a ventilator. She wanted the ventilator support withdrawn. The hospital refused to accede to her wishes. She went to court. Ultimately her claim was successful. She was held to have decision-making capacity and she thus had a right to refuse treatment – which included the right to refuse ventilation. Nominal damages were awarded against the hospital for continuing to treat her. Subsequently the ventilator support was removed and she died. This case has been juxtaposed with *Pretty*. Some commentators have seen this as an anomalous position. The cases can legally be distinguished in that Mrs Pretty would have required positive assistance to end her life whereas in the case of Ms B the medical staff would 'simply' be withdrawing 'treatment'. As Singer noted, although the cases were legally distinguishable,

❝ We have arrived at the absurd situation where a paralysed woman can choose to die when she wants if her condition means that she needs some form of medical treatment to survive, whereas another paralysed woman cannot choose to die when or in the manner she wants because there is no medical treatment keeping her alive in such a way that if it were withdrawn she would have a humane and dignified death.

Singer 2002

But is this an absurd situation – the fact that the law allows an individual to refuse treatment regardless of the consequences while at the same time it does not sanction euthanasia? That of course raises the question: Should we take that step and legalise euthanasia?

Should euthanasia be legalised?

As with abortion, euthanasia is an exceedingly emotive subject (Dworkin 1993). It has been argued that recognition of active voluntary euthanasia is simply a logical extension of the right to commit suicide, and that it is part of giving respect to the autonomy of the individual. Furthermore, it has been suggested that the present position, which sanctions the withdrawal of treatment while at the same time rejecting active euthanasia, is inconsistent and illogical. A number of unsuccessful attempts have been made over the years to legalise euthanasia in the UK. In other jurisdictions legislation has been introduced that has sanctioned some medical assistance in dying, although not without much controversy and debate. In Australia, the Northern Territory passed the Rights of the Terminally Ill Act 1995. This provided that a person could request assistance to terminate life. The request was to be voluntary, the patient must be of sound mind and over 18 and s/he had to be suffering from an illness that the medical practitioner believed would result in the death of the patient. The assessment of the need for euthanasia was to be confirmed by a second medical practitioner. The request was not to be effective if there were medically acceptable palliative care options. The legislation required notification of the criteria under the statute. During the period in which the Act was in force seven patients used the Act and four died under its provisions (British Medical Journal 1998). This statute proved controversial, was the subject of challenge in the Australian Federation and was struck down by Parliament in 1997. In the USA there was extensive media debate over the actions of Dr Jack Kevorkian in assisting patients to die (Brody 1999). The Oregon Death with Dignity Act 1997 allowed doctors to prescribe patients lethal drugs for self-medication. This statute was the subject of much heated debate. Finally the Pain Relief Promotion Act was passed in 1999. This had the effect that federally controlled substances – including morphine – could not be used for assistance in suicide and has had the effect that the Death with Dignity Act is ineffective.

In the Netherlands, while euthanasia itself was not recognised there was a policy of non-prosecution of doctors who followed a series of guidelines and also reported an assisted death to a regional committee comprised of doctors, lawyers and ethicists. Recently, legislation was passed giving legal effect to the existing position and legitimising assistance in dying. It came into force in October 2001 (De Haan 2002). The Termination of Life on Request and Assisted Review Procedure Act now provides that it is not a crime for a doctor to terminate the life of another person on their request if certain criteria are complied with. The doctor must satisfy a special review committee, set up on a regional basis, that the patient had made a voluntary and well-considered request, that he is convinced that the patient was suffering unbearably and hopelessly, that he had informed the patient about his situation and the prospect for improvement; that both he and the patient were agreed that the patient's condition was hopeless, that he had consulted one other independent doctor and that he has terminated life with all due care and attention. This law also applies to children. Persons over 16 may take the decision themselves. Those between 12 and 15 can seek euthanasia but the doctor must only act with parental consent. The doctor who administers euthanasia is required to inform the regional pathologist and must then report, without delay, to the regional review committee in his district. The task of the committee is to see whether the doctor has fulfilled the 'due care' criteria. Now the committee only has to send the case to the prosecutors if it believes that the criteria have not been satisfied.

The Netherlands approach was followed by similar legislation in Belgium in 2002. This applies to those who are conscious and who have an incurable illness. In contrast to the Netherlands, this legislation only applies to those persons over 18. In contrast to the Netherlands, each euthanasia case has to be reported to a national committee (Adams & Nys 2003). In recent years there has been some evidence of euthanasia tourism, with UK citizens travelling to Switzerland to receive assistance in dying. In January 2003 Reginald Crew, a 74-year-old patient with advanced motor neurone disease travelled with his wife and daughter to Zurich and ended his life by taking a drink laced with barbiturates (British Medical Journal 2003). In December 2004 a 65-year-old British woman with a degenerative brain disease, known only as Mrs Z committed suicide in a Zurich clinic after a High Court judge refused to intervene to stop her husband taking her abroad (British Medical Journal 2004; *Re Z (An adult's capacity)* [2004] EWMC 2817). Here the law limits those situations in which euthanasia is a crime. Thus, in contrast to the jurisdictions already discussed, life may be ended without the involvement of a doctor (Hurst & Mauron 2003). Article 115 of the Swiss penal code provides that assisting suicide is only a crime if the motive is selfish.

While it has been argued that recognition of voluntary euthanasia is something that accords respect to the autonomy of the individual patient, nevertheless, some strong voices have been raised in dissent. One fear is that of the 'slippery slope'. It is argued that it is easy to 'slip' from recognition of voluntary active euthanasia to involuntary euthanasia undertaken without an individual's consent, for convenience or other purposes. Critics of euthanasia point to the experience in the Netherlands, where claims have been made that procedures have not been complied with and that abuses have occurred (Keown 1991). The 'slippery slope' argument was one factor that influenced the Select Committee of the House of Lords to reject the introduction of euthanasia legislation in the UK (House of Lords Select Committee on Medical Ethics 1994). A further difficulty is, who would administer euthanasia? Should it be the same persons who normally care for patients? Were euthanasia to be introduced it would have considerable implications for the role of the nurse.

Recognition of active termination of life is opposed by those who see the function of health care as one of 'curing', not killing. In 2000 a special conference of the British Medical Association (BMA) into the question of the introduction of physician-assisted suicide held that 'It would alter the relationships between: doctors and patients; doctors and significant others; and doctors and society' (British Medical Association 2000a). During the previous year there had been considerable press coverage of the prosecution for murder, of Harold Shipman, a GP who had prematurely ended the lives of a large number of patients, predominantly elderly. There was no suggestion that these were 'mercy killings' but the ease with which the incidents had occurred and the length of time over which they took place without Shipman being detected, as well as the impact this had upon public confidence in the medical profession, suggested that, while the euthanasia debate was likely to continue in the UK, any alteration of the law to sanction active euthanasia appeared unlikely, at least in the near future.

However all this changed with the introduction by Lord Joffee of the Assisted Dying for the Terminally Ill Bill, originally in 2003. A revised version of this Bill was introduced in 2005. The Bill, if enacted, would give competent terminally ill patients with 'unbearable suffering' the right to request to be assisted to die. The Bill sets out procedural requirements, including ascertaining the patient's competence, an interview and the patient being informed of the availability of palliative care. At the time of writing the Bill is under consideration in the House of Lords.

Withdrawing treatment

While a health professional may not end a patient's life with a positive action, in some situations it is lawful to withdraw treatment in a hopeless case. This section considers the well-known case of Tony Bland and the situations in which treatment may legitimately be withdrawn. It should be noted here that 'withdrawal' includes not only the decision to, for instance, remove a feeding tube but also the decision not to administer a particular treatment should a relapse take place.

The Bland case

In the case of *Airedale NHS Trust* v. *Bland* ([1993] AC 879), Tony Bland was injured in the disaster at the Hillsborough football ground in 1989. His chest was severely crushed and as a result he suffered hypoxic brain damage. He entered a persistent vegetative state (PVS). He was fed through a nasogastric tube. After several years, during which he showed no noticeable sign of improvement, an application was made for a court order allowing the withdrawal of treatment. The order was granted. The judges in the House of Lords emphasised the fact that English law did not authorise euthanasia; however, there were situations in which there was no longer a duty to continue all treatment. The court recognised that there was a distinction in law between actions and omissions, and that failing to act was not usually culpable in criminal law. The House of Lords classed withdrawal of tube feeding where continued treatment was no longer in that patient's best interest as being an omission, not an act. In a case such as *Bland*, continued treatment was of no benefit to him as there was no prospect of his condition improving. What amounted to the patient's 'best interests' was to be assessed by reference to a responsible body of professional practice, the *Bolam* test (Ch. 2). While obtaining a court order is a civil procedure, in practice a successful murder prosecution involving medical staff who remove an artificial feeding tube after a court order has been obtained is highly unlikely. Indeed, an attempt to bring a prosecution after the death of Tony Bland was unsuccessful (*R v. Bingley Magistrates Court ex parte Morrow* 13 April 1994, unreported).

A duty to discontinue treatment?

The *Bland* case does not simply recognise that there may be a point at which it is legitimate to discontinue treatment and remove artificial feeding. It was suggested in the House of Lords that in some situations there may be a *duty* to do so. Lord Browne Wilkinson held:

> If there comes a stage where the responsible doctor comes to the reasonable conclusion (which accords with the views of a responsible body of professional medical opinion) that further continuation of a life support system is not in the best interests of the patient, he can no longer lawfully continue that life support system, to do so would constitute the crime of battery and the tort of trespass to the person.

The exact scope of this duty is yet to be determined. It should be noted that it may be in the patient's best interests to discontinue treatment even though the relatives believe that treatment should be continued (*Re G* [1995] 2 FCR 46). One emotive question that remains to be answered after *Bland* is whether spoon feeding will be classed along with feeding through a nasogastric tube as medical treatment.

Unauthorised termination of treatment

While a health-care professional may be authorised to remove a patient from life support systems, that does not mean that any person switching off such a machine will be held to have simply omitted to act. If a mother comes into the ward and turns off the life support system because she believes that her son has suffered enough, and has not obtained a court order, she may be prosecuted for murder.

Bland and the Human Rights Act 1998

The decision in *Bland* of course predated the Human Rights Act 1998. To what extent was the decision consistent with that legislation? This issue came before the courts in the case of *NHS Trust A v. M, NHS Trust B v. H* ([2000] 2 FLR 348). Here Butler-Sloss L.J. held that *Bland* was in accordance with the European Convention on Human Rights because withdrawal of treatment was an omission and not an act. There would only be a violation of Article 2, which protected the sanctity of life, if there was a positive obligation to preserve life and there was not such an obligation where a patient was in a persistent vegetative state. In a situation in which a decision was made to withhold treatment because it was no longer in a patient's best interests then there was no further obligation to take steps to safeguard life. There was also no violation of Article 3 – the prohibition on torture and inhuman and degrading and treatment. Butler Sloss L.J. held that Article 3 was inapplicable because it required that the individual be aware of the inhuman and degrading treatment.

In *Bland* the diagnosis was clear. The relatives and health-care professionals were in agreement. Nevertheless, the House of Lords noted that this was an exceptional case and that subsequent cases should be referred to the courts. In a number of later cases, withdrawal of treatment has been authorised but difficulties remain. In *Frenchay v. S* ([1994] 2 All ER 403), S had taken an overdose and suffered consequent brain damage. The consultant caring for him said that S was in a persistent vegetative state and had no chance of recovery. S was being fed through a gastronomy tube in the stomach wall. This tube became dislodged. The question was, should it be reinserted? The parents were divided as to whether treatment should be continued, while the health-care professionals caring for S were opposed to the continuation of treatment. On appeal, the Court of Appeal upheld the decision of the judge at first instance, supporting withdrawal of further treatment. The case of *Frenchay* differs from that of *Bland* in certain respects. In *Frenchay* there was no question of removing the feeding tube, as it had already become dislodged. In *Bland*, great emphasis was placed upon the fact that the patient was in an irreversible condition. One controversial aspect of *Frenchay* is that it was suggested that the diagnosis of PVS was by no means conclusive. In addition, the court in *Bland* had stated that there should be clear evidence as to the patient's medical condition, preferably from two doctors. Here, because the tube had become dislodged, the urgency of the case led to evidence being given by only one doctor. The *Frenchay* case may not be an isolated one. It is likely that many of these decisions concerning treatment withdrawal may arise in similar emergencies. This may be particularly problematic, since recent research has questioned the efficacy of diagnosis of PVS in many cases (Andrews et al 1996). It appeared that a considerable number of patients have, in the past, been the subject of misdiagnosis.

In *Bland* it was suggested that whether a patient had fallen into a hopeless condition was to be assessed by reference to the Bolam test – the view of a responsible body of professional practice. But in *Frenchay*, Sir Thomas Bingham M.R. indicated that the courts would be prepared to review the doctor's assessment as to what was in the patient's best interests. This is a different approach, which may involve considering factors such as the quality of life the patient would enjoy were treatment to be continued. It appeared to be a shift away from *Bland* in that the court is undertaking the task of determining what amounts to 'best interests' rather than leaving this as a matter of judgment by health professionals. As we noted in Chapter 6, today the courts, in interpreting the best interest test in relation to adults lacking mental capacity, are following such an approach and taking into account a wider range of factors when determining what constitutes 'best interests'. The Mental Capacity Act 2005, when it comes into force, will enable direct reference to be also made to broader criteria (see Ch. 6).

Withdrawing treatment from infants

Very difficult decisions concern withdrawal of treatment in a situation in which the patient is not in a PVS but is gravely handicapped and lacking mental capacity. Prior to *Bland*, a number of cases came before the courts concerning the decision to withhold treatment from handicapped children. If a child is born suffering from a serious handicap and after counselling the parents say they cannot cope and they do not want treatment to be continued, what can be done? This may be a situation in which it is sought to withdraw treatment. Such decisions are not to be taken lightly. Counselling should be given as to the nature of the handicap, prognosis and future survival rates. Handicaps can vary dramatically, from the Down's syndrome baby with a duodenal atresia where a simple operation to remove the complication can ensure that the child survives well into his/her 30s, to the anencephalic infant born without upper hemispheres of the brain whose lifespan is likely to be no more than a few weeks.

Where there is doubt as to whether treatment should be continued, it is advisable for an application to be made to the court to approve a course of non-active treatment. If such an order has been obtained then any subsequent criminal prosecution, if death results, would be unlikely. The court makes an order as to future treatment on the basis of what is in the child's best interests. At first sight this may be regarded as similar to the *Bland*-type case. But there are differences. In *Bland*, the situation was hopeless with no prospect of recovery. Ascertaining 'best interests' in the case of individuals who are incapacitated because of grave handicap may be more difficult. The court may be in effect assessing what is and what is not an adequate quality of life.

In *Re B* ([1981] 1 WLR 1421) a baby was born with Down's syndrome and a duodenal atresia. The parents did not want her to have an operation to correct the atresia. They believed that it would be better for her to die within the next few days. The hospital, however, informed the local authority. B was made a ward of court. The issue of whether to continue treatment was left to the court to determine. At first, the court authorised the operation. However, B was later removed to a different hospital where differences arose as to whether treatment should be given, and this led to the matter being referred back to the court. The Court of Appeal authorised the operation. Lord Justice Templeman said:

> " There may be cases, I know not, of severe proved damage where the future is so certain and the prognosis so uncertain and where the life of the child is so bound to be full of pain and suffering that the court might be drawn to a different conclusion, but in the present case the choice which lies before the court is this: whether to allow an operation to take place which may result in the child living for 20 or 30 years as a mongoloid or whether (and I think that this must be brutally the result) to terminate the life of a mongoloid child because she also has an intestinal complaint.

The court decided that the operation should go ahead, as once B had the operation she was perfectly capable of living a full life to the normal Down's syndrome lifespan. In a number of subsequent cases, the courts have shown themselves willing to approve an order not to pursue active treatment. These cases extend beyond the very young infant to include children of some 3 or 4 months old. In *Re C* ([1989] 2 All ER 782), the Court of Appeal approved an order in respect of an infant born prematurely, suffering from severe hydrocephalus with severe mental and physical handicaps. She was not gaining weight and the medical prognosis was that her condition was hopeless. On appeal, while the court approved the decision to cease active treatment, it said that the following words (in the original order of the judge): 'The hospital authority be at liberty to treat the minor to allow her life to come to an end peacefully and with dignity...' should be deleted because of the risk that misunderstanding would be caused by the phrase 'allow her life to come to an end'.

The meaning of 'best interests' was explored further in the case of *Re J* ([1990] 3 All ER 930). J was born nearly 13 weeks premature weighing only 1.1 kg. At birth, J was put on a ventilator and though later taken off the ventilator he suffered relapses and had to be reventilated. He was seriously brain-damaged and appeared also to be blind and deaf. In addition, it was likely that he would be totally paralysed. An application was made for an order to the effect that if J again suffered a collapse he should not be ventilated. The Court of Appeal made the order. Lord Donaldson M.R., referring to a Canadian case, suggested that, in deciding whether to withdraw treatment, 'the court must decide what the patient would choose if he was able to make a sound judgement'. This child endured a very poor quality of life. He had already been ventilated for very long periods and had an exceedingly unfavourable prognosis. In reaching his decision, Lord Donaldson emphasised the fact that mechanical ventilation was an invasive procedure that would cause the child distress. Lord Donaldson's approach has been criticised. As Wells et al (1990) comment, it is artificial to use a subjective test in relation to neonates and young children because there is no way of knowing what they would have wanted. Much uncertainty, however, remains in this area.

The nurse may play an important role in ensuring that any decision to withdraw treatment is carefully made. Any decision reached must be on the basis of the best interests of the child, as opposed to what may be convenient for parents or for health-care professionals. If the nurse believes that a child is not being given suitable care, this must be reported to the appropriate authorities.

Withdrawal of ventilator support

Withdrawal of treatment may also include withdrawal of ventilator support in a situation in which the patient has not been declared brain-stem-dead. Health-care professionals would need to assess whether withdrawal from the ventilator could be said to be in the patient's best interests. In 1996 the court authorised the withdrawal of ventilator support from an infant brain-damaged by meningitis. The girl was blind, deaf and unable to respond to her parents (*Re C (a baby)* [1996] FLR 43).

Conflicts between health-care professionals and parents in relation to treatment decisions at the end of life

The courts usually have upheld medical opinion over parental opinions in such situations. However an exception to this arose in the case of *Re T* ([1997] 1 WLR 242). Here the prognosis was that without the operation the child would not live for more than $2^1/_2$ years. A liver transplant operation had a good chance of success – success rates of 90% were quoted. Nonetheless in the Court of Appeal it was stated that here 'best interests' entailed respecting the mother's interest that the child should not undergo the pain/distress of this particular surgery. They emphasised that the child's welfare was dependent upon his mother. One doctor was of the view that there would be great problems in undertaking treatment without parental support. However this case may in many ways be regarded as exceptional. The parents were, at the time, living in another Commonwealth country and had to come to England for treatment to be undertaken. There was some suggestion that had a different approach been taken the parents would have moved outside the jurisdiction of the English courts.

What if the parents want treatment continued in the face of clinical opinion that the situation is hopeless? In *Re C (a minor)* ([1997] 40 BMLR), C was 16 months old and suffering from spinal muscular atrophy – a progressive condition with no curative treatment. The child was regarded as being in what was known as a 'no-chance' condition under the Royal College of Paediatricians guidelines. However the child was conscious – able to recognise the parents and smile. The child's parents, who were orthodox Jews, believed life should be preserved. It was proposed to remove the child from the ventilator. If she suffered a further relapse she would be left to die. While the parents supported the decision to see if the child could survive without a ventilator they wanted her to be attached to the ventilator if she relapsed. The courts indicated again that following the approach of the parents meant that the doctors would have been compelled to undertake a course of treatment, which they were unwilling to do. The court would not make an order requiring the doctors to treat. There has been some academic criticism of the case. Ian Kennedy commented that the guidelines from the Royal College of Paediatricians had been subject to a critical reception from the health-care professions and that 'Particular exception was taken to some of the language used to categories and the 'no chance" category was regarded as insensitive' (Kennedy 1997).

A very heated conflict arose with family members in *R v. Portsmouth Hospitals NHS Trust ex parte Glass* ([1999] Lloyd's Rep Med 367). Here D was 12 years old. He had been born with severe mental and physical disabilities, which included cerebral palsy, hydrocephalus and epilepsy. He was suffering from various postoperative infections and hospital staff were of the view that D was dying. They wanted to administer diamorphine with the aim of alleviating distress. The family were opposed to this and violent incidents in hospital followed. Criminal and civil proceedings were launched consequent upon this incident. D was discharged and was treated by his GP. The Trust wrote to the hospital and stated that should the child again fall ill it would be better for D to be treated in another hospital. An application was made for judicial review. One aspect of the claim was that they asked for a declaration regarding treatment/withdrawal of life-sustaining treatment. Judicial review was refused because of the fact that not only was this particular case not susceptible to judicial review but that also, in addition, it would be difficult to frame the action in meaningful terms in a hypothetical situation.

The *Glass* case ultimately was heard by the ECHR (*Glass* v. *UK* [2004] 1 FLR 1019). In the ECHR the Court held that to override the parental objection in this case in the absence of prior judicial approval constituted a violation of Article 8 of the European Convention on Human Rights.

A recent notable dispute between parents and health professionals arose in the case of Charlotte Wyatt (*Portsmouth NHS Trust* v. *Wyatt* [2004] EWHC 2243). The court ruled in favour of a non-resuscitation order in the case of baby Charlotte Wyatt, who was born 3 months premature and was brain-damaged, deaf and blind. Against the expectations of some medical experts, Charlotte survived. Subsequently in 2005 her parents attempted unsuccess-fully to obtain a variation of the order ([2005] 2 FLR 403); however, later Hedley J. was satisfied that her condition had improved enough to vary the order (*Re Wyatt* [2005] EWHC 2293). Recent press reports have indicated that Charlotte is now well enough to return home but sadly because of the circumstances of her family this may now not be possible.

Withdrawal of treatment from adult patients not in a persistent vegetative stage

After *Bland* there has been increasing judicial willingness to sanction with-drawal of treatment even though patients fall outside the PVS guidelines. In *Re D (Medical Treatment)* ([1998] 1 FLR 411), the patient, D, had suffered severe head injuries following a road accident. She had returned from hospital to live with her parents, who were caring from her. She was both physically and mentally disabled. She could communicate but when she realised that her condition could not improve further she became depressed and expressed serious dissatisfaction with her quality of life. She spoke about her death and funeral arrangements. In September 1995 she suffered an unexplained insult to the brain and in March 1996 she was diagnosed as being in PVS. She was kept alive by a tube providing artificial nutrition/hydration. On 18 March 1997 the tube became dislodged. A court order was sought. The Official Solicitor opposed this, saying that D did not come within the criteria as set out by the Medical Royal Colleges. The court granted the declaration. She did not fulfil the 1996 guidelines; for example, she could track objects with her eyes, exhibited a menace response and nystagmus occurred in response to ice water calories. But the judge did accept the view of the experts that she was indisputably in a PVS state. There was no evidence before the court that the defendant had any life whatsoever, she was suffering a living death and it was not in her best interests to be kept artificially alive. Subsequently in *Re H (a patient)* ([1998] 2 FLR 36), H had suffered serious brain damage in road traffic accident. He was 43 years old, kept alive via artificial feeding and was unaware of his environment. It was thought best for feeding to be withheld. The consultant clinical psychologist found that there was occa-sional visual tracing and believed that H could focus on an object and be aroused by clapping – in other words, not all Royal College of Physicians guidelines were fulfilled. But experts were of the view that H was in PVS. Sir Stephen Brown made the order. He indicated that the sanctity of life was not paramount: 'I am satisfied that it is in the best interests of this patient that the life-sustaining treatment should be brought to a conclusion'.

In *R (Burke)* v. *GMC* ([2005] EWCA 1003). Leslie Burke, a disability rights advisor, suffered from cerebellar ataxia, a progressively degenerative disorder that, as his condition worsened, would require treatment by artificial nutrition and hydration (ANH). The claimant would be likely to lose the ability to communicate his wishes but would retain full cognitive faculties right up to the end stage of his disease, at which point he would lapse into a coma, probably a few days before his death. He sought to challenge General Medical Council (GMC) guidance *Withholding and withdrawing life-prolonging treatments: good practice in decision-making* on the withdrawal of ANH, by way of judicial review, contending that it was incompatible with his rights under Articles 2, 3, 6, 8 and 14 of the European Convention for the Protection of Human Rights and Fundamental Freedoms 1950. In particular, he argued that the guidance had the effect that the doctors would be able to withdraw artificial nutrition and hydration at the stage when he would have mental awareness but would be unable to communicate his feelings. At first instance Mumby J. held that, where a patient possessed mental capacity, s/he could insist on receiving 'ordinarily available' life-sustaining treatment. The judgment of Mumby was notable for its breadth. In the Court of Appeal they were of the view that the declarations granted had extended considerably beyond what was required and that the doctors were not trying to withdraw artificial nutrition/hydration against Mr Burke's will. They also confirmed that there is no duty to obtain a court order before you can treat an adult who lacks mental capacity.

Living wills – advance decisions

> A patient is involved in a motorway crash and is brought unconscious into hospital. It appears that there are serious physical injuries and it is likely that, should the patient recover, he will be paralysed and severely brain-damaged. The relatives say that the patient has made a living will, and that this states that in such a condition the patient would not have wanted to have treatment continued. What should be done?

A living will is a statement made by the patient before s/he becomes incapable of making his/her own decision, stipulating what treatments the patient would not want pursued should s/he became incapacitated. In the past, judicial acceptance has been given to advance refusals of treatment (*Re T* [1992] 4 All ER 649). One common form of such advance refusal is the card carried by Jehovah's Witnesses. A living will is in some respects an extension of such a card. Although the common law did allow for advance refusals, in practice some in the health-care professions were unwilling to comply with them because of uncertainty over the legal position. Greater clarity will now follow the enactment of the Mental Capacity Act 2005. This Act, which comes into force in 2007, makes explicit statutory provision for advance directives – henceforth to be known as 'advance decisions' (Mental Capacity Act 2005 s24–26). One reason why the recommendations of the Law Commission regarding taking forward advance decisions took so long to reach fruition were expressed concerns that this was tantamount to sanctioning euthanasia. Section 62 of the Mental Capacity Act 2005 now explicitly states that the Act does not affect the existing law concerning assisted suicide or unlawful killing.

The Mental Capacity Act 2005 provides that advance decisions are valid where made by persons over the age of 18 who have the mental capacity to make that decision (s24(1)). Where the advance decision concerns the refusal of life-sustaining treatment this must be made explicitly and also must be in writing, signed and witnessed (s25(5)(6)). A patient can alter the advance decision at any point while they still have mental capacity to do so (s24(3)). In addition, an advance decision will not be valid where a patient has done 'anything else clearly inconsistent with the advance decision remaining his fixed decision' (s25(2)(c)).

While the recognition of advance decisions in the Mental Capacity Act 2005 may provide a useful guide as to what treatment should or should not be given, it is not unproblematic. The Act does not make the advance decision time-limited. Nonetheless one difficulty with the advance decision is that a person's view may change over time – what may seem a totally intolerable state of health at 20 years of age may not be regarded as intolerable at all at 75. The lapse of time between the advance decision being initially drawn up and later interpreted needs to be taken into consideration when applying it. Another issue is the applicability of an advance decision in the context of a woman who, when the issue of treatment and the validity of the living will arises, is pregnant. It has been suggested that before an advance decision is made, women of childbearing age are asked to consider the possibility of becoming pregnant (Law Commission 1995, para 5.24).

Drafting advance decisions – the role of the nurse

If advance decisions become commonly used the nurse may be involved in advising the patient as to how a living will should be drawn up and the implications of such a living will. The BMA (British Medical Association 1995) has stated that 'Hospital managers and GP practice managers need to consider how to respond to the increasing desire of patients to plan ahead on the basis of accurate health information and advice' (para 6.7). The BMA notes that some hospitals have specialist counsellors who provide support and information and that home visits are provided. It states that 'Hospice outreach services and community nurses may also become involved in carrying out such a role' (British Medical Association 1995, p. 22). This is in contrast with an earlier statement by the Royal College of Nursing (RCN) to the effect that the nurse should not be involved in drawing up living wills (Royal College of Nursing 1992). It is submitted that the RCN approach is preferable. If a patient wishes to draw up an advance decision, s/he should be able to seek advice for that purpose, but it should come from outside the clinical team. It is important to ensure that any decision is perceived to be wholly independent of any considerations of convenience in resource allocation.

Lasting powers of attorney

In some situations, although an advance decision may exist, it may not help the health professional. It may be insufficiently specific, it may have been made a number of years ago and doubts may be raised as to the extent to which this now reflects an individual's interests. One alternative is for a person to be appointed to make treatment decisions on behalf of the person lacking mental capacity. Such a person may be known as a 'treatment attorney' or proxy decision maker. At present, while a person may appoint another person to make decisions about his/her financial affairs, if s/he becomes incompetent, this does not apply to treatment (Enduring Powers of Attorney Act 1985). The Law Commission (1995, para 7.1) proposed that the law should be extended to recognise far more extensive use of proxy decision makers and to allow patients to nominate a person to act in their best interests when they themselves become incapable of making a decision. The government accepted the arguments in favour of the extension of powers of attorney in their document *Making Decisions* and provision is now made for lasting powers of attorney under the Mental Capacity Act 2005. Section 9 enables a lasting power of attorney to be created, conferring decision-making authority on a 'donee' that includes the power to make decisions about personal welfare. Donees are to be over the age of 18 (s10) and more than one person can be appointed as a donee and they may act jointly or separately (s10(4)). The power only applies once the donor lacks mental capacity (s11(2)(7)(a)); it is also subject to any existing advance decision (s11(7)(b)). A further safeguard is that it does not extend to consenting or refusing life-saving treatment unless specific provision to that effect has been made in the document creating the power of attorney (s11(6)(c)). Further discussion of the role of lasting powers of attorney is to be found in the draft Mental Capacity Act Code of Practice (Department of Constitutional Affairs 2006).

Recognition of proxy decision-making in the health-care context may bring its own problems. Not least is the fact that ascertaining a person's wishes may be difficult if it is a long time since they have exercised the power of appointment of the proxy decision-maker and is very much dependent upon how aware the proxy is of the patient's current views (British Medical Association 1995). Nevertheless, it may at least assist in providing some guidance regarding difficult treatment decisions.

'Do not resuscitate' orders

Hospital nurses will be familiar with the practice of placing a 'do not resuscitate' (DNR) order in the patient's notes. But on what basis should this decision be made? A joint BMA/RCN report considered the use of DNR orders (British Medical Association/Royal College of Nursing 1993). They recommended that use of a DNR order be considered if it is believed that cardiopulmonary resuscitation is unlikely to succeed, or if it is contrary to the patient's express wishes, or if, should a patient be resuscitated, s/he would be unlikely to have a quality of life that s/he would find acceptable. In ascertaining quality of life, the guidelines suggest that as far as possible the patient's views should be obtained, but if this is impossible then the patient's close relatives should be consulted. The guidelines leave the ultimate decision as to whether to make a DNR order in the hands of the consultant, although they do state that patient involvement in these decisions is 'valuable' and 'important'. While discussion is not mandatory, they suggest that careful enquiry should be made of those patients who are thought to be at risk and the results of these discussions should be included in the hospital notes.

But does this go far enough to safeguard the patient's interests? There is a danger that a patient is only involved in the process to ensure his/her compliance with the decision. While the guidelines recommend that consultations about DNR orders should be made with members of the clinical team, the ultimate responsibility for the decision is placed in the hands of the consultant. S/he has the task of assessing an individual patient's quality of life. However, as Schutz (1994) commented:

> " this is a highly subjective process which requires a depth of relationship that consultants are unlikely to achieve. Even though the consultant has legal responsibility for the patient's treatment in relation to resuscitation there needs to be more emphasis on the team approach.

Once a DNR order has been made the guidelines suggest that all members of the health-care team should be informed and that the order itself should be subject to a regular review.

The use of a DNR order has now been given judicial approval in principle in the case of *Re R* ([1996] 2 FLR 99). In this case, the court upheld a DNR order in relation to a 23-year-old man who had cerebral palsy, brain malformation and learning difficulties and, while not in PVS, was in what was termed a 'low awareness state'. Evidence was given that he was physically and neurologically deteriorating. The consultant treating R was of the view that it was in R's best interests to allow nature to take its course the next time he had a life-threatening incident. The judge made an order stating that it would be lawful to withhold the administration of antibiotics in the event of the patient suffering a life-threatening infection and to withhold cardiopulmonary resuscitation. The DNR order here was drawn up in line with the RCN/Department of Health guidance.

Despite the guidance, a study suggested that the guidance regarding DNRs is not being followed. In an audit of a hospital in north London it was found that only 9% of consultants were involved in DNR decisions and there were no records in any case of the issue being discussed with the patient (Hayes et al 1999). There was also considerable concern expressed in a report by Age Concern (2000) over evidence that decisions were not made with family consultation. Other countries, such as the USA, have legislation governing DNR orders, while up to now legislation on this matter has been rejected in the UK. It may be time for that position to be reconsidered. Meanwhile, the nurse may play an important role in monitoring the operation of DNR orders in his/her capacity as patient advocate.

DEATH

When are health-care professionals entitled to hold that a patient is dead? There is no statutory definition of death in English law. However, for many years clinical practice has recognised brain-stem death as the point at which death occurs (Royal College of Physicians, 1996). The courts have now confirmed this. In *Re A* ([1992] 3 Med Law R 303) the court held that a child who was being supported on a ventilator, and who had been declared brain-stem dead, was dead for all intents and purposes and thus a doctor who had disconnected the ventilator was not acting unlawfully. The House of Lords in *Bland* supported this approach. In that case their lordships confirmed that those patients in a state of 'cognitive death' with irreversible damage to the upper hemispheres of the brain and who were in a persistent vegetative state were not legally dead. Although the Human Tissue Act 2004 does not include any specific statement on the definition of death it did provide that the Human Tissue Authority (HTA) should produce a Code of Practice that included a definition of death for the purposes of the Act (s26(2)(d)).

Certification of death must be undertaken by a doctor (Births and Deaths Registration Act 1953 s22). It is not the role of the nurse to undertake this task. Certain deaths must be notified to the coroner by the doctor who is certifying death. These include death related to suspicious circumstances.

ORGAN TRANSPLANTS

Transplant technology has developed considerably over the past few decades. A wide variety of transplants of organs and tissues is increasingly undertaken, ranging from kidneys and bone marrow to heart and lungs and most recently face transplants. The nurse frequently plays an important part in the transplant process. The nurse may work as a transplant coordinator. S/he may counsel patients who are considering whether to undergo a transplant. S/he may also have to attend the patient's body after the removal of organs in the haemodialysis unit or intensive therapy unit. In this part of the chapter the regulation of organ transplantation is considered. The law concerning organ transplants has recently been the subject of radical revision as part of the reform of the law concerning the use of human material consequent upon the Alder Hey (Redfern 2001) and Bristol Interim Inquiries (Kennedy 2000) with the enactment of the Human Tissue Act 2004. This legislation repeals earlier legislation, including the Human Tissue Act 1961 and the Human Organ Transplants Act 1989. It covers the use of material from cadavers and from living donors. It also creates a new regulatory body, the Human Tissue Authority.

Cadaver transplants

A patient has been injured in a car crash and dies later in hospital. It is hoped that the patient's organs can be used for transplantation into a patient urgently awaiting a donor, but can they lawfully be used?

The Human Tissue Act 2004 now regulates transplantation from both live and cadaver donors. Guidance is also given by the Human Tissue Authority (2006) as to the transplantation process. The Act came into force on 1 September 2006.

Adults may make a decision to donate during their lifetime under section 3. The decision as to whether their organs are used after their death may also be entrusted to a 'nominated representative' under section 4 of the 2004 Act. If they have not, for example, executed a donor card or appointed a nominated representative, then consent may still be given by a person in a 'qualifying relationship'. In contrast to the previous legislation – the Human Tissue Act 1961 – which made reference to enquiries being made of 'surviving spouse/relative' of the deceased, the new Act now provides for a much more extensive list of persons from whom enquiries may be made. These are listed as being (a) the spouse or partner, (b) the parent or child, (c) brother or sister, (d) grandparent or grandchild, (e) niece or nephew, (f) stepfather or stepmother, (g) half-brother or half-sister, (h) friend of long-standing (s27(4)). In a situation in which there are two or more persons at the same level then the consent of one will be sufficient. A person may be disregarded if either they make clear that they do not want to make the decision or in a situation in which it is not reasonably practical to communicate with them during the time available (s27(8)).

Children and adults lacking mental capacity

In contrast to the previous law – the Human Tissue Act 1961 – specific provision is also made in the Human Tissue Act 2004 in relation to children under section 2 and to adults who lack mental capacity under section 6. Where children have decision-making capacity (satisfy the *Gillick* test) they may themselves consent to donate their organs for transplantation. Alternatively, the decision to donate may be made by the person with parental responsibility or by a person in a 'qualifying relationship' under section 27. In relation to adults lacking mental capacity, this is subject to the Human Tissue Act 2004 (Persons who lack capacity to consent and Transplants Regulations 2006; SI 2006 No. 1659).

Commercial dealing in organs

In the late 1980s there was a major scandal when it was discovered that individuals were being offered money to come to the UK from Turkey and sell their organs for transplantation. This led to disciplinary proceedings being brought against a number of doctors, with one being struck off the General Medical Council's register. One result of the scandal was the passage of the Human Organ Transplants Act 1989, which made it a criminal offence to pay persons to donate organs or to undertake any other commercial dealing in organs from live donors or from cadavers (s2). There has been some debate as to whether this situation should be altered (Radcliffe-Richards 1998). However there is firm opposition in the international community against trafficking in organs and organisations such as the World Health Organization (WHO 40 13J), and the Council of Europe in documents such as the Convention on Human Rights and Biomedicine (Article 22) have come down strongly against the commercialisation of the body and its parts. It was thus unsurprising that this approach is now followed in the Human Tissue Act 2004, which makes it an offence to traffic in human material for transplantation (s32), although there is an exception for expenses and loss of earnings (s32(7)).

Living organ donors

If it is sought to use living persons as organ donors, then the appropriate consent must first be given and additional provisions of the Human Tissue Act 2004 must be complied with. It appears generally accepted that organ transplantation from adults is the type of operation that may be lawfully undertaken. Nonetheless, it is doubtful whether a competent adult is capable of lawfully consenting to the removal of a vital organ with death as a consequence, if nothing else because such removal would lead to the surgeon being prosecuted for murder.

In addition, doubts have also been expressed as to the legality of transplantation of animal organs to humans because of the risk to the intended donor (Mason 1990). At present such transplants are not being undertaken on humans but this is now the subject of review by the Xenotransplantation Interim Regulatory Body (see discussion below; Fox & McHale 1997).

In some instances it may be sought to use a child as a donor. Although child patients are frequently bone marrow donors, use of child patients as solid organ donors is infrequent and it appears that surgeons are unwilling to use child patients as donors. In the Court of Appeal in *Re W (a minor)* ([1992] 3 WLR 758), Lord Donaldson said that the statutory right of children over 16 years to consent to treatment contained in the Family Law Reform Act 1969 did not apply to organ donation. Whether a child is able to consent to his/her organs being donated would have to be decided using the common law. Here, the only guidance available is the *Gillick* test that a child can consent to a procedure if s/he has sufficient maturity to consent to that procedure. In the case of a very young child, parental consent would be required. In practice, if donation is sought from a child patient, of whatever age, parental consent should be obtained. One particular difficulty may be in ensuring that consent is freely given, bearing in mind the very highly charged emotional situation in which such a decision would be made.

What if a child refuses a transplant? As we noted in Chapter 6 in the case of *Re M*, a teenager refused a transplant. She was unhappy with the procedure and with living with a transplanted organ from another person inside her. The court nevertheless went ahead and approved the conduct of the transplantation operation, in this particular case overriding her refusal. This case can be contrasted with that of *Re T* (1997; see above) where the court upheld the parent's decision to refuse a liver transplant for their child. In this case the prognosis for success of the procedure was exceedingly good. Nonetheless as was discussed in Chapter 6, this case may perhaps be distinguished not simply on the basis that here the parents were health-care professionals with long experience of caring for sick children but also the fact that the parents had to come to England for the surgery, which was unavailable in the jurisdiction in which they were working, and there were some suggestions that had a different judicial approach been taken the parents would have gone outside the jurisdiction of the English courts. The position in this area now needs to be seen in relation to the Human Tissue Act 2004, discussed below.

The old law – the Human Organ Transplants Act 1989 – made transplantation between genetically unrelated donors subject to special approval procedures. This was due to the concern that persons who were prepared to donate to a person who was not their relative might be motivated by commercial considerations. The principle of special regulation of transplantation from live donors is continued in the Human Tissue Act 2004. This Act now provides for specific regulation of transplants from (both genetically related and non-genetically related) living donors under section 33. Transplantation is made an offence unless those requirements that are to be set out in regulations issued by the Secretary of State have been complied with and that in addition the transplant has been authorised by the Human Tissue Authority.

The Human Tissue Authority replaces the body established under the 1989 Act – the Unrelated Live Transplants Regulatory Authority – and their approval will be necessary before transplants are undertaken from living donors. The draft Regulations define transplantable material as being organs (including kidney, heart, lung, liver, etc.), part-organs (as defined in the legislation), face or limbs (Human Tissue Act 2004 (Persons who lack capacity to consent and Transplants Regulations 2006; SI 2006 No 1659)). The regulations also require that before transplants are authorised the Human Tissue Authority is satisfied that no reward has been given in relation to the transplant. The Authority must also ascertain that valid consent has been given to the removal. Procedural requirements include a requirement for the donor and recipient to both be independently interviewed by a Human-Tissue-Authority-approved independent assessor (reg 3). Where it is proposed that a child or an adult lacking mental capacity will be a donor then this issue is to be considered on a case by case basis by a panel of Authority members.

Particular reference is also made to certain transplantation procedures in the code of practice –notably to 'paired donation' and 'pooled donation'. Pairing operates, for example, where a close relative is prepared to donate but his/her organ is not compatible. Pairing matches donor and recipient with a similar donor and recipient. Pooled donation arises where there are more than two pairs in this situation. The code of practice makes clear that, as this is a new system, to facilitate monitoring the approval of the HTA is required (Human Tissue Authority 2006, para 95). There is also recognition of the situation in which a person donates an organ for altruistic reasons where there is no designated recipient (Human Tissue Authority 2006, paras 98–102). This practice is known as 'non-directed altruistic organ donation'. As it is a new procedure it will require HTA approval. The code of practice makes clear that not only should there be explanation of the procedure but, in addition, under no circumstances would recipient or donor know each other's identity (Human Tissue Authority 2006, para 100). The code also refers to 'domino transplantation' (Human Tissue Authority 2006, paras 103–104). This refers to the situation in which a person receives a heart and lung transplant in a situation in which his/her lungs are failing. The heart is removed but can be suitable for transplantation into another person. As this is an already established procedure, specific HTA approval will not be required.

Reforming the system?

There is a grave shortage of organs and long transplant waiting lists. For example, at the end of March 2000 some 5354 persons were on the national transplant waiting list. Many proposals have been made for reform of the present system (e.g. New et al 1994, British Medical Association 2000a). These extend from clarification of the provisions of the Human Tissue Act 1961 to legislation allowing automatic removal of organs from the deceased save where the person had made an indication to the contrary before death. Below are set out some of the main suggestions for reform.

One option is the introduction of opting out legislation (New et al 1994, British Medical Association 2000a). It allows organs to be removed without express permission being obtained, unless a deceased person had expressed an objection before his/her death. There is some evidence that the introduction of such a scheme in countries such as Belgium has increased the supply of available organs. Opting-out legislation has been given support by the BMA (British Medical Association 2000). Nevertheless, proposals to introduce opting-out legislation into this country have met opposition. There are fears that persons may feel pressurised into not opting out. Opposition to such legislation may come from certain religious/cultural groups who are unhappy with transplantation or who do not accept brain-stem death. Opting out may also lead to relatives' wishes being ignored. In practice, however, in countries where opting out legislation has been introduced, the donor's relatives are still consulted. Indeed the BMA document suggests that in a situation in which a person has not expressed views on donation while they are alive but it is apparent in this situation that 'to proceed with the donation would cause major distress to a first-degree relative or long-term partner, the donation should not proceed' (British Medical Association 2000). While commendable in the sensitivity to feelings of relatives such an exception leads one to wonder whether the introduction of opting out legislation would lead to a radical increase in supply. The BMA does admittedly see opting out as one part of a wider strategy in relation to donation. It also proposes that there needs to be a comprehensive piece of legislation that governs all aspects of organ donation from live to cadaver. In 1999 the UK government, in response to the call in that year by the BMA for opting out (British Medical Association 2000b), indicated that it was not in favour of a change of the law to support the introduction of opting out at the present time.

Another alternative is that of 'required request', a practice used in the USA. There, hospitals are obliged to set up procedures enabling routine enquiries to be made of patients and their relatives as to whether organs may be used if the patient subsequently dies. Required request does not appear to have led to any dramatic increase in the number of organs available for harvest in the USA. This may be due, at least in part, to the fact that there have been practical problems with the operation of required request, not least the fact that in many hospitals the procedures have been badly established and operated. It has, however, been argued that required request can impose considerable burdens on hospital staff in having to make time-consuming enquiries of potential donors and relatives.

In the absence of legislative change there have been attempts to increase the supply of organs by improving the present system. For many years, members of the public have been encouraged to carry donor cards indicating their willingness to donate organs, although there has been some scepticism regarding the effectiveness of such a scheme (New et al 1994). A computerised organ donor register, the NHS Organ Donor Register, was introduced in 1994 that allows individuals to have their wishes regarding organ donation entered on to computer. Transplant coordinators can contact the Organ Donor Register as a means of identifying the donor's wishes. Intending donors may tick a box on their driving licence application form expressing their wish to donate organs, and this information will be entered on to the Organ Donor Register.

One method of facilitating the supply of organs for transplantation, which provoked considerable controversy, is a practice known as 'elective ventilation' (McHale 1995). Patients with an intracranial haemorrhage, in a hopeless condition and who were regarded as suitable donors, were transferred to intensive care units where they were ventilated to facilitate use of their organs for transplantation. This procedure was controversial in that when the patient is transferred to the intensive care unit s/he may not have been declared brain-stem dead. This practice was halted because it was stated to be illegal. While medical procedures can be performed upon a mentally incompetent patient if it is in their best interests, the extent to which this is applicable in relation to the mentally incompetent patient is uncertain. Elective ventilation is not undertaken for the patient's benefit but rather to benefit others. Indeed, it may be very much against the patient's interests if, as it has been suggested, it inhibits the patient's right to a peaceful and dignified end. The Law Commission left open the possibility that the question could be addressed in legislation (Law Commission 1995, 6.23–6.26). Should consensus be reached on this issue one option is for a person who is willing to have his/her organs used for transplantation and to be electively ventilated, to express this through some form of advance declaration. This could take the form of a donor card similar to the existing organ donor card but perhaps in a different colour or shape to avoid confusion. It remains to be seen whether elective ventilation will receive sufficient public support to lead to legislative reform.

It has also been suggested that there should be the enhanced use of live organs donors in relation to kidney transplantation. Living donor transplantation has better success rates. There are the risks of surgery, though some evidence suggest that kidney transplants have good safety records (Nicolson & Bradley 1999).

Transplantation technology in the future

New options have been suggested which may alter transplantation practice out of all recognition. The first is that of xenotransplantation, the second is the use of cloning of tissues and organs. At present xenotransplantation is regulated by the Xenotransplantation Interim Regulatory Authority, which was established following the recommendations of the Department of Health report, which was chaired by Professor Ian Kennedy (Fox & McHale 1997, 1998). This Advisory Group reviewed the acceptability of and ethical framework within which xenotransplantation may be undertaken (this followed an earlier report by the Nuffield Council on Bioethics). The Advisory Group approved the practice of xenotransplantation in principle, accepting that it is ethical to use animals as a source of organs, provided certain conditions are satisfied. The Group recognised that animals have rights in a minimal sense, namely that their interests in avoiding suffering must be considered in any assessment of the benefits and harms of any proposed course of action (para 4.22). It regarded xenotransplantation as having the potential for an unlimited and immediate supply of usable organs. But while xenotransplantation was approved in principle, the Group were concerned as to the prospect for disease transmission that could result from premature authorisation of such transplants. Its caution in delaying animal-human transplants is reflective of heightened public concern regarding the safety of certain animal products following the BSE crisis.

While the Advisory Group regards xenotransplantation as ethical, this view does not command universal support. The ethical issues are complex. In using animal organs, does this mean that we are treating them in a manner in which we would treat human subjects and if so does that mean that they are morally objectionable? In recognition of the fact that this is an ethically emotive area it has been suggested that health professionals should be given a statutory right of conscientious objection to participation in such procedures. They would be able to opt out without subsequent prejudice to career or employment (para 7.26). Were such a measure to be enacted, it would join only two other statutory provisions granting a right of conscientious objection to health professionals – section 4 of the Abortion Act 1967 and section 38 of the Human Fertilisation and Embryology Act 1990.

The Advisory Group stated that xenotransplantation should be the subject of statutory regulation and that a National Standing Committee should be established to regulate such procedures. The government accepted the Group's recommendations. A Xenotransplantation Interim Regulatory Authority was established to approve experiments and monitor progress. This is chaired by the former Archbishop of York, Lord Habgood, who has a background in pharmacology. It has declared a moratorium pending further research. If the Authority is prepared in the future to authorise such transplantations then a number of other issues require resolution. Currently, there is debate as to whether patients can lawfully consent to a procedure that is clinically risky, such as xenotransplantations (Mason 1992, Fox & McHale 1998). If the procedure is ultimately recognised as lawful in principle, then a matter that still has to be addressed is as to whether particular groups of individuals should become recipients. The Advisory Group was of the opinion that, at least in the first instance, the procedure should be confined to competent adults (para. 7.7). It recognised that recipients of xenotransplants should be afforded a high degree of information disclosure and counselling facilities as to the implications of the procedure (para 7.11). The sensitivity of the issue has led to the Group recommending that the fact that an individual chooses to refuse a xenotransplant should not inhibit their ability to subsequently become the recipient of a human organ (para 7.15).

The present situation represents a somewhat uneasy compromise. It remains to be seen whether such technology will be further developed into clinical applications. Ultimately one solution may arise through the development of therapeutic cloning. As we noted in Chapter 9, stem cell cloning has been sanctioned. There is the possibility that this tissue technology may lead to the growth of organs. The development of such technology in relation to solid organs may, however, take some time in the light of the fact that the growth of such organs will require exceedingly complex medical technology.

REFERENCES

Adams M, Nys H 2003 Comparative reflections on the Belgium Euthanasia Act 2002. Medical Law Review 11: 353–376

Age Concern 2000 Turning your back on us older people and the NHS. Age Concern England, London

Andrews K, Murphy L, Munday R, Littlewood C 1996 Misdiagnosis in a rehabilitative unit. British Medical Journal 313: 13–16

Brazier M 2003 Medicine, patients and the law, 3rd edn. Penguin, Harmondsworth.

British Medical Association 1995 Advance statements about medical treatment. BMA, London

British Medical Association/Royal College of Nursing 1993 Statement on cardiopulmonary resuscitation. BMA/RCN, London

British Medical Association 2000a Physician assisted suicide: a conference to promote the development of consensus. BMA, London. Available online at http://web.bma.org.uk

British Medical Association 2000b Organ donation in the 21st century:time for a consolidated approach. BMA, London

British Medical Journal 1998 Australian euthanasia law throws up many difficulties. British Medical Journal 317: 969

British Medical Journal 1999a News: GP on trial for murder. British Medical Journal 318: 1095

British Medical Journal 1999b News: British GP cleared of murder charge. British Medical Journal 318: 1306

British Medical Journal 2003 Briton ends his life at assisted suicide clinic. British Medical Journal 326: 180

British Medical Journal 2004 News roundup: High Court upholds right of woman to travel abroad for suicide. British Medical Journal 329: 1364

Brody H 1999 Kevorkian and assisted death in the United States. British Medical Journal 318: 953

De Haan J 2002 The new Dutch law on euthanasia. Medical Law Review 10: 57

Department of Constitutional Affairs 2006 Mental Capacity Act 2005. Draft Code of Practice. Department of Constitutional Affairs, London

Dworkin R 1993 Life's dominion: an argument about euthanasia and abortion. Harper Collins, London

Fletcher N, Holt J, Brazier M, Harris J 1995 Nursing law and ethics. Manchester University Press, Manchester

Fox M, McHale J 1997 Regulating xenotransplantation. New Law Journal 147: 115

Fox M, McHale J 1998 Xenotransplantation: the ethical and legal ramifications. Medical Law Review 6: 42

Hayes S, Henshaw D, Rai GS, Stewart K 1999 Audit of resuscitation decisions has little impact on clinical practice. Journal of the Royal College of Physicians of London 33: 348–350

House of Lords Select Committee on Medical Ethics 1994 HL Paper 21-I. HMSO, London

Human Tissue Authority 2006 Code of practice 2: Donation of organs and tissue for transplantation. HTA, London

Hurst S, Mauron A 2003 Assisted suicide and euthanasia in Switzerland: allowing a role for non-physicians. British Medical Journal 326: 271

Kennedy I 1997 Commentary. Medical Law Review 5: 102

Kennedy I 2000 Bristol Inquiry interim report: removal and retention of human material. Available online at http://www.bristol-inquiry.org.uk

Keown J 1991 Euthanasia in the Netherlands. Law Quarterly Review 108: 51

Law Commission 1995 Mental incapacity. Law Commission no. 231. HMSO, London

McHale JV 1995 Elective ventilation – some ethical and legal problems. Professional Negligence 11: 23–26

McHale J, Gallagher A 2004 Rights and the end of life. In: Nursing and human rights. Butterworth Heinemann, London, Ch 8

Mason JK 1900 Organ transplantation. In: Dyer C (ed.) Doctors, patients and the law. Blackwell Scientific, Oxford.

New B, Solomon R, Dingwall M, McHale JV 1994 A question of give and take. Research Report 18. Kings Fund Institute, London

Nicolson M, Bradley AJ 1999 Renal transplantation from living donors. British Medical Journal 318: 409–410

Radcliffe-Richards J, Daar AS, Guttmann RD et al 1998 The case for allowing kidney sales. Lancet 351 1950–1952

Redfern M 2001 Report of the Inquiry into the Royal Liverpool Children's Hospital (Alder Hey). (Alder Hey Report.) Available online at: http://www.rclinquiry.org.uk

Royal College of Nursing 1992 Living wills guidance for nurses. Ord. No. 00102. RCN, London

Royal College of Physicians 1996 Criteria for the diagnosis of brain stem death – review by a working group convened by the Royal College of Physicians. Endorsed by the Conference of Medical Royal Colleges and their Faculties. RCP, London

Schutz SE 1994 Patient involvement in resuscitation decisions. British Journal of Nursing 3: 1075

Singer P 2002 Ms B and Diane Pretty a commentary. Journal of Medical Ethics 28, 234–235

Wells C, Alldridge P, Morgan D 1990 An unsuitable case for treatment. New Law Journal 140: 1544

The NMC code of professional conduct: standards for conduct, performance and ethics

As a registered nurse, midwife or specialist community public health nurse, you are personally accountable for your practice. In caring for patients and client, you must:

- respect the patient or client as an individual
- obtain consent before you give any treatment or care
- protect confidential information
- cooperate with others in the team
- maintain your professional knowledge and competence
- be trustworthy
- act to identify and minimise risk to patients and clients.

These are the shared values of all the United Kingdom health-care regulatory bodies.

1 Introduction

1.1 The purpose of the NMC code of professional conduct: standards for conduct, performance and ethics is to:

▶ inform the professions of the standard of professional conduct required of them in the exercise of their professional accountability and practice

▶ inform the public, other professions and employers of the standard of professional conduct that they can expect of a registered practitioner.

1.2 As a registered nurse, midwife or specialist community public health nurse, you must:

▶ protect and support the health of individual patients and clients

▶ protect and support the health of the wider community

▶ act in such a way that justifies the trust and confidence the public have in you

▶ uphold and enhance the good reputation of the professions.

1.3 You are personally accountable for your practice. This means that you are answerable for your actions and omissions, regardless of advice or directions from another professional.

1.4 You have a duty of care to your patients and clients, who are entitled to receive safe and competent care.

1.5 You must adhere to the laws of the country in which you are practicing.

2 As a registered nurse, midwife or specialist community public health nurse, you must respect the patient or client as an individual

2.1 You must recognise and respect the role of patients and clients as partners in their care and the contribution they can make to it. This involves identifying their preferences regarding care and respecting these within the limits of professional practice, existing legislation, resources and the goals of the therapeutic relationship.

2.2 You are personally accountable for ensuring that you promote and protect the interests and dignity of patients and clients, irrespective of gender, age, race, ability, sexuality, economic status, lifestyle, culture and religious or political beliefs.

2.3 You must, at all times, maintain appropriate professional boundaries in the relationships you have with patients and clients. You must ensure that all aspects of the relationship focus exclusively upon the needs of the patient or client.

2.4 You must promote the interests of patients and clients. This includes helping individuals and groups gain access to health and social care, information and support relevant to their needs.

2.5 You must report to a relevant person or authority, at the earliest possible time, any conscientious objection that may be relevant to your professional practice. You must continue to provide care to the best of your ability until alternative arrangements are implemented.

3 As a registered nurse, midwife or specialist community public health nurse, you must obtain consent before you give any treatment or care

3.1 All patients and clients have a right to receive information about their condition. You must be sensitive to their needs and respect the wishes of those who refuse or are unable to receive information about their condition. Information should be accurate, truthful and presented in such a way as to make it easily understood. You may need to seek legal or professional advice or guidance from your employer, in relation to the giving or withholding of consent.

3.2 You must respect patients' and clients' autonomy – their right to decide whether or not to undergo any health-care intervention – even where a refusal may result in harm or death to themselves or a fetus, unless a court of law orders to the contrary. This right is protected in law, although in circumstances where the health of the fetus would be severely compromised by any refusal to give consent, it would be appropriate to discuss this matter fully within the team and with a supervisor of midwives, and possibly to seek external advice and guidance (see clause 4).

3.3 When obtaining valid consent, you must be sure that it is:
- ▶ given by a legally competent person
- ▶ given voluntarily
- ▶ informed.

3.4 You should presume that every patient and client is legally competent unless otherwise assessed by a suitably qualified practitioner. A patient or client who is legally competent can understand and retain treatment information and can use it to make an informed choice.

3.5 Those who are legally competent may give consent in writing, orally or by cooperation. They may also refuse consent. You must ensure that all your discussions and associated decisions relating to obtaining consent are documented in the patient's or client's health-care records.

3.6 When patients or clients are no longer legally competent and have lost the capacity to consent to or refuse treatment and care, you should try to find out whether they have previously indicated preferences in an advance statement. You must respect any refusal of treatment or care given when they were legally competent, provided that the decision is clearly applicable to the present circumstances and that there is no reason to believe that they have changed their minds. When such a statement is not available, the patients' or clients' wishes, if known, should be taken into account. If these wishes are not known, the criteria for treatment must be that it is in their best interests.

3.7 The principles of obtaining consent apply equally to those people who have a mental illness. Whilst you should be involved in their assessment, it will also be necessary to involve relevant people close to them; this may include a psychiatrist. When patients and clients are detained under statutory powers (mental health Acts), you must ensure that you know the circumstances and safeguards needed for providing treatment and care without consent.

3.8 In emergencies where treatment is necessary to preserve life, you may provide care without consent, if a patient or client is unable to give it, provided you can demonstrate that you are acting in their best interests.

3.9 No-one has the right to give consent on behalf of another competent adult. In relation to obtaining consent for a child, the involvement of those with parental responsibility in the consent procedure is usually necessary, but will depend on the age and understanding of the child. If the child is under the age of 16 in England and Wales, 12 in Scotland and 17 in Northern Ireland, you must be aware of legislation and local protocols relating to consent.

3.10 Usually the individual performing a procedure should be the person to obtain the patient's or client's consent. In certain circumstances, you may seek consent on behalf of colleagues if you have been specially trained for that specific area of practice.

3.11 You must ensure that the use of complementary or alternative therapies is safe and in the interests of patients and clients. This must be discussed with the team as part of the therapeutic process and the patient or client must consent to their use.

4 As a registered nurse, midwife or specialist community public health nurse, you must cooperate with others in the team

4.1 The team includes the patient or client, the patient's or client's family, informal carers and health and social care professionals in the National Health Service, independent and voluntary sectors.

4.2 You are expected to work cooperatively within teams and to respect the skills, expertise and contributions of your colleagues. You must treat them fairly and without discrimination.

4.3 You must communicate effectively and share your knowledge, skill and expertise with other members of the team as required for the benefit of patients and clients.

4.4 Health-care records are a tool of communication within the team. You must ensure that the health-care record for the patient or client is an accurate account of treatment, care planning and delivery. It should be consecutive, written with the involvement of the patient or client wherever practicable and completed as soon as possible after an event has occurred. It should provide clear evidence of the care planned, the decisions made, the care delivered and the information shared.

4.5 When working as a member of a team, you remain accountable for your professional conduct, any care you provide and any omission on you part.

4.6 You may be expected to delegate care delivery to others who are not registered nurses or midwives. Such delegation must not compromise existing care but must be directed to meeting the needs and serving the interests of patients and clients. You remain accountable for the appropriateness of the delegation, for ensuring that the person who does the work is able to do it and that adequate supervision or support is provided.

4.7 You have a duty to cooperate with internal and external investigations.

5 As a registered nurse, midwife or specialist community public health nurse, you must protect confidential information

5.1　You must treat information about patients and clients as confidential and use it only for the purposes for which it was given. As it is impractical to obtain consent every time you need to share information with others, you should ensure that patients and clients understand that some information may be made available to other members of the team involved in the delivery of care. You must guard against breaches of confidentiality by protecting information from improper disclosure at all times.

5.2　You should seek patients' and clients' wishes regarding the sharing of information with their family and others. When a patient or client is considered incapable of giving permission, you should consult relevant colleagues.

5.3　If you are required to disclose information outside the team that will have personal consequences for patients or clients, you must obtain their consent. If the patient or client withholds consent, or if consent cannot be obtained for whatever reason, disclosures may be made only where:

▶ they can be justified in the public interest (usually where disclosure is essential to protect the patient or client or someone else from the risk of significant harm)
▶ they are required by law or by order of a court.

5.4　Where there is an issue of child protection, you must act at all times in accordance with national and local policies

6 As a registered nurse, midwife or specialist community public health nurse, you must maintain your professional knowledge and competence

6.1　You must keep your knowledge and skills up to date throughout your working life. In particular, you should take part regularly in learning activities that develop your competence and performance.

6.2　To practise competently, you must possess the knowledge, skills and abilities required for lawful, safe and effective practice without direct supervision. You must acknowledge the limits of your professional competence and only undertake practice and accept responsibilities for those activities in which you are competent.

6.3　If an aspect of practice is beyond your level of competence or outside your area of registration, you must obtain help and supervision from a competent practitioner until you and your employer consider that you have acquired the requisite knowledge and skill.

6.4　You have a duty to facilitate students of nursing, midwifery and specialist community public health nursing and others to develop their competence.

6.5 You have a responsibility to deliver care based on current evidence, best practice and, where applicable, validated research when it is available.

7 As a registered nurse, midwife or specialist community public health nurse, you must be trustworthy

7.1 You must behave in a way that upholds the reputation of the professions. Behaviour that compromises this reputation may call your registration into question even if is not directly connected to your professional practice.

7.2 You must ensure that your registration status is not used in the promotion of commercial products or services, declare any financial or other interests in relevant organisations providing such goods or services and ensure that your professional judgment is not influenced by any commercial considerations.

7.3 When providing advice regarding any product or service relating to your professional role or area or practice, you must be aware of the risk that, on account of your professional title or qualification, you could be perceived by the patient or client as endorsing the product. You should fully explain the advantages and disadvantages of alternative products so that the patient or client can make an informed choice. Where you recommend a specific product, you must ensure that your advice is based on evidence and is not for your own commercial gain.

7.4 You must refuse any gift, favour or hospitality that might be interpreted, now or in the future, as an attempt to obtain preferential consideration.

7.5 You must neither ask for nor accept loans from patients, clients or their relatives and friends.

8 As a registered nurse, midwife or specialist community public health nurse, you must act to identify and minimise the risk to patients and clients

8.1 You must work with other members of the team to promote health-care environments that are conducive to safe, therapeutic and ethical practice.

8.2 You must act quickly to protect patients and clients from risk if you have good reason to believe that you or a colleague, from your own or another profession, may not be fit to practise for reasons of conduct, health or competence. You should be aware of the terms of legislation that offer protection for people who raise concerns about health and safety issues.

8.3 Where you cannot remedy circumstances in the environment of care that could jeopardise standards of practice, you must report them to a senior person with sufficient authority to manage them and also, in the case of midwifery, to the supervisor of midwives. This must be supported by a written record.

8.4 When working as a manager, you have a duty toward patients and clients, colleagues, the wider community and the organisation in which you and your colleagues work. When facing professional dilemmas, your first consideration in all activities must be the interests and safety of patients and clients.

8.5 In an emergency, in or outside the work setting, you have a professional duty to provide care. The care provided would be judged against what could reasonably be expected from someone with your knowledge, skills and abilities when placed in those particular circumstances.

9 Indemnity insurance

9.1 The NMC recommends that a registered nurse, midwife or specialist community public health nurse, in advising, treating and caring for patients/clients, has professional indemnity insurance. This is in the interests of clients, patients and registrants in the event of claims of professional negligence.

9.2 Some employers accept vicarious liability for the negligent acts and/ or omissions of their employees. Such cover does not normally extend to activities undertaken outside the registrant's employment. Independent practice would not normally be covered by vicarious liability, while agency work may not. It is the individual registrant's responsibility to establish their insurance status and take appropriate action.

9.3 In situations where employers do not accept vicarious liability, the NMC recommends that registrants obtain adequate professional indemnity insurance. If unable to secure professional indemnity insurance, a registrant will need to demonstrate that all their clients/ patients are fully informed of this fact and the implications this might have in the event of a claim for professional negligence.

Glossary

Accountable   Responsible for something or to someone.

Care   To provide help or comfort.

Competent   Possessing the skills and abilities required for lawful, safe and effective professional practice without direct supervision.

Patient and client   Any individual or group using a health service.

Reasonable   The case of *Bolam v. Friern Hospital Management Committee* (1957) produced the following definition of what is reasonable. 'The test is the standard of the ordinary skilled man exercising and professing to have that special skill. A man need not possess the highest expert skill at the risk of being found negligent... it is sufficient if he exercises the skill of an ordinary man exercising that particular art'. This definition is supported and clarified by the case of *Bolitho* v. *City and Hackney Health Authority* (1993).

Summary

As a registered nurse, midwife or specialist community public health nurse, you must:

- respect the patient or client as an individual
- obtain consent before you give any treatment or care
- cooperate with others in the team
- protect confidential information
- maintain your professional knowledge and competence
- be trustworthy
- act to identify and minimise the risk to patients and clients

Index

A

Abortion, 211–217
Abuse of mentally ill patients, 135–136
Abused children, 128
Access to justice, 12–14
Accident victims
 consent to treatment, 106, 107, 117
 duty of care and, 26–28
 police enquiries, 152
Accidents, 25–26
Accountability, professional, 20–24, 64
 expanded role nursing, 72–73, 74–76, 77
 nurse prescribing, 95
Acts of Parliament (statutes), 8–9, 12
Advance decisions, 234–236
Advance directives *see* Advance decisions
Advanced nursing practice *see* Expanded
 role nursing
Adverse drug reactions, 94–95
Adverse outcomes
 supplementary prescribing, 95
 Woolf reforms, 7
AIDS patients, 108, 144
Algorithms *see* Clinical guidelines
Animal organs, transplantation, 172, 240,
 243–245
Animal research, 173
Artificial feeding, 227, 228, 229, 233, 234
Assisted reproduction, 157–158, 197–199,
 203–204, 213–214
Assisted suicide, 223–224, 226–227, 235
Association of British Pharmaceutical
 Industries (ABPI), 188
At-risk children, 128

B

Balance of probability test, 38–39
Battery, 105, 106–107, 178, 208–209
Best interests test, 102–103, 104–105, 194,
 207, 229, 230–231
Bills, 8

Birth plans, 205–208
Births, registration, 217–218
Bland case, 227–229
Blood case, 200
Blood transfusions, 107, 120, 127, 205–206
Bolam test, 29–30, 31, 36–37, 82, 109
Bolitho case, 31–32, 36–37, 83
Brain-stem death, 237–238
Breach of confidence, 3
 see also Confidentiality
Breach of duty of care, 26, 29–35
 congenital disability, 211
 criminal liability, 44–45
 damage caused by, 35–37, 114–115
Bristol Inquiry (Kennedy Report), 112
British Medical Association (BMA)
 advance decisions, 235
 assisted suicide, 226–227
 delegation, 76
 surrogacy, 203
'But for test', 35

C

Cadaver transplants, 238–239
Caesarean sections, 205–210
Caldicott review, 166–167
Capacity
 access to records and, 166
 advance decisions, 235, 236
 confidentiality and, 146
 consent to research, 180–184, 185
 consent to treatment, 100–105
  abortion, 214
  child patients, 118–119, 124–126, 214
  mentally ill patients, 128, 139, 140
  pregnant women, 206–208, 214
  sterilisation operations, 194–196
 organ transplants, 239, 241
Case law, 9–10
Causation, 35–39, 114–115
Central Office for Research Ethics
 Committees (COREC), 174, 190

Chancery Division, High Court, 4
Child destruction, 216
Childbirth, 204–211
Children
  abortion, 214
  access to records, 166
  clinical research, 180–181, 185
  confidentiality, 145–146
  congenital disability, 211
  consent to research, 180–181
  consent to treatment, 117–128, 214, 240
  contraceptive advice/treatment, 118–119,
    145–146, 194–195
  court orders, 119–123, 126
  end of life, 220, 221, 226, 229–231
  organ donation, 239, 240, 241
  protection policies, 128
  wardship, 119
  withdrawing treatment from
    handicapped, 229–233
Circumcision, 118, 124
Civil courts, 4
Civil Justice Council, 5
Civil justice system, 5–8, 13–14, 46
Civil law, 2–3
Civil law liability
  confidentiality, 152
  consent to treatment, 106–115
Civil Procedure Rules Committee, 5
Clinical governance, 15–16
Clinical guidelines, 80–85
  see also Protocols, nurse prescribing
Clinical management plans, 93–94
Clinical Negligence Scheme for Trusts
  (CNST), 42
Clinical pathways see Clinical guidelines
Clinical practice
  keeping up to date with, 33–35, 84
  reasonable differences of opinions on,
    30–32
  see also Expanded role nursing; Nurse
    prescribing
Clinical research, 171–190
  adults lacking mental capacity, 181–184,
    185
  animal research, 173
  anonymisation of information, 154
  children, 180–181, 185
  compensation for injury, 188
  compulsory participation, 179–180, 181
  confidentiality, 153–154
  consent to, 175, 176–177, 178, 180–184,
    185, 186
  duty to inform, 178–179
  ethics committees, 174–175, 176–177, 180,
    184–185, 188–189, 190
  human tissue samples, 185–187
  inducements to participate, 175–176

information provision, 177–179
innovative therapies, 173
medicines, 173, 174, 177–178, 181, 184–185
monitoring, 188, 189–190
negligence, 178–179, 187–189
non-therapeutic, 178, 179, 180, 181, 182,
  183, 188
nurses' liability, 188–189
randomised controlled trials, 177–178
regulatory framework, 171–173
review process reform, 190
unethical, 189
ward care and, 187–188
Clinical trials see Clinical research
Cloning, 197, 200–202, 245
Code of Professional Conduct see NMC Code of
  Professional Conduct: Standards for
  Conduct, Performance and Ethics (the
  Code)
Commission for Health Improvement, 15
Commission for Social Care Inspection, 16
Common law, 9–10
Communicable diseases, 108, 153
Community Legal Service, 13
Community Legal Services Fund, 13
Community, treatment in, mentally ill
  patients, 137–138, 139, 140
Compensation
  culture of, 35
  liability for paying, 41–44
  no-fault schemes, 46
  research subjects, 188
Competence
  developing, 33–35
  expanded role nursing, 77, 78–80
  to consent to treatment see Capacity
Complaints
  patients, 7, 53, 54–65
  whistleblowers, 159–161
Compulsory care, 108
  caesarean sections, 205–210
  child patients, 118, 124, 125–126, 181
  mentally ill patients, 129–130, 131,
    132–133, 134–135, 139, 140
Compulsory participation in research,
  179–180, 181
Conditional fee system, 13–14
Conditions of practice orders, 23
Conduct and Competence Committee,
  NMC, 22–23
Confidence, breach of, 3
  see also Confidentiality
Confidentiality, 143–144
  adults lacking mental capacity, 146
  after patient's death, 147
  children, 145–146
  general obligations, 144–145
  grounds for disclosure, 146, 147–157, 168

Confidentiality *(cont'd)*
  law reform, 168–169
  negligence, 152, 156–157, 168
  security of records, 166–167
  statutory obligations, 153, 157–158
  whistleblowing, 158–163
Congenital disability, 211
Conjoined twins case, 122–123
Conscientious objection
  abortion, 215–216
  reproductive treatment, 200
  xenotransplantation, 244
Consent to information disclosure, 146,
  147–148
Consent to organ donation, 239
Consent to research, 175, 176–177, 178,
  180–184, 185, 186
Consent to treatment, 99–116
  capacity, 100–105, 118–119, 124–126, 128,
    139, 140, 194–196
  children, 117–128, 214, 240
  civil law liability, 106–116
  compulsion *see* Compulsory care
  consent forms, 99–100
  criminal law liability, 105–106
  express, 100
  implied, 100
  information provision, 100–101, 105–116,
    127–128, 133
  mentally ill patients, 128–141, 208–210
  non-therapeutic, 114, 118
  public health powers, 108
  refusal to give, 101–102, 107–108
    by children, 124–128, 214, 240
    by mentally ill patients, 138
    by parents, 120–124, 126–128
    by pregnant women, 205–210, 214
    end of life, 224–225
  sterilisation, 193, 194–196
Consent to use of stored embryos, 199–200
Consent to use of stored sperm, 200
Contingency fee system, 14
Continuing professional development
  (CPD), 75
Contraceptive advice/treatment, 118–119,
  145–146, 193–196
  see also Sterilisation operations
Contracts
  definition, 3
  employment, 78
Coroners' courts, 8
Corporate manslaughter, 45
Cot-sides, 30
County Courts, 6, 12
Court of Appeal, 4, 9
Court appearances by nurses, 3, 152
Court orders, treatment of children,
  119–123, 126, 127

Court structure, 4
Courts, types of, 4, 6, 8
Criminal courts, 4
Criminal Defence Service, 13, 14
Criminal law, 2
Criminal liability, 44–45
  abortion, 216
  consent to treatment, 105–106
  end of life, 219–237
Crown Courts, 4
Crown reviews, nurse prescribing, 86–87,
  88–90
Cumberlege report, 85, 205

D

Damage, tort of negligence, 26, 35–37
Damages
  definition, 3
  liability for paying, 41–44
  for loss of chance, 38–39
Data protection, 163–165
Death
  access to patient's records after, 166
  certification of, 238
  definition, 237–238
  patient confidentiality after, 147
  posthumous conception, 200
Declarations, 3
Declarations of incompatibility, 12
Delegation, 75–76
Department of Health, 14
Dependent (supplementary) prescribing,
  89–90, 92–95
Direct liability, 43–44
Disciplinary proceedings
  confidentiality and, 150–151, 159
  whistleblowers, 159, 161
Disclosure of information
  clinical research, 177–179
  confidentiality, 146, 147–157, 167, 168
  consent to treatment, 108–116
  whistleblowing, 158–163
Discretionary orders, 3
Dispute resolution mechanisms, 5–6
DNA, research involving, 185, 186
Do not resuscitate (DNR) orders, 123,
  236–237
Domino transplantation, 241
Donor cards, 243
Double-effect doctrine, 123, 222
Drugs
  clinical research, 173, 174, 177–178, 181,
    184–185
  nurse prescribing, 85–95
  pain-killing, 220, 221–222, 225
Duty of care, 26–28

Index

Duty of care (*cont'd*)
  breach of, 26, 29–35
    congenital disability, 211
    criminal liability, 44–45
    damage caused by, 35–37, 114–115
  expanded role nursing, 78–80
Duty of confidence, 3, 144, 145
Duty to inform, clinical research, 178–179

E

Education
  patient expectations, 51–52
  post-registration, 74–75
Elective ventilation, 243
Electroconvulsive therapy (ECT), 134, 135
Electronic patient records, 164, 166–167
Embryo research, 172, 197, 202
Embryo storage, 199–200
Emergencies
  abortion, 213
  compulsory care, 108, 129–130, 131, 135, 207
  consent to treatment, 106–107, 117, 129–130, 131, 135
  duty of care and, 26–28
  mentally ill patients, 129–130, 131, 135
  police enquiries, 152
  pregnant women, 207
Employment contracts, 78
  confidentiality obligations, 144
Employment law, whistleblowers, 161–163
End of life, 219–245
  advance decisions, 234–236
  consent to treatment, 123
  definition of death, 237–238
  do not resuscitate orders, 123, 236–237
  legalisation of euthanasia, 225–227
  living wills, 234–236
  organ transplants, 238–245
  pain-killing drugs, 220, 221–222, 225
  parents' obligations to children, 221
  refusal of treatment, 224–225
  suicide, 222–224, 226–227
  whistleblowers, 220–221
  withdrawal of treatment, 227–234
Ethics committees
  clinical research, 174–175, 176–177, 180, 184–185, 188–189, 190
  infertility treatment, 198
European Convention on Human Rights (ECHR), 11, 12
European Court of Justice (ECJ), 11, 19, 20
European law, 10–11, 19–20
Eusol, 31
Euthanasia, 219–220, 223–227, 234–235
Evidence-based clinical guidelines, 84–85

Evidence-based practice, 31, 32
Evidence in court, confidentiality, 152
Ex-RHAs Scheme, 42
Existing Liabilities Scheme (ELS), 42
Expanded role nursing, 69–85
  clinical guidelines, 80–85
  clinical negligence, 77, 78–80, 82–85
  definitions, 71–75
  delegation, 75–76
  problems with codes, 76–77
  professional misconduct, 77
  standards of care, 78–80, 83
  stress at work, 78
  see also Nurse prescribing
Expert evidence, 7–8, 32

F

Families
  consent to research, 180–182
  genetic information, 155–156
  of mentally ill patients, 130, 136, 137, 146
  see also Parents
Family balancing, sex selection, 203
Family Division, High Court, 4
Family law courts, 8
'Fast-track' courts, 6
Female circumcision, 118
Fetus
  capability of live birth, 216, 217
  status in law, 206–207, 209
Financial resource allocation, 17–20
First aid, 28
Fitness to practice, 21–24
Foundation Hospital Trusts, 15
Freedom of the press, 150

G

GAfREC (Governance Arrangements for NHS Research Ethics Committees), 174, 177, 180, 189
Gagging clauses, 162–163
Gender reassignment surgery, 18–19
Gene therapy, clinical research, 172
General Medical Council (GMC)
  consent to treatment, 112
  delegation, 75, 76
Genetic information, 154–156
Gillick competence, 118–119, 125, 146
Good Samaritan acts, 26–27, 28
Government legislation, 8, 9
Gross negligence, 44–45
Guardians of health care information, 166–167
Guardianship orders, 137

Guidelines
  clinical, 80–85
  clinical research, 172
  whistleblowing, 159–161
  see also Protocols, nurse prescribing

H

Health-care records
  confidentiality, 144, 148–149, 150,
    151–152, 153
  patient access, 163–166, 168
  patient retention of, 168
  police access, 151–152
  security, 166–167
  supplementary prescribing, 94
Health Committee, NMC, 22–23
Health Service Commissioner *see* Health
    Service Ombudsman
Health Service Ombudsman (HSO)
  complaints system, 62–65
  whistleblowing, 160
Health service provision, failure of, 16–20
Healthcare Commission, 15–16
  complaints system, 59–62
High Court, 4, 12
HIV-positive patients, 108
  confidentiality, 150, 154, 158
  consent to treatment, 121–122
Hormones, surgical implantation, 134, 135
Hospital(s)
  abortion in, 214–215
  admission of mentally ill patients,
    128–131
  births in, 205
  detention of mentally ill patients, 131–132
    emergencies, 135
    monitoring, 138–139
    nurses' powers, 132–133
    pregnant woman, 208–209
    proposed new powers, 140
    seclusion, 135–136
    transfers, 136
    treatment, 133–135
  discharge of mentally ill patients,
    136–138
  NHS structure, 15
House of Lords, 4, 9, 12
Houses of Parliament, 8
Human Fertilisation and Embryology
    Authority (HFEA), 172, 197–198, 200,
    201–202, 203
Human rights, 11–12
Human tissue, 185–187, 203, 238
  see also Organ transplants
Human Tissue Authority, 185–186, 203, 238,
    241

I

Indemnity insurance, 41–42, 95, 188
Independent complaints advocacy services
    (ICAS), 56
Independent prescribing, 88–92, 93
Infertility treatment, 157–158, 165, 197–200,
    213–214
Information Commissioner, 164
Information disclosure
  confidentiality, 146, 147–157, 167, 168
  whistleblowing, 158–163
Information provision
  clinical research, 177–179
  consent to treatment, 100–101, 105–116,
    127–128, 133
Informational privacy, 143
  see also Confidentiality
Injunctions
  confidentiality, 144
  definition, 3
Innovative therapies, 173
Insurance, 41–44, 95, 188
Interferon, 18
Investigating Committee, NMC, 22
IVF treatment, 157–158, 197–199, 213–214

J

Jehovah's Witnesses, 107, 120, 127–128, 234
Judicial review, 3
Juries, 4
Justice, access to, 12–14

K

Kennedy Report (Bristol Inquiry), 112
Knowledge, updating professional, 33–35

L

Lasting powers of attorney, 235–236
Law Lords, 4
Law sources, 8–12
Legal aid, 12–13
Legal Services Commission, 13, 14
Liabilities to Third Parties Scheme (LTPS), 42
Life support systems, 228
Litigation claims, 6–7, 45–46, 52–55
Living organ donors, 240–241, 243
Living wills, 234–236
Lord Chancellor, 4, 5
Lord Chief Justice, 4
Lord Justices of Appeal, 4
Loss of chance, 38–39

M

Magistrates courts, 4
Maim, 105–106
'Man must be mad' test, 130–131
Manslaughter, 44–45, 175, 217, 221
Master of the Rolls, 4
Media, disclosures to, 150, 161–162
Medical Care Practitioners, 76
Medical negligence *see* Negligence
Medical Research Council, 188
Medicines
  clinical research, 173, 174, 177–178, 181, 184–185
  nurse prescribing, 85–95
  pain-killing, 220, 221–222, 225
Mental capacity
  access to records and, 166
  advance decisions, 235, 236
  confidentiality and, 146
  consent to research, 180–184, 185
  consent to treatment, 100–105
    abortion, 214
    child patients, 118–119, 124–126, 214
    mentally ill patients, 128, 139, 140
    pregnant women, 206–208, 214
    sterilisation operations, 194–196
  organ transplants, 239, 241
Mental disorder, definition, 130–131
Mental Health Act Code of Practice, 132–133
Mental Health Act Commission, 16, 138–139
Mental health review tribunals, 136–137, 139
Mentally ill patients
  confidentiality, 148–149, 156–157
  consent to treatment, 128–141
    children, 125–126
    pregnant women, 208–210
Mercy killings, 221–222
Morning after pill, 216
Mothers' conduct during pregnancy, 204–211
'Multi-track' courts, 6
Murder, 217, 220

N

National Health Service (NHS)
  culture, 51–52
  structure, 14–20
National Health Service Litigation Authority (NHSLA), 42, 52
National Institute for Health and Clinical Excellence (NICE), 15, 16, 20
  clinical guidelines, 80–82, 84, 85
  technology appraisals, 173
National Patient Safety Agency (NPSA), 49, 50–51
National Reporting and Learning System (NRLS), 49, 50
Necessity doctrine, 122–123, 129
Neglected children, 128, 221
Negligence, 25–46
  in childbirth, 210–211
  clinical research, 178–179, 187–189
  costs and claims of, 52–55
  criminal liability, 44–45
  expanded role nursing, 77, 78–80, 82–85
  for failure to inform, 106, 108–116
  liability in tort, 25–41
  no-fault schemes, 46
  nurse prescribing, 95
  patient confidentiality and, 152, 156–157, 168
  payment of compensation, 35, 41–44, 46
  product liability, 44
  reform proposals, 45–46
  Woolf reforms, 6–7
Negotiated confidentiality, 157
NHS trusts, 15, 42
Nightingale oath, 143
NMC *Code of Professional Conduct: Standards for Conduct, Performance and Ethics* (the Code), 25, 247–253
  Clause 1, 27, 29, 247–248
  Clause 2, 248
  Clause 3, 99, 102, 248–250
  Clause 4, 250
  Clause 5, 144, 148, 251
  Clause 6, 33–34, 71, 80, 92, 171, 251–252
  Clause 7, 92, 252
  Clause 8, 26–27, 28, 158–159, 252–253
  Clause 9, 41–42, 95, 253
No-fault schemes, 46
Non-delegable duties, 43
Non-directed altruistic organ donation, 241
Notifiable diseases, 108, 153
Nurse consultants *see* Expanded role nursing
Nurse practitioners *see* Expanded role nursing
Nurse prescribing, 85–95
Nursing and Midwifery Council (NMC), 20–24
  code of conduct, 21
    see also NMC *Code of Professional Conduct: Standards for Conduct, Performance and Ethics* (the Code)
  fitness to practice, 21–24
  professional register, 21, 23, 75
  role expansion, 71, 75, 80
Nursing negligence *see* Negligence

O

Obiter dictum, 10
Observational studies
    consent to, 182
    ward care, 187–188
Occupational health, 154
Opting out legislation, organ donation,
    242
Organ transplants, 238–245

P

Pain-killing drugs, 220, 221–222, 225
Paired organ donation, 241
Parents
    consent to research, 180–181
    consent to treatment, 117, 119–124
        child's refusal and, 124–128, 214
        organ donation, 240
    end-of-life treatment decisions, 231–233
    obligations to children, 221
    see also Families
Parliament, 8, 12
Patient access to records, 163–166, 168
Patient Advice and Liaison Service (PALS),
    56
Patient expectations, 51–52, 53–54
Patient group directions (PGDs), 87–88
Patient retention of records, 168
Patient safety, 49–52
Patient's Charter, 15, 53
Persistent vegetative state (PVS), 227, 229,
    233, 238
Personality disorders, 140
Pink, Graham, 158, 159
Placebo effect, 177
Police enquiries, 151–152
Politics of uncertainty, 52
Pooled organ donation, 241
Post-registration Education and Practice
    (PREP), 74–75
Posthumous conception, 200
Postnatal care, 210
Powers of attorney, 235–236
Practice parameters see Clinical
    guidelines
Pre-action protocols, 7
Precedent system, 9–10
Pregnant women, 204–211, 214, 235
Prescribing by nurses, 85–95
Press, disclosures to, 150, 161–162
Primary Care Trusts (PCTs), 15, 42
Privacy, 143, 145
    see also Confidentiality
Private Members' Bills, 8
Product liability, 43–44

Professional accountability, 20–24, 64
    expanded role nursing, 72–73, 74–76, 77
    nurse prescribing, 95
Professional indemnity insurance, 41–42, 95
Prohibited steps orders, 119
Property Expenses Scheme (PES), 42
Prostaglandin abortions, 215
Protocols, nurse prescribing, 85, 86–88, 89–90
    see also Clinical guidelines
Proximate cause see Remoteness
Proxy decision makers, 236
Prudent patient test, 179
Psychiatric treatment, 128–130, 131–133,
    134–135, 137–139, 140
Psychopathic disorder, 130, 131
Psychosurgery, 134, 135
Public health disclosure requirements, 153
Public health powers, 108
Public interest exceptions, confidentiality,
    148–150, 156–157
Public law, 3

Q

Queen's Bench Division, High Court, 4

R

Randomised controlled trials, 177–178
Ratio decendendi, 10
Rationing, 17–20
Records see Health-care records
Refusal of treatment, 101–102, 107–108
    by children, 124–128, 214, 240
    by mentally ill patients, 138
    by parents, 120–124, 126–128
    by pregnant women, 205–210, 214
    end of life, 224–225
Regional Health Authorities, Ex-RHAs
    Scheme, 42
Register of nurses and midwives, 21, 23, 75
Registration of births and stillbirths,
    217–218
Regulatory Authority for Tissues and
    Embryos, 203
Relatives see Families
Religious beliefs
    abortion, 215–216
    consent and, 107, 120, 126–128, 205–206
    parents' obligations to children, 221
Remedial orders, 12
Remoteness, tort of negligence, 26, 37–39
Reproductive choices, 193–218
    abortion, 211–217
    contraceptive advice/treatment, 118–119,
        145–146, 193–196

Reproductive choices (cont'd)
   registration of births, 217–218
   registration of stillbirths, 217–218
   reproductive technology, 157–158, 165,
      197–204, 213–214
   women's conduct during pregnancy,
      204–211
Reproductive technology, 157–158, 165,
   197–204, 213–214
Required request, organ donation, 242
Res ipsa loquitur principle, 39–41
Research see Clinical research
Resource allocation, 17–20
Review systems, 84
   supplementary prescribing, 94
Richardson Review, 139–140
Risk assessment, 32
   clinical research, 175
   mentally ill patients, 140
Risk disclosure
   consent to clinical research, 178–179
   consent to treatment, 108–116
Risk minimisation, 33
Risk Pooling Scheme for Trusts (RPST), 42
Role expansion, 69–85
Royal College of Nursing (RCN), advance
   decisions, 235
RU486, 214–215, 216

S

Safety of patients, 49–52
Seclusion, use in mental hospitals, 135–136
Secretary of State for Health, 14, 15, 16–17
Settlements, 14
Sex selection, 203
Sexually transmitted diseases, 158
Shipman, Harold, 227
Sidaway test, 109
Skills, updating professional, 33–35
'Small claims' courts, 6
Social services
   child protection, 128
   guardianship orders, 137
Social workers, approved, 130, 137
Sotos' syndrome, 194
Specialist courts, 8
Specialist nurses see Expanded role nursing
Specific issue orders, 119, 120, 126
Standards of care
   clinical governance, 15–16
   clinical guidelines, 80–85
   differences of opinion on, 30–32
   expanded role nursing, 78–80, 83
   making public concerns about see
      Whistleblowing
Statutes, 8–9, 12

Statutory instruments, 9
Statutory interpretation, 9
Statutory orders, 3
Stem cells, 202, 203, 245
Sterilisation operations, 106–107, 193,
   194–196
Stillbirths, registration, 217–218
Strategic Health Authorities (SHAs), 14–15
Stress, work-related, 78
Striking-off orders, 23
Suicide, 222–224, 226–227, 235
Supervision in the community, 138
Supplementary (dependent) prescribing,
   89–90, 92–95
Surrogacy, 203–204
Suspension orders, 23

T

Thalidomide, 211
Therapeutic privilege, 113
Tissue see Human tissue
Torts
   definition, 3
   nursing negligence, 25–41
   privacy, 145
Transplants, 238–245
Treatment
   advance decisions, 234–236
   compulsion see Compulsory care
   consent to see Consent to treatment
   innovative therapies, 173
   mentally ill patients, 128–130, 131–135,
      137–139, 140
   parents' obligations to children, 221
   refusal of consent to, 101–102, 107–108
      by children, 124–128, 214, 240
      by mentally ill patients, 138
      by parents, 120–124, 126–128
      by pregnant women, 205–210, 214
      end of life, 224–225
   withdrawal, 227–234
Treatment attorneys, 236
Trials see Clinical research
Tribunals, 8
   mental health, 136–137, 139

U

UK Ethics Committee Authority, 175, 184
United Kingdom Central Council for
   Nursing, Midwifery and Health
   Visiting (UKCC)
   duty of care, 27, 28
   role expansion, 71–72, 74
Updating, professional, 33–35, 84

V

Venereal disease, 158
Ventilator support, 224, 231, 243
Viagra, 18
Vicarious liability, 42–43

W

Waiting lists, 19–20
Wardship, 119, 204
Warnock Committee, 197, 203–204
Whistleblowing, 158–163
    end of life, 220–221

Withdrawal of treatment, 227–234
Woolf reforms, 4, 5–7, 46

X

Xenotransplantation, 172, 240, 243–245

Y

Yellow card scheme, 95